WORKING WITH SPIRITUAL STRUGGLES IN PSYCHOTHERAPY

Working with Spiritual Struggles in Psychotherapy

FROM RESEARCH TO PRACTICE

Kenneth I. Pargament
Julie J. Exline

THE GUILFORD PRESS
New York   London

The authors have checked with sources believed to be reliable in their efforts to provide
information that is complete and generally in accord with the standards of practice that are
accepted at the time of publication. However, in view of the possibility of human error or
changes in behavioral, mental health, or medical sciences, neither the authors, nor the editor
and publisher, nor any other party who has been involved in the preparation or publication
of this work warrants that the information contained herein is in every respect accurate or
complete, and they are not responsible for any errors or omissions or the results obtained from
the use of such information. Readers are encouraged to confirm the information contained in
this book with other sources.

Library of Congress Cataloging-in-Publication Data

Names: Pargament, Kenneth I. (Kenneth Ira), 1950– author. | Exline, Julie
    J., author.
Title: Working with spiritual struggles in psychotherapy : from research to
    practice / Kenneth I. Pargament, Julie J. Exline.
Description: New York : The Guilford Press, [2022] | Includes
    bibliographical references and index.
Identifiers: LCCN 2021025563 | ISBN 9781462524310 (hardcover)
Subjects: LCSH: Psychotherapy—Religious aspects. | Spirituality. | BISAC:
    PSYCHOLOGY / Psychotherapy / Counseling | RELIGION / Psychology of
    Religion
Classification: LCC RC489.S676 P373 2022 | DDC 616.89/14—dc23
LC record available at *https://lccn.loc.gov/2021025563*

To my grandchildren—
Emmy, Oliver, Hudson, Noah—
and all who bring hope
for a world of greater wholeness
—K. I. P.

To my mom and dad, Audrey and Jon Juola,
who provided me with great love and care, a strong
spiritual foundation, and openness to the idea that
growth often comes through struggle
—J. J. E.

About the Authors

Kenneth I. Pargament, PhD, is Professor Emeritus of Psychology at Bowling Green State University. He has pioneered studies on the vital role of religion and spirituality in coping with stress and trauma. A clinical psychologist, Dr. Pargament has been a leading figure in the effort to integrate research on religion and spirituality into clinical practice. He has received the William James Award from Division 36 (Society for the Psychology of Religion and Spirituality) of the American Psychological Association (APA), the Oskar Pfister Award from the American Psychiatric Association, and the Outstanding Contributor to the Applied Psychology of Religion and Spirituality Award from APA Division 36, of which he was the inaugural recipient.

Julie J. Exline, PhD, is Professor in the Department of Psychological Sciences at Case Western Reserve University. Her primary research interests focus on spiritual struggles and supernatural attributions. Dr. Exline is a clinical psychologist and was certified as a spiritual director through the Ignatian Spirituality Institute at John Carroll University. She is a past president of the Society for the Psychology of Religion and Spirituality (Division 36 of the APA) and is a recipient of the Society's Margaret Gorman Early Career Award, Virginia Sexton Mentoring Award, and William James Award, in recognition of her research in the psychology of religion and spirituality.

Preface

We were coming down the home stretch, putting the final touches on this book, when, within the space of what seemed to be just a few days, the world descended into the COVID-19 pandemic. Plagues, many of us had thought, were a thing of the distant past. Yet, here we were facing our own modern-day plague. COVID-19 posed an existential crisis, threatening and destroying the lives of people all over the world, throwing our economies into a tailspin, disconnecting people from their webs of support, forcing major disruptions of many hopes and dreams. But COVID-19 was more than an existential crisis. For many of us, it was a spiritual crisis as well—shaking, damaging, or destroying those things we hold most sacred.

With the onset of COVID-19, our book on spiritual struggles took on more immediacy. We believe this book has much to say about the deeper impact of the traumas and transitions we encounter in life. More than that, it offers some insights into how we can understand spiritual struggles and how we can help people move through their times of struggle to find greater wholeness and growth.

The book is the culmination of over 20 years of thinking and research on spiritual struggles by us and many other researchers who have delved into this important area of study. Research on spiritual struggles has increased dramatically over this time period, with now literally hundreds of studies published and many more in the works. We know a lot about struggles now, though many, many questions remain. Our hope is that this book, which captures the current state of research and practice on this topic, will provide a foundation and framework to help people who are struggling, and to encourage future studies.

Our book is the outgrowth of several years of collaboration between us. We have long shared an interest in spiritual struggles, studying them, writing about them, and at times experiencing struggles of our own. But we brought different backgrounds to our studies and approached the topic somewhat differently. Ken Pargament, a Jewish clinical psychologist, became interested in spiritual struggles through his research on religious coping with major life stressors. His measure of religious coping assessed not only many types of positive religious resources but also (what were then called) negative religious coping methods that reflect stress and strains around religious and spiritual matters. To his surprise, he found that, in comparison to positive religious coping, negative religious coping was generally more strongly and consistently related to psychological adjustment and well-being. Negative religious coping, later relabeled spiritual struggles, appeared to have real power. At the same time, Ken also became more sensitive to signs of struggle in his clinical work with psychotherapy clients. Few came to therapy complaining of spiritual struggles, yet struggles were at times not far beneath the surface of the problems clients brought to treatment and seemed to call for attention. Ken's interest was piqued. But his interest in this area has been more than scholarly and professional. Over the years, he himself has struggled with many of the issues that are described in this book.

Julie Exline was raised within the Christian tradition but has been a "moving target" in terms of religious affiliation. After spending her first 15 years in a fundamentalist Baptist church, she has twice been a member of charismatic/Pentecostal congregations (one Assemblies of God, one nondenominational). She also attended Catholic churches for several years and eventually became an Ignatian spiritual director through a local Jesuit university. Consistently self-identifying as spiritual but not always as religious, Julie is currently a member of an Episcopalian church, but she identifies most strongly with a mystical, universal spirituality focusing on love and interconnectedness. Over the course of her life, Julie has experienced many personal struggles around her religious faith, which long preceded her academic interest in the topic. After spending a few years working in the computer science field, Julie went to graduate school in psychology with the hope of studying spiritual struggles, although this label did not exist at the time. Although her training in clinical and social psychology was more traditional, she continued to seek out opportunities to do research on spiritual struggles.

Though we both approached struggles from different backgrounds and angles, we long admired each other's work, liked each other, and felt that a collaboration would make good sense. With Julie serving as the principal investigator, we applied for and received a grant from the John Templeton Foundation to conduct numerous studies on spiritual struggles. Drawing on the findings from this initiative, we also took on the task of writing this book, with Ken taking the lead. What followed were several years of brainstorming, data analysis and interpretation, half-day meetings in northern Ohio locales, and the shared sense of excitement that we were building an important body of knowledge together. We have been enriched personally and professionally through our collaboration.

While the process of writing this book has been rewarding in many ways, it has also been challenging in several respects. First, we want our work to reach both researchers from the health and social sciences, and practitioners from psychology, psychiatry, social work, counseling, pastoral care, health care, and chaplaincy. We firmly believe that the rapidly accumulating body of knowledge about spiritual struggles can and should inform clinical practice. Conversely, the experiences of clients and therapists can shed new light on spiritual struggles and point to new and important questions for systematic investigation. We hope we have found a good blend of research and practice that will appeal to both of our audiences.

The book has been challenging to write for a second reason. Most mental health practitioners do not receive any graduate training in the area of religion and spirituality. In addition, researchers and practitioners in the social sciences and mental health fields tend to be more secular than the general population. Our task was to welcome our readers to what may be a new area of research and a dimension of mental health care that is often overlooked in treatment. It is time, we feel, to integrate spirituality more fully into science and practice. Our hope is that this book contributes to this goal.

A third challenge comes from our desire for the book to be relevant to people from a variety of traditional and nontraditional religious and spiritual backgrounds (including atheists who may also encounter spiritual struggles). Toward that end, we sought out research studies from cultures outside the United States and from religious groups that include but also go beyond Christians and Jews. In addition, we looked for stories of spiritual struggle from diverse religious traditions, and developed composite cases of clients who come from a variety of religious backgrounds. Even so, in spite of our best efforts, we suspect that our book continues to reflect a Western perspective. We eagerly await more contributions to the study of spiritual struggles from other cultures and traditions.

Finally, the topic of spiritual struggles itself is also a new and challenging one. Like the spices of a wonderful dish that go unidentified but are a critical part of the recipe, spiritual struggles are an often hidden but integral part of life. They can be found in the cracks and crevices of the problems people bring to treatment. This is not to say that spiritual struggles should be treated as psychopathology or signs of spiritual immaturity. Although struggles are often accompanied by distress and disorientation, we maintain that they are a natural and normal part of life. We try to convey that the job of the practitioner is not to cure struggles with a pill, on the one hand, or disregard them, on the other. The challenge is, instead, to help clients move through their struggles toward greater wholeness and growth rather than brokenness and decline.

We have been very fortunate to have been able to work with a wonderful set of graduate students and colleagues over the years who have stimulated, challenged, supported, and enriched our own thinking. Ken would like to thank Jim Nageotte and Jane Keislar of The Guilford Press for their guidance, support, and encouragement in the development and completion of this book, as well as Anna Nelson for her help in the production process. He is grateful to his graduate student Serena Wong for her many insights, her sensitive and astute reading of much of the manuscript, and her patient and expert help with the modern-day technology of writing a book. Carmen Oemig Dworsky also provided invaluable feedback and perspective on earlier drafts of several of the chapters. Thanks also go to his former graduate students (now colleagues) who extended research on spiritual struggles in new and exciting directions: Hisham Abu-Raiya, Gene Ano, Ethan Benore, Margaret Bockrath, Brenda Cole, Jeremy Cummings, Kavita Desai, Carol Ann Faigin, Melissa Falb, Meryl Reist Gibbel, Allie Hart, William Kooistra, Elizabeth Krumrei, Steve Lucero, Gina Magyar-Russell, Aaron Murray-Swank, Nichole Murray-Swank, Russell Phillips Jr., Julie Pomerleau, David Rosmarin, Aaron Sedlar, Nalini Tarakeshwar, and Kelly Trevino. In addition, Ken would like to acknowledge colleagues who have been valuable sources of wisdom, encouragement, and support. These include Jon Allen, Jeffrey Bjorck, Sian Cotton, Richard Cowden, Joseph Currier, Carrie Doehring, George Fitchett, Nick Gibson, Daniel Grossoehme, Josh Grubbs, Gail Ironson, Samuel Karff, Stephen King, Harold Koenig, Neal Krause, James Lomax, Annette Mahoney, Douglas Oman, James Pawelski, Michelle Pearce, Heidi Pedersen, Kate Piderman, Judith Ragsdale, Katia Reinert, Pninit Russo-Netzer, Kimon Sargeant, Tor Torbjørnsen, Vitaliy Voytenko, and Josh Wilt. And, above all, Ken feels very fortunate to have had the chance to work on this project with such a wise and wonderful collaborator and friend: Julie. Finally, Ken is deeply grateful to his wife, Aileen, who buoyed his spirits, offered her always honest feedback, assisted with the references, nourished him with wonderful meals, kept him connected to the real world after days in the office, and (with reasonably good humor) tolerated times in the middle of the night when he would jump out of bed to write down an idea.

Julie would like to thank her many mentors and teachers, collaborators, graduate students, and postdocs who have shared their insights, efforts, and energy to contribute to a deeper understanding of spiritual struggles. Although this list is woefully incomplete, she would like to thank Marci Lobel, Roy Baumeister, Dave Myers, Joan Nuth, Barbara Fields, and Dottie Rieman for their roles as mentors, teachers, and guides—and Bob Boice, of course, for helping her learn to see writing as an enjoyable journey. She is thankful for the ongoing support from her family, friends, and colleagues, as well as her graduate students from over the years: Anne Zell, Mickie Fisher, Alyce Martin, Eric Rose, Briana Root, Josh Grubbs, Steffany Homolka, David Bradley, Valencia Harriott, Alex Uzdavines, Seyma Saritoprak, Jessie Kusina, Will Schutt, and Kathleen Pait. Of course, Josh Wilt, Nick Stauner, and Matt Lindberg all played pivotal roles in this work, as did Dorothy Yun, Crystal Park, Ann Yali, Maryjo Prince-Paul, Todd Hall, Ellen Teng, Melinda Stanley, and Chris Smith. A big thank you to the IRPS group, the teachers at Centering Space and the Jesuit Retreat House, and of course all of her School of Rock friends, who have patiently tolerated many spiritually oriented conversations at the Loco Leprechaun. Finally, Julie is *especially* grateful to the John Templeton Foundation (Grants 36094 and 59916), and, in particular, to our program officer, Nick Gibson. Most of all, Julie is grateful to Ken for his friendship, his collaboration, and his huge role in taking the lead on this book. Julie has cherished the opportunity to work with Ken on this book and all of their joint projects. It has been a privilege and a joy!

Contents

PART I. UNDERSTANDING SPIRITUAL STRUGGLES

CHAPTER 1   Introducing Spiritual Struggles   3

CHAPTER 2   A Conceptual Model of Spiritual Struggles   25

CHAPTER 3   Where Do Spiritual Struggles Come From?   38

CHAPTER 4   Do Spiritual Struggles Lead to Decline?: The Painful Side   61

CHAPTER 5   Do Spiritual Struggles Lead to Growth?: The Brighter Side   84

CHAPTER 6   What Shapes the Outcomes of Spiritual Struggles?   104

PART II. CLINICAL CHALLENGES OF SPIRITUAL STRUGGLES

CHAPTER 7   How to Address Spiritual Struggles in Clinical Practice   137

CHAPTER 8   Divine Struggles   162

CHAPTER 9   Struggles of Ultimate Meaning   189

CHAPTER 10   Struggles with Doubt   213

CHAPTER 11   Moral Struggles   241

CHAPTER 12   Demonic Struggles   270

CHAPTER 13   Interpersonal Struggles   298

CHAPTER 14   Concluding Thoughts   323

              References   329

              Author Index   374

              Subject Index   383

PART I

UNDERSTANDING SPIRITUAL STRUGGLES

CHAPTER 1

Introducing Spiritual Struggles

In my security I said I shall never be shaken.
—PSALM 30

The call came in after dinner. One of Nancy's fellow coworkers at the emergency room spoke to her in a strained voice: "You need to get over here right away. Your daughter has been shot." The rest of that night seemed like a series of snapshots to Nancy, burning images seared into her mind: the look of pity in the doctor's eyes as he delivered the news that her daughter had been shot in her car and was in very serious condition; her adult daughter, her precious Lilly, so frail and helpless, lying on a table ensnared in a spider's web of medical lines; and the bleakness of the cold white room where Nancy sat holding her daughter's limp hand until death came.

Before that unforgettable night, Nancy's 52 years had been rich and rewarding, filled with more than she could have hoped for. Her daughter, a surprise after many years of infertility, had been a special blessing. "You're my gift from God," she had often told Lilly. "I had a hand in choosing my career and your father, but you just came to me, like a miracle. And on top of that, you became my best friend."

The days, weeks, and first months after Lilly's death passed in a blur. She knew she had to keep herself going, if not for herself, for the sake of Lilly's two small children who Nancy and her husband would now be raising. One foot in front of the other, one foot in front of the other, she told herself. But it was all an act. She felt as if she had been thrown into the middle of an ocean, totally disoriented, at the mercy of waves, tides, and the weather. She was familiar with the symptoms of posttraumatic stress disorder (PTSD), and she knew she met the criteria: those awful flashbulb-like memories of her daughter in the hospital; her futile efforts to avoid anything that reminded her of the tragedy; and then the tears, nausea, and rage that would sweep over her at the most unexpected times.

As painful as Nancy's psychological symptoms were, it was the feeling of being lost at sea, with nothing solid to grab on to, nothing to ground her, and nowhere to go, that was even more distressing. Adding to her pain were the

3

questions that rushed in to fill the void left by Lilly, agonizing questions that overwhelmed her every time she thought about the death of her daughter. Nancy had always believed that if she lived a good life, God would spare her from this kind of suffering. Now she found herself repeatedly asking, Why, why had God taken away the special gift he had given her? Nancy couldn't stop thinking about that bullet, that mini guided missile that had honed in on Lilly with such perfect precision. So many hundreds of small events had to come together to create this horror. The police had been unable to find a shooter and had attributed it to "a stray bullet, a random act of violence." It didn't feel random to Nancy, though. Why would the God who had created the miracle of Lilly undo it all through this "antimiracle"? Or perhaps it was the act of evil, demonic forces in the universe that had singled her daughter out for an attack? Nancy had never given much thought to the idea of evil but now she found herself preoccupied by it. At other times, Nancy wondered whether she was being punished for sins she had committed. Had she failed to live the good life she had imagined she was living? Nancy had been far less than perfect, but what could she have done that merited the death penalty for her precious Lilly? And what kind of God would be so cruel? God, she had been taught, would never give her more than she could handle, but this was way more than she could handle. Perhaps the God she had believed in was just a child's fantasy.

When she sought out comfort from her church, she was met with sentiments that only made matters worse. "Remember that God called Lilly to Him for his own purpose," one friend told her. "You have to trust in God's plan," said another. Nancy knew these remarks were well intended, but they only infuriated her. How could God need Lilly more than she and Lilly's young children did? What kind of divine plan was this? This was no plan; that bullet flying through the night was surely a sign of sheer chaos in the universe. Going to church only increased Nancy's sense of unease and alienation. But who could understand? She herself used to offer similar bromides to members of the church who had lost loved ones. Nancy was adrift, cut off from other people, cut off from herself. After much prompting by her husband and friends, Nancy scheduled an appointment with a psychotherapist.

The prospect of working with Nancy would make many practitioners uneasy. After all, Nancy's nightmare-come-to-life raises our own deep-seated fears. Don't we, like Nancy, assume a basic level of security in our world? Don't we also live by some implicit expectation that we can manage to avoid our own fateful calls in the night? Nancy poses a challenge to our own positive illusions. If the unthinkable could happen to her, why couldn't it happen to us as well?

But the uneasiness of working with clients like Nancy could be due to another reason as well. Nancy was experiencing more than PTSD, more than a purely psychological or psychiatric problem. Her trauma was made especially torturous because she had lost the most precious part of her life. Not only the loss itself—but the manner of the loss—had thrown her most basic values, assumptions, actions, and beliefs into confusion, leaving her bewildered and disoriented, shaken to the core. And in the midst of this upheaval, Nancy found herself grappling with profoundly spiritual questions. In short, she was experiencing spiritual struggles, formidable struggles that were the source of her greatest pain.

While many clinicians might be tempted to try to sidestep Nancy's struggles and focus purely on her psychological symptoms, the reality is that Nancy's psychological problems and spiritual struggles were deeply intertwined. Attempting to disentangle the two would be as futile as trying to pull apart the black and white threads of a gray sweater. And to overlook Nancy's spiritual struggles would, we believe, impede her recovery and opportunity to move from her place of brokenness to greater wholeness. Instead, Nancy's psychological recovery and growth would require attention not only to her symptoms but also to her spiritual tensions and conflicts.

Although Nancy's personal story is unique, she is not alone in her spiritual struggles. As we will see, spiritual struggles are interwoven into many of the problems people bring to therapy. How can practitioners understand these struggles and help individuals like Nancy? Unfortunately, the reality is that most of us are ill equipped to recognize, understand, and assist people facing spiritual struggles—and with good reason: Most mental health professionals have not received any kind of training on how to address religious and spiritual issues, including spiritual struggles, in their graduate education (Saunders, Petrik, & Miller, 2014). And yet, training in spiritual competencies has been shown to enhance the knowledge, skills, and attitudes of practitioners (Pearce, Pargament, Oxhandler, Vieten, & Wong, 2020). As we will see, a significant body of research is emerging on spiritual struggles. And this research, we believe, can be of tremendous value to practitioners looking for guidance in their work. To be of greatest help to clients like Nancy who seek us out in the midst of their suffering, we have to draw on theory, research, and clinical example, integrating a deeper understanding of spirituality in general, and spiritual struggles in particular, into our clinical perspective and practice. This book is designed largely to enhance the ability of practitioners to understand and help people who come to us shaken to the core—however, we hope that the theory and research presented here serves as an up-to-date and useful resource for researchers as well. In this chapter, we begin by considering the defining characteristics of spiritual struggles and why they deserve attention from practitioners and researchers.

WHAT ARE SPIRITUAL STRUGGLES?

Though many of us might wish for smooth, predictable lives, our days are punctuated occasionally by change, transition, and turmoil. Struggle is part and parcel of life. Certainly, not all struggles are on the order of Nancy's. We can struggle with less momentous issues—the struggle to get out of bed, the struggle to lose weight, the struggle to adjust to a new job. Spiritual struggles are among the deepest of all conflicts. They can shake us to the heart of our being. More formally, we define spiritual struggles as experiences of tension, conflict, or strain that center on whatever people view as sacred (Exline, 2013; Pargament, Murray-Swank, Magyar, & Ano, 2005).

As is true of many definitions, this one needs a little unpacking. In particular, what do we mean by "sacred"? The term *sacred* refers not only to traditional understandings of God or higher powers but also to any other aspect of life that is perceived to hold divine-like qualities (Pargament & Mahoney, 2005). What first comes to mind for most people when they think about the sacred are images of divinity, be they God, Allah, the Holy Spirit, Jesus, Brahman, Yahweh, or Jehovah. But the sacred is not limited to the divine. People can perceive sacredness within any part of life. In fact, the world's major religious traditions do all they can to encourage their adherents to perceive a presence of the divine in life. Most traditions teach that, because life comes from God, it carries a spark of the divine. To care for ourselves, care for one another, and care for the world then become spiritual imperatives.

Even those who are not traditionally religious or theistic may perceive sacredness in aspects of their lives, by attributing to them divine-like qualities, such as transcendence, ultimacy, and boundlessness. Consider a few examples. A marriage can be seen as a legal contract, but it can be much more. In most wedding ceremonies, the love and commitment binding a couple are described as everlasting and eternal. Work too can take on a deeper meaning. For some, a job is simply a way to put food on the table and pay the bills. For others, though, work is less a job than it is a calling or a vocation, a source of ultimate purpose in life. Music, dance, poetry, and painting can also be perceived with greater depth— through the arts many people feel they experience something of essential and timeless truth. In short, the capacity to see domains of life such as these through a sacred lens, imbuing them with deeper divine-like character and significance, may be the essence of spirituality. And it is not a rarity. Empirical studies have shown that many people do, in fact, instill life, in part or in its entirety, with sacred status (Mahoney, Pargament, & Hernandez, 2013). For instance, in one national survey in the United States (Doehring & Clarke, 2002), 75% of individuals agreed or strongly agreed that they "see God's presence in all of life," and 76% indicated that they "experience something more sacred than simply material existence."

Spiritual struggles involve a process of grappling with questions and concerns that involve whatever is held sacred. The questions and concerns embedded in spiritual struggles are often existential in nature: Who am I? Why am I here? How should I live my life? Is the world safe and trustworthy? Am I alone in the universe? Am I loved? What is true? How can I make sense of and deal with suffering? How do I come to terms with my own frailties and finitude? Of course, these questions may not be explicitly linked to spiritual matters. Existential writers have produced wonderful books on the topic with little mention of the sacred (e.g., Yalom, 1980). Nevertheless, the fact is that life's most fundamental existential questions often do become fraught with sacred power and significance. And when they do, struggles become spiritual struggles. Questions of meaning become struggles with whether the universe is chaos or cosmos (cf. Karff, 1979), whether the individual has a divine purpose, and whether there are absolute truths to live by. Questions of identity turn into battles over whether the person can live up to his or her spiritual values, whether the individual has a soul, or whether the person is being influenced by demonic or evil forces. Questions about one's place in the world become worries over whether the person can be part of a sacred community in which he or she is truly known and affirmed by others, whether there is a loving God (or a God of any kind), and how best to relate to that God. In their spiritual struggles, people wrestle with not just any set of questions, but questions replete with sacred significance, questions that have to do with the ultimate destinations of life and the pathways to get there.

THE DIVERSITY OF SPIRITUAL STRUGGLES

Because people can struggle with the sacred in any of its expressions, spiritual struggles can take many forms. Spiritual struggles may focus on gods, demons, or other supernatural entities; on relationships with individuals, families, groups, organizations, or institutions; or on one's own internal beliefs, values, feelings, and practices. In short, spiritual struggles may be supernatural, interpersonal, or intrapersonal. They encompass not only struggles with elements of organized religious life, such as religious dogma, religious institutions, God, and the demonic, but struggles with other sacred dimensions of human experience. And different types of spiritual struggles can raise different sets of existential questions. Thus, spiritual struggles can be found in surprising places, including conflicts and tensions around seemingly secular parts of life.

Different kinds of struggle are not mutually exclusive; people may encounter more than one struggle at the same time. For example, Nancy was dealing with anger and confusion about God, questions about the place of evil in the universe, feelings of alienation from her church, doubts about her faith, guilt that she had perhaps failed to live up to her own highest standards, and fear that she would never be able to fill the vacuum created by the loss of the most sacred part of her life. In fact, Nancy's struggles fed into one another like individual logs fueling a larger fire.

Over the last 20 years, researchers have begun to measure spiritual struggles more systematically. A number of scales have been developed that focus on particular kinds and contexts of struggle. For example, the Penn Inventory of Scrupulosity (Abramowitz, Huppert, Cohen, Tolin, & Cahill, 2002) assesses fears about having committed sins and being punished by God. Piedmont (2012) created the four-item Religious Crisis Scale to assess conflicts and difficulties individuals may experience with God and their religious community. The Inventory of Complicated Spiritual Grief (Burke et al., 2014) measures spiritual struggles with the divine and other people in the context of bereavement. Exline, Yali, and Sanderson (2000) devised a Religious Strain Scale that measures alienation from God, religious rifts with others, and fear/guilt (see Table 1.1).

The most widely used measure of spiritual struggles, the negative subscale of the Brief Religious Coping scale (Brief RCOPE; Pargament, Smith, Koenig, & Perez, 1998), consists of seven items (see Table 1.1). As you can see, the majority of the items assess the degree to which people feel punished or abandoned by God and question God's power and love for them. These items can be referenced to the ways people respond to specific life stressors or to their lives and situations more generally. Although the terms *negative religious coping* and *spiritual struggles* are often used interchangeably, we now prefer the term *spiritual*

TABLE 1.1. Scales Related to Spiritual Struggle from Our Research Teams

Items from the Religious Strain Scale (Exline, Yali, & Sanderson, 2000)

Alienation from God

  1. Feeling that God is far away
  2. Feeling abandoned by God
  3. Feeling that your faith is weak
  4. Difficulty trusting God
  5. Difficulty believing God exists

Fear/guilt

  6. Belief that you have committed a sin too big to be forgiven
  7. Fear of evil or of the devil
  8. Belief that sin has caused your problems
  9. Fear of God's punishment

Religious rifts

10. Bad memories of past experiences with religion or religious people
11. Disagreement with a family member or friend about religious issues
12. Disagreement with something that your religion or church teaches
13. Feeling lonely or different from others because of your beliefs

Negative religious coping items from the Brief RCOPE
(Pargament, Smith, Koenig, & Perez, 1998)

  1. Wondered whether God had abandoned me
  2. Felt punished by God for my lack of devotion
  3. Wondered what I did for God to punish me
  4. Questioned God's love for me
  5. Wondered whether my church had abandoned me
  6. Decided the devil made this happen
  7. Questioned the power of God

struggles for two reasons: (1) the coping methods that were previously labeled negative do not always lead to negative outcomes; and (2) by using the language of spiritual struggle, we convey the possibility of growth as people work through these conflicts.

These measures have helped to bring spiritual struggles into sharper focus. However, the scales assess a very limited range of spiritual struggles, and the field has lacked a standard metric for assessing these tensions and conflicts. This makes it difficult to form general conclusions about spiritual struggles across different studies and samples.

Six Types of Spiritual Struggle

In an effort to examine spiritual struggles more comprehensively (though not exhaustively) and establish a more standard measure, our research group (Exline, Pargament, Grubbs, & Yali, 2014) delineated six types of spiritual struggles that tap into the supernatural, intrapsychic, and interpersonal domains:

1. *Divine struggles* take the form of anger or disappointment with God, and feeling punished, abandoned, or unloved by God.
2. *Demonic struggles* involve worries that problems are caused by the devil or evil spirits, and feelings of being attacked or tormented by the devil.
3. *Interpersonal spiritual struggles* reflect conflicts with other people and institutions about sacred issues; anger at organized religion and feeling hurt, mistreated, or offended by others in relation to religious or spiritual issues.
4. *Struggles with doubt* are marked by feeling confused about religious/spiritual beliefs and feeling troubled by doubts or questions about religion/spirituality.
5. *Moral struggles* take the form of tensions and guilt about not living up to one's higher standards and wrestling with attempts to follow moral principles.
6. *Struggles of ultimate meaning* involve questions about whether one's life has a deeper meaning and whether life really matters.

We went on to create a set of items to assess these six types of struggle (Exline, Pargament, Grubbs, & Yali, 2014) and administered these items to two samples of adults and one large sample of college students (see Table 1.2 for items). Through factor analyses, we found solid support for the distinctiveness of these six types of struggle. It is important to add that the six types of spiritual struggle were moderately intercorrelated with one another, meaning that those who experienced one form of struggle were more likely to experience other forms of struggle as well. As a group, spiritual struggles share something

TABLE 1.2. Religious and Spiritual Struggles Dimensions and Items

Divine struggles

1. Felt as though God had let me down
2. Felt angry at God*
3. Felt as though God had abandoned me*
4. Felt as though God was punishing me*
5. Questioned God's love for me

Demonic struggles

6. Felt tormented by the devil or evil spirits
7. Worried that the problems I was facing were the work of the devil or evil spirits*
8. Felt attacked by the devil or by evil spirits*
9. Felt as though the devil (or an evil spirit) was trying to turn me away from what was good

Interpersonal struggles

10. Felt hurt, mistreated, or offended by religious/spiritual people*
11. Felt rejected or misunderstood by religious/spiritual people
12. Felt as though others were looking down on me because of my religious/spiritual beliefs
13. Had conflicts with other people about religious/spiritual matters*
14. Felt angry at organized religion*

Moral struggles

15. Wrestled with attempts to follow my moral principles*
16. Worried that my actions were morally or spiritually wrong
17. Felt torn between what I wanted and what I knew was morally right
18. Felt guilty for not living up to my moral standards*

Struggles of ultimate meaning

19. Questioned whether life really matters*
20. Felt as though my life had no deeper meaning*
21. Questioned whether my life will really make any difference in the world
22. Had concerns about whether there is any ultimate purpose to life or existence

Doubt-related struggles

23. Struggled to figure out what I really believe about religion/spirituality
24. Felt confused about my religious/spiritual beliefs*
25. Felt troubled by doubts or questions about religion or spirituality*
26. Worried about whether my beliefs about religion/spirituality were correct

Note. Based on Exline, Pargament, Grubbs, and Yali (2014).

*Items included in the RSS-14 (Exline, Pargament, Wilt, Grubbs, & Yali, 2021).

in common: the experience of grappling with matters of profound significance. However, each form of struggle is also distinctive in some respects. (We take a closer look at specific spiritual struggles in the second half of this book.)

Other Variations in Spiritual Struggles

Spiritual struggles vary along other dimensions as well. For some people, spiritual struggles are relatively short-lived experiences—the fleeting feeling that an illness might be a divine punishment, or perhaps the momentary unease that one's own core religious beliefs might simply be fantasies or human inventions. For example, following the death of his wife after only 3 years of marriage, Christian writer C. S. Lewis (1961) described how his painful struggles with his wife's illness came to a head one evening:

> What chokes every prayer and every hope is the memory of all the prayers H. and I offered and all the false hopes we had. . . . Step by step we were "led up the garden path." Time after time, when He seemed most gracious He was really preparing the next torture. (p. 27)

The next morning, however, his intense pain and anger toward God gave way to more reflective thought: "I wrote that last night. It was a yell rather than a thought. Let me try it over again. Is it rational to believe in a bad God? Anyway, in a God so bad as all that? The Cosmic Sadist, the spiteful imbecile?" (p. 27).

Although spiritual struggles can be relatively brief for some, others experience spiritual struggles over a period of years. For example, Dennis, a 50-year-old veteran dealing with depression and anxiety, had been a special operations officer in Vietnam where he had killed a number of civilians and combatants. As a soldier, he had begun to question his actions, but he had kept his doubts to himself. A Roman Catholic, Dennis believed he had committed a set of sins that placed him beyond the realm of forgiveness and condemned him to eternal hell. For almost 25 years, Dennis had been struggling with an unrelenting sense of guilt, a dread of the divine punishment to come when he died, and the belief that none of this could be changed. His spiritual struggles, he believed, were intractable. Studies suggest that many people, like Dennis, face long-lasting spiritual struggles in the wake of serious negative life events. For instance, 40% of parents of children with Down syndrome indicated some level of spiritual struggle 11 years after the birth of their children (Mussett, 2012). Among survivors of hematopoietic cell transplant, 30% reported some degree of spiritual struggles up to 33 years later (King et al., 2018).

While some people may experience only one episode of spiritual struggle over the course of their lives, others encounter spiritual struggles at many points in the lifespan. In his classic but heart-wrenching book *Night,* Elie Wiesel (1972) described the spiritual struggles he encountered as an adolescent with his father in Auschwitz. The cruelty and immensity of suffering he witnessed was of such breathtaking scale that it was difficult to put into words. Yet, Wiesel was able to offer a bitterly powerful lamentation of rage toward the God who could allow such an event to happen:

> Why, but why would I bless him? Every fiber in me rebelled. Because He caused thousands of children to burn in His mass graves? Because He kept six crematoria working day and night, including Sabbath and the Holy Days? . . . How could I say to Him: Blessed be Thou, Almighty, Master of the Universe, who chose us among

all nations to be tortured day and night, to watch as our fathers, our mothers, our brothers end up in the furnace? (p. 85)

This is a God Wiesel must accuse. This is a God Wiesel (1979) finds guilty, as we see literally enacted in his later play *The Trial of God*. However, although Wiesel must rebel against this God, he cannot abandon Him. In the concentration camp and later, Wiesel continues to pray for himself, his parents, and the world. And he commits himself to a remarkable life of writing, teaching, and political activism in which he bears witness against the atrocities he experienced.

Yet even a man with the tremendous maturity and humanity of Wiesel was not immune to subsequent spiritual struggles in his life. At the age of 82, he suddenly faced the need for life-threatening quintuple bypass surgery. In his account of his surgery and recovery, *Open Heart,* Wiesel (2012) once again grapples with profound spiritual questions and tensions. At one point, he briefly wonders whether his disease is a divine retribution: "Evidently, I have prayed poorly, lacking concentration and fervor; otherwise, why would the Lord, by definition just and merciful, punish me in this way?" (p. 14). Later, reminiscent of his struggles with the Holocaust, Wiesel returns to the questions of "why," now in the context of his illness: "Why this illness? These pains, why did I deserve them . . . for what purpose?" (p. 66). As he had over 70 years earlier, Wiesel leaves the reader with this sentiment: "I confess to having rebelled against the Lord, but I have never repudiated Him" (p. 68). Wiesel's example is instructive. The struggles experienced at one age and the resolutions people reach in response to these struggles do not preclude the possibility of similar or different struggles at a later time in life.

In sum, as we look more closely at spiritual struggles, we see that they are far from uniform. They are multidimensional human experiences that vary in type, duration, intensity, and frequency.

CHARACTERISTICS OF SPIRITUAL STRUGGLES

In spite of their differences, spiritual struggles share some important characteristics, characteristics that underscore why struggles deserve attention from practitioners and researchers. We suggest that spiritual struggles are often pervasive, painful, and pivotal.

Spiritual Struggles Are Pervasive

Spiritual struggles are an essential part of the personal journeys of the world's religious exemplars. In the Hebrew Bible, "complaint with God co-mingles with communion with God" (Beck, 2007, p. 72). For example, we read about Job's bitterness and bewilderment resulting from the cataclysm that has befallen him.

How, he asks God, can a man of piety and faith suffer the loss of family, home, health, riches, and security? His struggle with "why the righteous suffer" is a question that echoes down through the ages. In the New Testament, we listen to Jesus's final anguished plea and expression of abandonment on the cross: "My God, my God, why hast thou forsaken me?" (Matthew 27:46). Within Islam, we hear of the struggles of the Prophet Muhammed to establish a new religion against the backdrop of the ruling elite of Mecca and the larger polytheistic culture. Within Buddhism, we read of Siddhartha Gautama's search for enlightenment. Before he becomes the Buddha, Gautama rests beneath a fig tree where he is confronted by the demon Mara who presents him with the greatest worldly temptations: the desires to give in to fear and rage, to lust, and to pride. More recently, we have witnessed the Dalai Lama's struggle to withstand the efforts of the Chinese regime to stifle Buddhist thought and expression in Tibet. Of course, there is more to the great religious traditions than spiritual struggle. But a religious tradition missing these stories of struggles would lack power and drama, and might never reach the level of greatness because these moving accounts of turmoil set the stage for the profoundly inspirational insights and transformations that follow.

Stories of spiritual struggle are not limited to religious scriptures or seminal religious figures. They are easy to find in the great literature of the world as well. *Beowulf,* the oldest long poem in Old English, written at least 1,000 years ago, describes the epic struggle of the King of the Geats, Beowulf, against an array of supernatural beasts, demons, and dragons. *Crime and Punishment,* Dostoevsky's masterpiece, focuses on the moral struggle and spiritual alienation of the protagonist after he commits acts of murder. In *The Bridge of San Luis Rey,* Thornton Wilder raises the question of how to find a larger meaning in the capriciousness of a world in which five innocent people lose their lives in a bridge collapse.

Spiritual struggles and the ways people come to terms with them are also central to the life stories of many well-known people, past and present. Over 400 years ago, Galileo conducted telescopic observations that led him to conclude that the Earth revolved around a stationary Sun. These conclusions also precipitated a decades-long struggle with the Catholic Church, ultimately resulting in his conviction for the heresy of "heliocentrism" and imprisonment in his house for the remainder of his life (Finocchiaro, 1989). Before he developed his theory of evolution, Charles Darwin was, in fact, an orthodox Christian. His observations about the workings of the natural world, as well as personal losses in his life, including the death of his beloved daughter, gradually led him to profound religious doubts and eventually a loss of belief in a personal God (Pleins, 2013). After he had already accumulated wealth and achieved success as a writer, Leo Tolstoy (1983) experienced a life-threatening midlife crisis of ultimate meaning that prompted the question "Is there any meaning in my life that couldn't be destroyed by the death that inevitably awaits me?" (p. 35). Beatles' guitarist

George Harrison faced a similar struggle. The material success, fame, and highs of drugs and sex left him wondering whether that is all there is to life, a question that propelled him toward a more spiritual path in his music and his lifestyle (Greene, 2007).

Struggles repeatedly emerge as a theme in the lives of remarkable people, so much so, that one might wonder whether spiritual struggles are part of the price people pay for greatness. Research, however, suggests that ordinary people face spiritual struggles, too. We sprinkle many personal accounts throughout this book to illustrate this point. Here we present just a few statistics. In a study of over 17,000 adults in the United States, participants were asked how often they had experienced each of the six types of spiritual struggle identified by Exline, Pargament, and Grubbs (2014) over the past few weeks. A sizable minority of the sample reported that they had recently experience some level of the various struggles: divine (32%), demonic (31%), interpersonal (35%), moral (49%), doubt (35%), and ultimate meaning (43%). If we ask about how often people have faced spiritual struggles over the course of their lifetimes, the percentages go even higher. For example, in one national survey of over 1,000 adults, approximately 75% reportedly experienced most of the types of spiritual struggle at some time in their lives (Exline, Pargament, & Grubbs, 2014).

As high as these figures are, they may still be underestimates, for our method of asking people to report whether they have experienced spiritual struggles assumes that people are aware of these tensions and conflicts, and willing to admit them to others (Exline & Grubbs, 2011). Yet as we will see, spiritual struggles may bubble beneath the surface of an individual's consciousness. Moreover, there can be guilt, shame, and stigma associated with the expression of spiritual struggles. In any case, though, it seems clear that spiritual struggles are far from unusual.

Research also shows that spiritual struggles can be found in any particular group, any particular situation, or any particular time. Spiritual struggles are reported by men and women, all ages, all ethnicities, and all religious groups that have been studied so far (e.g., Roman Catholic, Protestant, unspecified Christians, Eastern Orthodox, Jewish, Buddhist, Hindu, Muslim, Spiritual not Religious; see Abu-Raiya, Pargament, Exline, & Agbaria, 2015; Abu-Raiya, Pargament, Weissberger, & Exline, 2016; Mercadante, 2020; Phillips et al., 2009; Saritoprak, Exline, & Stauner, 2016; Tarakeshwar, Pargament, & Mahoney, 2003). Spiritual struggles unfold across diverse life situations, ranging from the experiences of mental and physical illness to natural disaster to marital and family conflict. For example, in one study of family caregivers for loved ones with dementia, spiritual struggles were frequently reported, especially moral struggles (64.5%), ultimate meaning struggles (61.6%), and doubt-related struggles (48.0%; Wong & Pargament, 2019). In another study of older patients with cancer in outpatient palliative care centers, 66% reported some spiritual struggle and 20% indicated quite a bit or a great deal of struggle (Damen et al., in press). And, it is important to add, spiritual struggles are commonplace among people seeking help for psychological problems. For example, 50% of older adults with depression reported spiritual struggles (Murphy, Fitchett, & Emery-Tiburcio, 2016), as did 47% of outpatients in treatment for a mood disorder (Rosmarin, Malloy, & Forester, 2014). Among college students in campus counseling centers, one-third reported spiritual struggles (Johnson & Hayes, 2003).

It may seem counterintuitive, but even atheists may run into spiritual struggles. Family members, friends, coworkers, or strangers may deride, confront, or challenge atheists about their unbelief. Atheists may also have their own unresolved tensions regarding their religious stance. In one survey of atheist and theist college students and Internet respondents, atheists reported lower levels of spiritual struggles than theists, unsurprisingly (Sedlar et al., 2018). Even so, the atheists still manifested spiritual struggles, particularly interpersonal, moral, and ultimate meaning struggles. Along similar lines, Bradley, Exline, and Uzdavines (2015, 2017) have conducted studies that show that some people who do not believe in God still have negative emotion around the idea of God. These may be, as Rabbi Samuel Karff (1979) put it, "atheists with an ache" (p. 5).

In short, spiritual struggles can be found among people from past and present, from diverse religious and nonreligious groups, from the most ordinary to the most exemplary, from all walks of life, from all cultures, and among those facing the full range of life experience, including individuals with psychological problems. Later, we see that spiritual struggles are more common among some groups and in some situations than others. Taken as a whole, however, the stories and studies we briefly described here all lead to the same strong conclusion: spiritual struggles are a pervasive human experience.

Spiritual Struggles Are Painful

Pain is built into spiritual struggles. Because they can shake and shatter our most fundamental beliefs, values, practices, and relationships, spiritual struggles can yield a great deal of heartache. Consider the true story recounted by Joan Chittister (2003) in her powerful book *Scarred by Struggle, Transformed by Hope*. Chittister, a teacher and member of a Roman Catholic religious order, was looking forward to pursuing her dream of becoming a writer of fiction. It seemed as though her dream would come true. With the encouragement of her superior and religious order, she had applied and won admission to the prestigious master's of art writing program at Iowa State University. However, just a few weeks before she was to leave for Iowa, she received another call from her superior. Inexplicably, Chittister was told that she had to withdraw from the program. She was, her superior said, not "ready for a Master's degree" (p. 6). Chittister was shaken to the core: "It was life-altering to me. It was cataclysm in the midst of calm. It was the end of the dream, the loss of the hope. It was forced change at the center of my personal universe. It was impossible" (p. 7). She goes on to describe her spiritual struggle:

> God had become a question mark, not a certainty. Religious life had become cruel, not fulfilling. As I tried to pray, shaken, isolated, and in darkness, I could feel the dust of my soul under my tongue. . . . My body went on living but my soul had died in a darkness so thick I could not see through it. (p. 39)

And her struggle was accompanied by a wave-like pain not unlike that experienced by Nancy:

> Suddenly without warning . . . I would find myself swimming in a sea of black, my arms and legs heavy and lifeless, tears in my eyes. The frustration of it all swept over me like waves on a beach, pulling me under, upending me in deep water, washing me out away from a firm emotional shore. Day after day, the struggle raged. (p. 91)

Chittister refuses to sentimentalize her spiritual struggles. "Struggle," she concludes, "is never done without cost. Real struggle marks us for life" (p. 81).

Throughout this book, we provide examples of the potent links between spiritual struggles and many signs of emotional distress. We will see that spiritual struggles can be embedded in the full range of psychological problems. A study led by researcher Kelly Trevino (formerly McConnell) provides one initial illustration. They surveyed a national sample of people in the United States about their symptoms of psychopathology and spiritual struggles (McConnell, Pargament, Ellison, & Flannelly, 2006). Symptoms of virtually every form of psychopathology—anxiety, phobias, depression, paranoid ideation, obsessions–compulsions, and somatization—were associated with higher levels of spiritual struggles. These findings are consistent with what clinicians often hear in therapy: descriptions of psychological and physical symptoms comingled with statements of spiritual tension, conflict, and confusion. The client dealing with bipolar illness blurts out how she fears God has abandoned her. The abusive father of a young child admits that he feels he is battling with the devil for his child's soul. The depressed older man in treatment for cancer wonders whether his life has had any real purpose and why he should bother to go on. Comments such as these illustrate how physical and mental health problems are often profoundly disturbing to the client's most basic values, beliefs, and assumptions about life. And the spiritual struggles triggered by psychological trauma and pathology may, in turn, exacerbate the client's psychological functioning and undermine progress in treatment (Evans et al., 2018; Magyar-Russell, Pargament, Trevino, & Sherman, 2013; Pomerleau, Pargament, Krause, Ironson, & Hill, 2020). Studies have shown spiritual struggles to be risk factors for poorer treatment outcomes

(Currier, Holland, & Drescher, 2015; Medlock et al., 2017). There are many good reasons, then, to attend to spiritual struggles in clinical practice.

A caveat is needed here. Distressing though they are, spiritual struggles are not signs of weakness, pathology, immaturity, or weak faith. As we saw above, even the greatest of religious figures experienced their periods of spiritual storm and stress, and through their struggles underwent powerful transformations that shaped not only their lives but the course of history. Rather than signs of pathology, spiritual struggles are a natural part of the lifelong search for significance. They are embedded in the human condition. Beneath the pain, turmoil, and conflict of spiritual struggles, we find people striving to find and realize their most important goals and purposes. We elaborate on this important point in the following chapter.

Struggles, spiritual and nonspiritual, play a key role in development and offer the potential for growth. Without them, how could we ever learn new ways of thinking about ourselves, other people, and the world? Without struggle, how could we find our way through seemingly impassable thickets and discover new pathways to our goals or abandon lost destinations for new ones? This notion is, of course, central to many psychological theories, such as the work of Jean Piaget (1954) and Erik Erikson (1998).

Thinking about spiritual struggle in this way forces us to shift out of the mindset of weakness and pathology. Spiritual struggles are certainly painful and can lead to problems, but they are not medical illnesses or even symptoms. For that reason, we selected the term *spiritual struggles* rather than other related terms in the literature—*spiritual injury, spiritual distress, spiritual trauma, spiritual crisis, spiritual emergency, spiritual wounding*—because spiritual struggles connote not only pain but also active possibility and potential. The language of spiritual struggles, we believe, discourages strugglers from seeing themselves as spiritually deficient or wanting (Santiago & Gall, 2016). In fact, spiritual struggles offer the potential for growth, as well as decline. They are, in short, pivotal experiences.

Spiritual Struggles Are Pivotal

Nancy, the woman who had lost her beloved daughter in a shooting, comes to therapy at a pivotal time in her life. Her future holds many possibilities: she could start drinking, medicating herself, or engaging in a series of extramarital affairs in an effort to fill the spiritual void in her life; she could deaden her emotions by placing herself on automatic pilot, going through the day-to-day motions disconnected from any feelings; she could explore dramatic changes and try to turn her life around through a new job, a new career, a new faith, a rejection of religious commitments, a move to another community or country; she could decide that her situation calls for soul-searching and introspection, and use this time to become more aware of herself and the sources of her suffering. The options are almost endless for Nancy. In short, Nancy is coming to treatment at a pivotal time in her life, a time in which she finds herself at the junction of a multiforked road.

Spiritual struggles are often momentous. Like nuclear energy, they are fraught with power and possibility (Griffith, 2010). They are periods when "destiny is hanging in the balance," as Anton Boisen (1955, p. 116), founder of pastoral counseling, once said. On the one hand, spiritual struggles create the potential for transcendence and growth. Most religious traditions present powerful stories of the greatest of figures—from Moses to Jesus to Muhammed—strengthened, tempered, and transfigured by their spiritual trials. From a religious perspective, struggles are opportunities for spiritual regeneration. Theologian Martin Marty (1983) writes, "Brokenness and wounding do not occur in order to break human dignity but to open the heart so God can act" (p. 123).

On the other hand, even though spiritual struggles can indeed lead to greater wholeness and growth, we will see in later chapters that this outcome is far from guaranteed. Suffering builds character, the old saying goes, but like many old sayings it can be misleading. Suffering can build character, some of the time. Nevertheless, if spiritual struggles have the capacity to "make," they also have the capacity to "break" (cf. Boisen, 1955).

The stark reality is that spiritual struggles lead many people down a dark road to despair and brokenness. Of course, even then, possibilities for recovery, wholeness, and growth remain. However, we review a number of sobering studies that point to the destructive, even deadly consequences of spiritual struggles. Some people, it appears, do not find their way back once they have gone down this painful spiritual path.

What determines the outcomes of these pivotal times: whether spiritual struggles make or break an individual, or perhaps some measure of both? Later, we try to provide some answers to this central question by drawing on research and clinical practice. These answers help us respond, in turn, to the questions of greatest concern for practitioners: How do we work with spiritual strugglers, like Nancy, who have come to us at a fork in the road in their lives? How do we help them bear and survive their struggles? How do we help them find paths to greater wholeness and growth rather than brokenness and decline?

THE PURPOSE OF THIS BOOK

In her pioneering book *Trauma and Recovery,* Judith Herman (1992/1997) describes how, historically, mental health professionals overlooked the role that trauma played in many of the psychological problems that clients presented in treatment. Although Freud initially believed that his hysterical patients' reports of abuse, assault, and incest were true, later he shifted to seeing these stories as fabrications and fantasies based on the desires and needs of his patients rather than their real-world experiences. Similarly, Herman notes, for much of the 20th century, practitioners attributed the psychological problems of soldiers who had broken down in combat to moral and character weakness rather than to the actual horrors of the battlefield. Through the screen of television, the Vietnam War brought home the life-shattering reality of combat itself and stimulated the growth of study on trauma leading, eventually, to the term *posttraumatic stress disorder*. The field of mental health had overlooked a dimension of psychological suffering that, with all the wisdom of hindsight, appears rather obvious.

The same might be said of spiritual struggles. Helping professionals have not generally paid close attention to the spiritual dimension of problems that people bring in to treatment, though there are signs of change (e.g., Doehring, 2015; Griffith, 2010; Jones, 2019; Pargament, 2007; Park, Currier, Harris, & Slattery, 2017; Rosmarin, 2018). The point may apply at times even to chaplains and clergy. Herman (1992/1997) cites an apt illustration from the work of Norman (1989), who recounts the following interaction between a soldier and a priest:

> I could not rationalize in my mind how God let good men die. I had gone to several . . . priests. I was sitting there with this one priest and said, "Father, I don't understand this: how does God allow small children to be killed? What is this thing, this war, this bullshit? I got all these friends who are dead. . . . " That priest, he looked me in the eye and said, "I don't know, son, I've never been in war." I said, "I didn't ask you about war, I asked you about God." (p. 55)

The lack of attention to spiritual concerns may come with costs. Balboni and colleagues (2011) conducted a study of patients at the end of life that speaks to this point. Although they did not measure spiritual struggles directly, they found that patients who did not feel their spiritual needs were being met had considerably higher costs of treatment, received less hospice care, spent more time in an intensive care unit (ICU), and experienced more ICU deaths. These effects were especially strong among minorities and people who look to their faith for help in coping.

To avoid the topic of spiritual struggles is to miss an important opportunity for change. Because spiritual struggles represent critical crossroads, conversations about these struggles can have powerful, long-lasting consequences for the trajectory of the individual's life. By broaching spiritual struggles in treatment, then, practitioners may be better able to arrest decline, heal brokenness, and foster wholeness and growth. In fact, efforts to address spiritual struggles explicitly in therapy have yielded promising results in evaluative studies, as we discuss later (Dworsky et al., 2013; Harris et al., 2011).

This book shines a light directly on spiritual struggles. It is designed, in part, for researchers interested in a thorough (though not exhaustive), up-to-date review of what we have learned from studies of spiritual struggles. It is also designed to help mental health professionals recognize, understand, and address spiritual struggles in treatment. As coauthors of this book, we are aware that the work of practitioners is already very demanding. And we do not want to complicate that work further by adding yet another issue to consider in psychotherapy. Yet, because spiritual struggles are pervasive, painful, and pivotal, they do call for clinical attention.

Many clients themselves would like the chance to discuss spiritual matters, including spiritual struggles, in their mental health care. For example, in a study of 253 patients with psychiatric issues, over half (58%) expressed at least some desire to integrate spirituality into their psychotherapy. Interestingly, a significant percentage of patients (37%) with no religious affiliation also voiced interest in talking about spirituality in treatment (Rosmarin, 2018). Clients experiencing spiritual struggles and strain have shown even greater interest in integrating spirituality in their mental health care (Exline et al., 2000). However, it is important to recognize that some clients may be hesitant to talk about their spiritual struggles because these conflicts may elicit feelings of guilt, shame, or fear of stigmatization (Currier, McDermott, Hawkins, Greer, & Carpenter, 2018; Exline & Grubbs, 2011).

Even though spiritual struggles can be a sensitive topic for clients, we believe the reluctance to broach this topic in practice often comes from clinicians. Several forces have led practitioners to steer clear of spirituality: the history of antireligious bias among several of the founding figures in the field; the tendency of mental health professionals to underestimate the importance of spiritual and religious issues, perhaps as a result of their own lower levels of religiousness (Shafranske & Cummings, 2013); fears about overstepping appropriate professional boundaries; and perhaps most importantly, and, as we noted earlier, the lack of training about spirituality in graduate professional education (Oxhandler, Parrish, Torres, & Achenbaum, 2015; Saunders et al., 2014).

It is time to break the silence. Spirituality is too important to be ignored in treatment. Like any other issue relevant to the client's mental health and goals in therapy, spiritual matters can and should be a part of the therapeutic dialogue. Spiritual struggles in particular deserve far greater attention. More than that, we believe that addressing spiritual struggles is a key element of spiritually competent mental health care (Pearce, Pargament, Oxhandler, Vieten, & Wong, 2019). We will see that, like other sensitive topics, spiritual struggles can be discussed in ways that are respectful of clients and of the professional boundaries and competence of practitioners.

In this chapter, we have stressed that spiritual struggles are a natural part of the human journey. There are no signs of that changing. People today continue to feel the powerful effects of a bewildering array of disorienting biological, social, and cultural forces: pandemics, militarism, terrorism, ethnic hatreds, misogyny, economic disparity, racial discrimination, weapons proliferation, sociopolitical conflict, ecological destruction, family breakdown, and genocide. In this world in flux, Chittister (2003) notes, "there is no such thing as a noncombatant" (p. 11). We strongly suspect that this bubbling caldron of elements will continue to produce the more immediate experiences—the stray bullet that took the life of Nancy's daughter, Lilly—that throw sacred values and beliefs into confusion and turmoil. All the more reason then for mental health professionals to better understand and help people as they struggle with life's most sacred matters in their search for significance.

THE APPROACH OF THIS BOOK

No group or profession can lay exclusive claim to the topic of spiritual struggles. They are of interest to many people, including clergy, chaplains, theologians, mental health and medical professionals, artists, scientists, scholars, and the general public. Each group has important insights that help illuminate spiritual struggles. This book draws on the wisdom and contributions of people from many traditions, disciplines, and backgrounds. Thus, the substance of this book includes not only findings from research but also stories, anecdotes, symbols, and metaphors; we believe that the subject matter calls for them. Empirical studies provide invaluable, at times, surprising insights into spiritual struggles, and we review this burgeoning literature here. Even so, spiritual struggles cannot be fully captured by the methods of science. Like spirituality more generally, spiritual struggles can be ineffable (cf. James, 1902)—that is, hard or even impossible to put into words. Grasping spiritual struggles sometimes requires nonlinear modes of thought and expression. Spiritual struggles, like spirituality more generally, can often be best understood by asking people to tell the story of their struggle; struggles seem to be encoded by the mind in narrative form. There are other aspects of spiritual struggles that can be best understood from the corner of the eye or, as Emily Dickinson (Johnson, 1960) put it poetically, on the "slant" (p. 1129). Admittedly, ours is an ambitious approach; we run the risk of producing our own hodgepodge of ideas—a discordant composition on spiritual struggles that is just plain hard to listen to.

The harmony and balance in the book, we believe, comes from its psychological orientation. Although the material included consists of many notes, tones, and rhythms, it is all written in the key of psychology, a psychology inclusive of many methods and theories to be sure, but a psychology nevertheless, one defined by values of curiosity, tentativeness, skepticism, clear and critical thinking, and rigor. This psychology is not to be confused with theology. Psychology has nothing to offer when it comes to finding the "ultimate truth," but it can speak in volume to perceptions of truth and their effects on peoples' lives—the footprints left by faith (cf. Batson, Schoenrade, & Ventis, 1993). We hope that our approach is of value to researchers and practitioners from a variety of fields, backgrounds, and orientations.

What does a psychological approach mean in the context of a book that touches on beliefs about supernatural entities, including a God or gods; the devil, demons, or supernatural evil forces; and spirits of people who have died? It means that we primarily use a *psychological lens* to view these supernaturally focused beliefs and experiences. Using this lens, practitioners would typically frame client reports about supernatural phenomena, adaptive or maladaptive, in terms of normal psychological processes, such as development, temperament, motivation, experience, learning, and socialization, without taking a stance on whether or not the associated supernatural beliefs or perceptions are based in reality. However, it is important to note that a psychological approach is not the only one that people might find valuable in framing such experiences. Depending on their own personal beliefs, prior experiences, and professional practice settings, some professionals might opt to use what we term a *mental illness lens* (framing the belief or experience as a sign of medical or mental illness) or a *supernatural lens* (framing the experience as an actual result of supernatural activity).

Imagine, for example, that a client described an experience that was seen as a personal message from God or a departed loved one. Some professionals, perhaps especially those with materialistic worldviews or who work in psychiatric settings, might readily adopt a mental illness lens: They would want to examine whether this experience might be the result of a hallucination or a delusion, perhaps due to serious mental illness, or a neurological or another medical condition. Others, perhaps especially those with strong beliefs in a personal, relational God or an afterlife, might easily take up a supernatural lens, one that would allow them to seriously consider and perhaps even adopt a supernatural explanation for a client's experiences. Some practitioners might choose to address the supernatural angle directly—perhaps by praying with a client, encouraging the client to actively seek out messages, or consulting with a religious or spiritual professional (e.g., a member of the clergy, a spirit medium, a shaman) who would try to address the issues within a supernatural framework that is shared by the client. A professional might opt to use any or all of these lenses. In this book, we address the role that mental illness can play as one potential cause and consequence of spiritual struggles. Nevertheless, we view supernatural beliefs and experiences primarily through the psychological lens, with its emphasis on normal psychological processes.

As psychologists, we place a priority on trying to recognize the ways our own particular biases and commitments may shape our work, knowingly or unknowingly. This recognition is especially important when we move from research to practice and face the risks of imposing our own beliefs and values on our clients. Readers, too, should be aware of the backgrounds and biases of the authors they are studying. This book is written by one Jewish psychologist

(K.I.P.) and another psychologist—a spiritual seeker from a Christian background (J.J.E.). We joined forces in our research and worked on this book as a result of our common interests, the feeling that we could deepen and enrich our understanding through collaboration, and the fact that we like and respect each other a lot. Though we come from Jewish and Christian traditions, respectively, we share a deep interest in and appreciation of other religious traditions. We have both sought out research collaborations focusing on a diverse range of worldviews, including a wide variety of religious perspectives (Jewish, Christian, Muslim, Hindu, Buddhist), as well as viewpoints that are secular or spiritual without being religious. In addition, K.I.P. has worked extensively with people from diverse religious traditions, including his graduate students and clients. J.J.E. also has a broad, enduring interest in learning more about the world's religious and spiritual traditions, as reflected in Buddhist meditation retreats, yoga practice, and study of the Hebrew and Arabic languages. Nevertheless, we recognize that this book comes out of the perspectives of two psychologists who have lived their lives in a Western context and are familiar first and foremost with the religions of Judaism and Christianity. It also becomes apparent that both of us are eclectic in our orientations to change, and draw on the valuable resources of many therapeutic perspectives to meet the diverse needs of clients. Likewise, we hope that our work on spirituals struggles is helpful to practitioners who come from a wide range of mental health-related disciplines and hold a wide range of therapeutic orientations. Undoubtedly, our own backgrounds and biases have shaped the ideas that run through these pages.

We believe spiritual struggles represent one of the most complex topics in our field. Spiritual struggles do not lend themselves to quick fixes or how-to manuals. Though it might be tempting to try to provide a few simple recommendations for addressing spiritual struggles in mental health care, we do not do so, for simple solutions to complex problems are likely to be ineffective at best and harmful at worst. Instead, we offer readers some ways to think about spiritual struggles in the context of the larger human search for significance, and then some tools to help clinicians recognize spiritual struggles and respond to them in treatment. This book is a work in progress. It reflects the youthful stage of a developing area of study. Yet, we have already learned a great deal about spiritual struggles. We share this body of knowledge with readers as one of the first rather than last words on spiritual struggles. Our hope is that this initial work opens the door to further conversations and study that advance our ability to understand and assist clients who come to us shaken to the core.

This book is divided into two parts. Part I rests on the assumption that before we can help people who are experiencing spiritual struggles, we have to understand them. Each chapter takes up an important question. In this first, introductory chapter we asked, "What are spiritual struggles?" and described why they are a vital part of clinical care and practice. The following chapter places spirituality and spiritual struggles in the larger context of a theoretical model or way of understanding the search for significance. In Chapter 3, we consider "Where do spiritual struggles come from?" The next two chapters zero in on the question of whether spiritual struggles really matter and, if so, how. Chapter 4 focuses on the dark side of the answer to this question, along with the links between spiritual struggles and distress, disorientation, and decline. Chapter 5 looks at the bright side of the response to this question—namely, the possibility that spiritual struggles may be related to growth. This leads to the critical question of what determines whether spiritual struggles lead to decline or growth. Chapter 6 asks, "What shapes the outcome of spiritual struggles?"

Building on this understanding of spiritual struggles, Part II focuses on the ways that practitioners can respond to the clinical challenges that arise when spiritual struggles enter into psychotherapy. Chapter 7 provides a general framework and set of tools to answer the question "How can practitioners address spiritual struggles?" We then shift the focus from spiritual struggles in general to six specific spiritual struggles and the distinctive challenges they raise and the responses they call for in practice. These six chapters bridge research and practice. The first half of each chapter focuses on practically relevant theory and research, and the second half of each chapter builds on that body of knowledge to consider how practitioners can help people facing divine struggles (Chapter 8), struggles of ultimate meaning (Chapter 9), struggles with doubt (Chapter 10), moral struggles (Chapter 11), demonic struggles (Chapter 12), and interpersonal struggles (Chapter 13). In our final chapter, we offer some brief concluding thoughts.

Let's get started!

CHAPTER 2

A Conceptual Model of Spiritual Struggles

To be able to understand and address spiritual struggles, practitioners and researchers must first have a way to think about spiritual struggles. In this chapter, we lay the foundation for the book by introducing a conceptual model of spiritual struggles, and with it, a set of terms and themes that appear throughout the chapters that follow. Our model places spiritual struggles within the larger context of spirituality and the search for significance (see Figure 2.1). Spiritual struggles are, we believe, a natural outgrowth of the desire to find, hold on to, and, at times, transform the things that are most significant to us. The presentation of our model is admittedly brief—we unpack it further in the chapters to come. For a more extended discussion, readers can look into Pargament's (1997, 2007) earlier writings. We organize the overview by seven premises about the search for significance.

PEOPLE SEEK SIGNIFICANCE

We are, in part, reactive beings, shaped by our early developmental experiences, our social and cultural environments, and our genetics and biology. This is not the full story, however. We are also intentional beings, able to envision and plan for the future. As Rabbi Jonathan Sacks (2016) wrote, "Like our bodies, our souls were not made for sitting still. We were made for moving, walking, traveling, learning, searching, striving, growing" (p. 4). But these actions are not random; we are drawn to things that offer us a purpose, what has been called "significance" (Pargament, 1997). Psychologist Gordon Allport (1950b) wrote, "Starting fairly early in our lives we are propelled . . . not by instincts, but interests" (p. 155). In the search for significance, we try to discover what matters, conserve or hold on to what matters once we have found it, and when necessary, transform

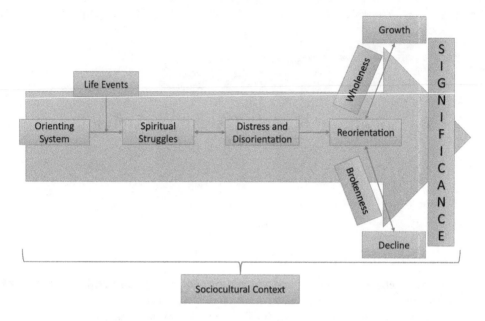

FIGURE 2.1. A framework for understanding spiritual struggles.

our relationship with what matters. Significance then becomes a magnet, the attractor that draws us forward and shapes the direction of our lives. It is both objective, the "what" we seek out of life, and subjective, the sense of purpose that often accompanies having meaningful goals to pursue.

There is of course a diverse array of significant ends, motives, goals, and values that people can hold, as psychologists from Murray (1938) to Maslow (1970) have described. Which among these is the most important motivating force? Theorists have long debated this question. Sigmund Freud (1927/1961) insisted that people are fundamentally motivated to reduce tension in their lives. Emile Durkheim (1915) countered with the argument that people are guided by a need for social connectedness. Erich Fromm (1950) emphasized the human motivation for growth. And Clifford Geertz (1966) held that people are motivated by the need to make meaning or sense out of the world.

Although theorists have often tried to explain the diversity in human behavior through singular motivations, empirical studies suggest that there is no need to choose a single winner. People can and do pursue many different sets or configurations of significant goals: material (e.g., money, houses), physical (e.g., fitness, good health), psychological (e.g., meaning, growth, avoiding discomfort), and social (e.g., intimacy, social justice; Emmons, 1999; Ford & Nichols, 1987). It is important to add that not all significant ends are necessarily constructive; clinicians are well aware that people can devote the same determination to the pursuit of destructive goals (e.g., drugs, violence, suicide, abusiveness) as constructive ones. Thus, the purposes people seek out of life have tremendous implications for the trajectory their lives will follow.

SPIRITUALITY IS EMBEDDED
IN THE SEARCH FOR SIGNIFICANCE

Curiously, however, until recently researchers and practitioners largely overlooked one powerful source of significance for many people: spirituality. Many scholars have attempted to explain why people are spiritual or religious in terms of presumably more basic motivations (Pargament, 2013). Spirituality has been said to be, at its root, a way to find peace and comfort in life, a way to achieve interconnectedness with others, a means of controlling one's own impulses, a way to make meaning out of life, and a way to stay healthy. Though there is certainly some truth to each of these explanations, they run the risk of attempting to explain spirituality away.

We prefer to think of spirituality in a nonreductionistic way, as a particular kind of search for significance, one directed to whatever people hold sacred. To put it more succinctly, spirituality is "a search for the sacred" (Pargament, 1999, p. 12). This is not a new idea. Scholars past and present have written about the human yearning for something of ultimate value and meaning, of something that takes us beyond our material selves, of something that represents a deeper reality. Saint Augustine (1960) captured this longing quite poignantly: "our heart is restless until it rests in you" (p. 43). Theologian Paul Tillich (1957) spoke to this motivation more broadly, defining faith as "the centered movement of the whole personality toward something of ultimate meaning and significance" (p. 123). Similarly, Bakan (1966) described a fundamental human impulse that "presupposes that the manifest is but the barest hint of reality . . . and that the function of the impulse is to reach out toward the unmanifest" (p. 5). In more recent years, the motivation for self-transcendence has continued to figure large in the research and writings of several psychologists (e.g., Cloninger, Svrakic, & Przybeck, 1993; Piedmont & Wilkins, 2013).

The human propensity to seek out the sacred is the heart and soul of spirituality. It can occur within an established institutional context (e.g., churches, temples, synagogues, mosques, fellowships), in which case we would also apply the word *religious* (Pargament, Mahoney, Exline, Jones, & Shafranske, 2013). Or the search for the sacred can unfold outside of a traditional setting. Moreover, the sacred destination can take the form of traditional theistic goals or seemingly secular purposes that have been imbued with sacred significance. This point is worth elaborating. When people are asked to list their major strivings in life, many respond with goals related to God, such as "to seek God's will for my life" and "to increase my faith in God" (Emmons, Cheung, & Tehrani, 1998). Spiritual strivings do not have to center around God, however. In a study of a community sample, Mahoney and colleagues (2005) had participants articulate their major strivings and then rate the degree to which they perceived each one to be a manifestation of God or imbued with sacred qualities, including transcendence, ultimacy, and boundlessness. The participants viewed a wide range of strivings as sacred, including those that might not seem to be spiritual at first glance, family, helping others, and well-being.

It is important to add that the ability to envision and seek out something sacred is not limited to traditionally religious individuals or theists. Even though Albert Einstein (1956) did not believe in a personal God, he did perceive a deeper, sacred dimension to his scientific quest, as we hear in the following words:

> A knowledge of the existence of something we cannot penetrate, of the manifestations of the profoundest reason and the most radiant beauty—it is this knowledge and this emotion that constitute the truly religious attitude; in this sense, and in this alone, I am a deeply religious man. (p. 7)

Thus, the search for the sacred is not an esoteric pursuit or one restricted to those who attend a religious congregation. Many people, theists and nontheists, religious and nonreligious, search for the sacred in their lives. Of course, they do so in a variety of ways—because the sacred can take so many forms, the spiritual journey itself unfolds in an almost limitless set of directions, including those that are not necessarily positive. To echo James (1902), where the individual's "centre of energy" lies has important implications for the search for significance.

The search for sacred forms of significance is likely to have special power. People feel a particularly strong magnetic attraction to whatever they hold sacred. Allport (1950a) noted that, even though spiritual motivation may grow out of its association with more basic hungers, fears, and needs, it can become "functionally autonomous" of these motives. Empirical studies suggest that this kind of spiritual motivation represents another distinctive dimension of personality. For example, Piedmont (1999) found that his measure of spiritual transcendence formed a sixth factor independent of the often-used five-factor model of personality.

Having a spiritual motivating "magnet" can provide energy and direction even in discouraging times that may otherwise sap an individual's energy and hope. It can also be a source of powerful spiritual emotions. In his classic book *The Idea of the Holy,* theologian Rudolf Otto (1917/1928) wrote about the fascinating and overpowering emotions, what he called the mysterium, that accompany experiences of the divine. In support of Otto's theory, sacred experiences have been linked with emotions of awe and elevation (Haidt, 2003), gratitude (Emmons & Crumpler, 2000), and happiness and joy (Mahoney et al., 2005). Sacred experiences also have the capacity to soothe, comfort, and empower (LaMothe, 1998; Yaden, Haidt, Hood, Vago, & Newberg, 2017). Why? Perhaps because they place life in a larger transcendent context, one that generates greater meaning and purpose, connects people to the past and the future, and creates enduring bonds between people who share common ways of understanding the sacred. Consistent with this explanation, researchers have found that the pursuit of the sacred is accompanied by several benefits. In their review of this literature, Mahoney et al. (2013) cite several relevant findings. Individuals who perceive their strivings in life as sacred rate their goals as more meaningful. People who define their work as a vocation rather than a job report greater satisfaction with their work. And individuals who view their marriages and sexuality as sacred report greater satisfaction with their marriages and sex lives. Thus, in striving for the sacred, people may be more able to sustain themselves in good times and bad.

In short, the quest for the sacred has an especially important place in the search for significance. Mental health practitioners can ill afford to overlook the role of spirituality and spiritual struggles in the search for significance because the spiritual dimension is a vital part of clients' lives, including the problems they bring to treatment and the solutions to these problems.

PEOPLE ARE GUIDED IN THE SEARCH FOR SIGNIFICANCE BY AN ORIENTING SYSTEM

If significance provides the destination we seek in life, then how do we get there? Where do we find a map or a compass to point us in the direction we would like to go? In the search for significance, we are guided by an orienting system (cf. Pargament, 1997), a system of general beliefs, attitudes, habits, experiences, practices, coping skills, and personality characteristics, as well as a network of social relationships that provide a sense of direction and stability. An orienting system is like the knapsack we carry with us in life. It contains a map and compass to guide us, and the necessary food and drink to sustain us, as well as the tools to solve the problems that arise along the way. But the knapsack can also hold burdens that weigh us down and make the trek all the more difficult. Not all orienting systems are alike. Some are stronger, more capable of orienting people and grounding them in their search for significance than others. Thus, some of us are better equipped than others to handle the journey. Even so, the reality is that no one can ever be fully equipped to handle all of the surprises, challenges, and troubles, large and small, that we may encounter.

Note that the term *orienting system* has much in common with other psychological terms, such as *worldviews, working models, assumptive worlds, cognitive schemas, philosophies of life, plausibility structures,* and *meaning systems.* However, while these latter terms have a cognitive focus, the notion of an orienting system goes beyond the ways individuals think about themselves and their world, important as they are. The orienting system also encompasses the ways people generally behave, their general health status, their emotional styles, and their social connections. The orienting system is in this sense biopsychosocial.

The orienting system is more than that, though—it also has a spiritual dimension. We can think of the spiritual orienting system as a subset of the larger general orienting system. The spiritual orienting system includes relatively stable patterns of belief, practice, emotion, and relationship linked to the sacred that guide the individual along preferred pathways to significant destinations. Spiritual orientations take a remarkable variety of forms. Many spiritual orientations are nested within established religious institutions. In fact, when asked to select among four options—spiritual but not religious, spiritual and religious, religious and not spiritual, not religious and not spiritual—most people (48%) in the United States label themselves as spiritual *and* religious (Pew Research Center, 2017a). However, spiritual orientations can also develop outside of established religious institutions. There are many nontraditional paths to the sacred: yoga, meditation, knitting, gardening, social action, music, and the list goes on. The percentage of people who label themselves "spiritual but not religious" in the United States appears to be growing (27%), though it remains a minority (Pew Research Center, 2017a). Some among this group, Hood (2003) adds, are not simply nonreligious; they are rebelling against organized religious life.

Spiritual orientations have also been differentiated according to the motivations underlying religious and spiritual involvement. For example, Allport and Ross (1967) contrasted intrinsically oriented people, who are motivated to live according to their faith, with extrinsically oriented people, who use their faith to achieve nonreligious ends, such as social status and psychological comfort. To this scheme, Batson et al. (1993) added the concept of quest orientation, which involves a search for truth, meaning, and answers to life's deepest questions through religious involvement. Even this list likely underestimates the full range of spiritual orientations (Pargament, 1997). Other spiritual orientations may vary according to whether they are held lightly or intensely, flexibly or inflexibly, literally or symbolically, and consciously or unconsciously. It may also be useful to differentiate among people whose spiritualities are largely experiential or emotion centered, belief centered, practice centered, or relationship centered (Hood, 2003). We can make even finer distinctions among spiritual orientations. These include differences in spiritual coping resources (Pargament, 1997) and differences in the theodicies people hold—that is, the ways in which they reconcile pain and suffering in the world with beliefs in God (Hale-Smith, Park, & Edmondson, 2012; Wilt, Exline, Grubbs, Park, & Pargament, 2016).

A few more points about the spiritual orienting system are relevant here. Like the orienting system more generally, spiritual orienting systems vary in the degree to which they are well integrated and whole, capable of helping people weather life's ups and downs and find some sense of significance. It is also important to recognize that people often become deeply attached to their preferred spiritual pathways, be it going to a particular type of religious service, practicing mindfulness meditation, committing to core tenets of a faith tradition, spiritual coping methods, or attending a 12-step program. Spiritual orientations can then be instilled with a spiritual significance of their own and turn into sacred pursuits in their own right.

THE SEARCH FOR SIGNIFICANCE IS TYPICALLY NEITHER SMOOTH NOR STRAIGHTFORWARD

The search for significance is a process that unfolds over the lifespan, but it is not necessarily easy or uniform. At times, obstacles arise from within or outside of ourselves that block us from discovering, attaining, or living according to what matters most. At other times, we simply lose our way. The search for significance is then marked by ebb and flow, starts and stops, wrong turns and dead ends, and periods of stability and of remarkable transformation.

In short, no journey through life is stress-free. "Be kind," an anonymous saying goes, "for everyone you meet is fighting a hard battle." Of course the battles vary in number, type, and intensity. Although a singular trauma as devastating as the Holocaust, the 9/11 terrorist attacks, or most recently the COVID-19 pandemic can upend the security and stability of most anyone, the gradual accumulation of smaller hassles and stressors over time can also take their toll. We can distinguish among historical stressors, such as experiences of physical and sexual abuse as a child; ongoing stressors, such as discrimination and systemic racism; and life stressors that have occurred within the last few months or year. Some stressors come from within, reflecting the challenges that arise in developmental transitions from one phase of life to another, and other stressors come from outside of ourselves, as in the case of sexual harassment. Stressors can be experienced firsthand or vicariously—for example, therapists are regularly exposed to secondhand stress in listening to their clients' stories. It is also useful to differentiate between anticipated, on-time events, such as the death of a grandparent, and unanticipated, off-time events, such as the loss of a young child. Stressful events can be grouped into different content categories: sociocultural (e.g., war), physical (e.g., experiencing a stroke), relational (e.g., marital conflict), moral (e.g., committing a crime), occupational (e.g., unemployment), or religious (e.g., a congregation closing, clergy sexual abuse). And stressful events can be distinguished according to whether the cause is attributed to oneself, others, natural forces, accident or chance, karma, the divine, or something mysterious (e.g., Exline, Wilt, et al., in press).

Although stressful life events and transitions are often unwelcome, they play an important role in the search for significance by creating instability that can lead to struggle and change, including opportunities for positive growth and transformation.

SPIRITUAL STRUGGLES GROW OUT OF THE INTERPLAY OF SIGNIFICANCE, THE ORIENTING SYSTEM, AND LIFE EVENTS AND TRANSITIONS

As depicted in Figure 2.1, spiritual struggles are the product of three key processes that guide the search for significance: (1) the significant purposes the individual seeks in life, (2) the nature of the person's orienting system, and (3) the life events and transitions the individual experiences along the journey. First, spiritual struggles can grow out of disruptions to the person's significant purposes in living. As we noted earlier, a large body of theory and research points to the vital importance of having a set of meaningful life goals. Sacred pursuits are especially powerful: Rather than simply framing them as goals, people often think of them as missions, vocations, or destinies. As such, they often land at the top of the list of what people hope to achieve and what they strive for (Emmons, 1999). But more than that, sacred strivings frequently serve as an overarching, defining force in people's lives. By knowing an individual's most sacred values, we discover a great deal about who that person is and is not. To learn that someone is committed to living as a devout Muslim, Jew, or Christian can tell us more about his or her daily habits and practices, social connections, and core beliefs and values than knowing his or her age, gender, occupation, education, or political affiliation. Sacred purposes also help place lower-order goals and values into a larger, more unified whole. In Emmons et al.'s (1998) research on strivings, people were asked to list what they were striving for in life. Those who included more sacred strivings in their list also reported more coherence and less conflict within their system of goals. Sacred pursuits thus appear to be particularly powerful sources of self-definition, social identity, and integration, factors that may help people maintain their balance through life's ups and downs, and experiences of spiritual struggle.

Perhaps not surprisingly, then, people can go to remarkable lengths to preserve and protect their most sacred values. In his description of Jewish life during the Holocaust, Berkovits (1979) captured the extraordinary measures people sometimes take to protect their sacred identities. In one instance, a mother and father were interrupted by the Gestapo in the midst of the ritual circumcision of their newborn son. The mother cried out, "Hurry up! Circumcise the child. Don't you see? They have come to kill us. At least let my child die as a Jew" (p. 45). Individuals preserve and protect sacred parts of their lives in more ordinary, day-to-day ways as well. Mahoney and colleagues (2013) conducted several studies relevant to this point. They found that when nature is perceived as sacred, people are more likely to invest in environmental causes. When the body is seen as sacred, people eat and drink more sensibly, wear a seat belt, and engage in more physical exercise. When marriage is perceived as sacred, spouses are less likely to engage in destructive forms of marital communication. These findings make good sense—because sacred objects are precious objects that provide organization and definition to our lives, they elicit the greatest devotion, protection, and care. There is, however, an important corollary: When people are unable to preserve and protect their sacred values and purposes, they are more likely to experience spiritual struggle, turmoil, and pain.

Spiritual struggles can also be rooted in the individual's orienting system. We stressed that people are not empty-handed when they face challenges in living. They are equipped with an orienting system of beliefs, practices, experiences, and relationships that can assist them in their efforts to pursue their significant purposes. But not all orienting systems are alike. Some are stronger and better able to orient people to their goals than others. This helps to explain how individuals can respond so differently to virtually the same life stressor. In their study of severely burned patients, Silver and Wortman (1980) observed:

> One patient is crying, moaning, complaining, demanding that more be done for him; another appears completely comfortable and unconcerned; another appears intensely preoccupied and seems to make very little contact with the observer; still another appears sad and troubled but friendly, responding with a weak smile to any approach made to him; and so it goes from one bed to the next. (p. 300)

Differences in the individual's spiritual orienting system can also help explain how the same life experience leaves one person's faith unaffected, another person shaken and struggling spiritually, and yet another person completely disenchanted with religious life.

Finally, spiritual struggles are shaped by stressful experiences. Few people go through their lives without encountering a major negative event of one kind or another. In one survey of the general population within 24 countries, over 70% reported that they had experienced at least one major traumatic event (Benjet et al., 2016). The most common traumas were witnessing death or serious injury, the unanticipated death of a loved one, being mugged, and having a life-threatening illness or injury. Major stressors of all types can have powerful psychological, social, and physical effects, as extensive research has shown (Folkman, 2011). Difficult life situations have a way of disrupting our life journeys. They can leave us without an ultimate sense of purpose. Not only that, stressful events can shake the guiding beliefs, practices, and experiences that orient us toward our goals. Janoff-Bulman (1992) vividly describes how experiences of the most traumatic kind are able to shatter the inner assumptive world of victims:

> Overwhelming life experiences split open the interior world of victims and shatter their most fundamental assumptions. . . . Rather than feel safe, they feel intensely vulnerable. . . . Suddenly the victim's inner world is pervaded by thoughts and images representing malevolence, meaninglessness, and self-abasement. They are face to face with a dangerous universe. (p. 63)

Stressful life events can impact people spiritually, as well as psychologically, socially, and physically. For example, one Iranian woman describes how her diagnosis of cancer disoriented her spiritually, and precipitated struggles about God's role in her illness: "I used to think that sinners get cancer; however, I was diagnosed with this illness and it was a blow to me. I did not hurt a soul. Why did I get this disease? I am still wondering why God did this to me" (Ghaempanah, Rafieinia, Sabahi, Hosseini, & Memaryan, 2020, p, 12). Stressful life events and transitions create conditions that are ripe for spiritual struggles.

These three processes—significant purpose, the orienting system, and stressful life events and transitions—are not fully independent of one another; they interact dynamically in ways that make spiritual struggles more probable. People are particularly likely to struggle spiritually when they encounter life events that reach out to shake their deepest sources of significance or overwhelm their orienting systems. None of this is to say that spiritual struggles should be equated with human weakness or pathology. Under the right conditions, anyone could experience a spiritual struggle. Spiritual struggles are a normative aspect of development and change, a natural part of the quest for significance. For some, as we will see, spiritual struggles can even be a preferred way of life.

SPIRITUAL STRUGGLES CAN LEAD TO GROWTH, DECLINE, OR BOTH

Spiritual struggles are fundamentally disorienting. Embedded in these struggles are disturbing questions about the individual's sources of significance and the most basic beliefs, practices, experiences, and connections that have guided and oriented the individual's efforts to realize his or her dreams. Because they can be so disruptive, spiritual struggles are likely to be accompanied by signs of pain, confusion, distress, and disorientation at multiple levels: emotional, cognitive, behavioral, relational, biological, and spiritual.

Distressing as spiritual struggles may be, they also create opportunities for development and growth. This point has been well established with respect to struggles in other domains of development, from the cognitive development of children (Piaget, 1954) to the formation of character. For example, lifespan psychologist Erik Erikson (1998) maintained that every phase of life comes with its own psychosocial crises and developmental tasks—how people negotiate these challenges has key implications for the shape of personality. Does the infant develop a sense of trust and security in others or come out of infancy with the feeling that other people and life itself cannot be trusted? Does the adolescent find a clear and compelling personal identity or leave adolescence with confusion about his or her place in the world and role in life? Does the older adult look back on life with a sense of meaning, fulfillment, and wholeness, or with feelings of despair and regret about a life that was not well lived? Each of these developmental crises can be painful, but each is necessary—we are forged by struggles, for better or worse.

In the spiritual area, struggles are accompanied by disorientation and disequilibrium, but they also signal the need for a reorientation, as shown in Figure 2.1. This reorientation may involve a conservational process of getting back on track by strengthening the orienting system and commitment to the pursuit of significant goals. It could also involve a transformation of purpose and orientation in which the person discovers and pursues new forms of significance, hopefully with new tools and resources better suited to the journey. If successful, the individual may realize profound growth. If not, the end result may be serious breakdown and decline. This is why we describe spiritual struggles as pivot points, forks in the road that hold powerful implications for the individual's trajectory in life. We explore both the potentially darker and brighter sides of spiritual struggles in Chapters 4 and 5, respectively.

THE TRAJECTORY OF SPIRITUAL STRUGGLES IS SHAPED BY ATTRIBUTES OF HUMAN WHOLENESS AND BROKENNESS

Whether spiritual struggles lead to growth or decline depends on the individual's degree of wholeness and brokenness. In speaking about wholeness and brokenness, we turn away from the possibility of discovering a single key to well-being and, instead, wrestle with life in its entirety and complexity (Pargament, Wong, & Exline, 2016). The language of wholeness includes terms such as *breadth and depth, life affirmation,* and *cohesiveness.* The converse of wholeness—brokenness—also calls for its own language, including terms such as *shallowness, narrowness, harshness, imbalance,* and *rigidity.* Wholeness and brokenness speak to life in toto—that is, every aspect of the human search for significance, including the destinations we strive toward and the pathway or orienting system that guides us toward these ends. When you come right down to it, the concepts of wholeness and brokenness have to do with how well we put our lives together.

Spirituality can also contribute to wholeness and brokenness. It may seem counterintuitive that spirituality could be a source of wholeness to people dealing with spiritual struggles, but it is important to keep in mind that spiritual struggles are not equivalent to spiritual disengagement or abandonment. In times of struggle, spirituality is often very much alive. Moreover, struggles may occur in one area of spirituality and leave other aspects of spiritual life unaffected. The individual's spiritual sources of significance, beliefs, practices, experiences, methods of coping, and relationships can reflect and foster wholeness, brokenness, or some blend of both. Several points about wholeness and brokenness deserve some emphasis.

First, wholeness and brokenness aren't end points in the search for significance, because the search itself is never finished. In Figure 2.1, you can see that the arrows from reorientation to wholeness and to brokenness point in both directions. It is true that reorientation can lead toward brokenness and decline, but brokenness can also lead back to reorientation and a shift toward greater wholeness and growth. We can be broken, but the damage is not irreparable. In this vein, Polish psychiatrist Kazimierz Dabrowski (1964) developed a theory of "positive disintegration" in which he suggested that disintegration may, in fact, be an important precursor to greater wholeness and ultimately growth toward higher ideals and values. On the other hand, the achievement of greater wholeness does not preclude the possibility of brokenness later in time. Though people can be remarkably resilient, even the strongest among us cannot be fully protected against the stressors and ruptures that life can bring our way.

Second, wholeness and brokenness are not mutually exclusive. (Figure 2.1 does not fully capture this complexity.) Even though it is useful to contrast the elements of wholeness and brokenness, the reality is that each of us is to some extent whole and to some extent broken. Full wholeness is impossible because we always remain human, finite, and, in part, flawed. Instead, we might speak of "net wholeness." Pargament, Wong, and Exline (2016) note that "the challenge in the search for significance is to become as whole as possible in the context of our human woundedness, limitations, frailties, and struggles. Wholeness and brokenness then are not two black-and-white options for living" (p. 382). This point is nicely illustrated by a Japanese ceramic art form, kintsugi, which rests on the philosophy that beauty is created by embracing flaws and imperfection. In kintsugi, broken pottery is repaired by re-fusing the shattered pieces into a new whole, with powdered gold or silver as the visible glue. Rather than attempting to conceal the brokenness, the reconstructed ceramic becomes a work of art by revealing simultaneously the brokenness and wholeness of the object (see the front book cover for an example).

Finally, it is important to recognize from the outset that wholeness and brokenness are highly value-laden constructs. Evaluation, however, is unavoidable in efforts to help people; it is an essential part of the work of practitioners. Psychologist Stanton Jones (1994) wrote, "One cannot intervene in the fabric of human life without getting deeply involved in moral and religious matters" (p. 197). Some kind of evaluative frame of reference is needed to assess clients' strengths and weaknesses, identify reasonable goals for treatment, and determine progress toward growth or decline. The notion of complete neutrality and impartiality in clinical work may simply be impossible, as Allen Bergin (1991) has maintained. We agree with Bergin, who argued that in the attempt to achieve complete objectivity, the therapist runs the risk of becoming a subtle manipulator of the client's values. That risk is reduced when practitioners are more open about their underlying system of values while remaining sensitive to the client's ultimate right to choose his or her life direction. In Chapter 6, we take a close look at the attributes of wholeness and brokenness that shape the trajectory of spiritual struggles. This discussion has important implications for the rest of this book, in which we consider how to address spiritual struggles in clinical practice.

CONCLUSIONS

In this chapter, we set the stage for our in-depth focus on spiritual struggles by presenting a brief overview of our way of thinking about spiritual struggles in the context of spirituality and the search for significance. Before moving on, it is important to stress that the search for significance does not occur in a vacuum. It plays out in a larger sociocultural context that has a key role of its own in shaping the search, including what we hold significant, our guiding orientations to life, and the challenges we are likely to experience along the way, including spiritual struggles. Therapists, too, become part of this larger context when they work with clients who are struggling spiritually. To be effective in this task, therapists have to be conversant with spiritual struggles and their roles in clients' lives. Until this point, we have considered what spiritual struggles are and their place in the search for significance. We turn now to a key foundational question: Where do spiritual struggles come from?

CHAPTER 3

Where Do Spiritual Struggles Come From?

Gary hadn't left his dorm room for 3 days. He was too embarrassed to be seen on campus. He might run into someone who noticed him when he got drunk and somehow ended up naked and hungover in a strange woman's apartment. But Gary also knew he couldn't remain holed up in his room forever. He couldn't afford to miss any more classes, let his grades drop, and put his scholarship at risk. If he did that, everything would crumble. He would have failed his family, God, and his church. One of his father's sayings kept running through his mind like a broken record: "Let down and let us down."

Gary's father was a man of unbending principle, and he had raised Gary with the same values: "God gives us what we deserve"; "No excuses, period"; "Don't get on the wrong side of God"; and "Put your faith in family and church." Gary's mother had left the family when Gary was a toddler. A ghost in his life, Gary never saw her again and his father had never spoken of her.

A shy, nervous boy who never wanted to risk his father's disapproval, Gary did his best to become his equal in discipline and focus. Gary was talented in science and mathematics and enjoyed losing himself in challenging problems. He could, like his father would say, "find the problem and solve it."

In middle school, Gary didn't fit in. Overweight, introverted, and socially awkward, he was teased and bullied by several of his classmates. Church, for Gary, was a refuge. There, he could avoid the harassment and gain some reassurance from the message that God would reward him if he didn't stray from the teachings of his church.

Things started to get better for Gary in high school. He excelled in his studies and found a few fellow "geeks" who shared his interest in science and math. Gary received a full scholarship to a prestigious school of engineering. When he was about to leave home, the church threw him a special "good-bye" luncheon with a banner saying, "You make us proud." His father's words were "Remember, don't let up."

At college, Gary felt as though he had entered a totally different universe: so many people from other countries, practicing other faiths or no faith at all, and living different lifestyles. Even though he was often bewildered by the differences he encountered, Gary found that he enjoyed meeting and talking to the people who inhabited his new world. And much to his surprise, they seemed to like Gary, too, for his scientific talents and his goofy but sweet nature. A few young women began to pay some attention to him. But with the words of his father ("Don't let up") in mind, Gary remained focused on his studies.

Although Gary was doing well at school, the courses were becoming increasingly challenging and the competition with his fellow students was getting tougher. In the second semester, Gary received a D on a test in mechanical engineering—a first; he had never received a grade below a B. Many others in his class had failed the test, but that was little consolation to Gary, who feared that his dreams were now in jeopardy. That night when his friends asked him once again to go out for a drink, Gary agreed. With little experience drinking, Gary quickly became drunk and the next morning he woke up naked in a strange woman's apartment with no memories of what had happened the night before.

Pushed by a friend, Gary left his dorm room and met with a counselor. Gary talked about the almost immobilizing anxiety he felt: a general sense of apprehension and dread punctuated by panic attacks in which he was convinced he was dying. These symptoms were intertwined with clear signs of spiritual struggle: intense fear that his whole life was about to be plunged into an abyss of ultimate meaninglessness, terrible guilt that he had failed to live up to the values of his father and church, and dread that he would face punishments from and perhaps abandonment by God, church, and family as a result of his transgressions.

Any therapist working with Gary would need to help him address not only his psychological symptoms but also his spiritual struggles. How, though? Unfortunately, we cannot offer a quick-and-easy answer. In fact, we believe the quick-and-easy approach to handling spiritual struggles would be ineffective at best or harmful at worst. Instead, effective help grows out of a deep understanding of spiritual struggles—what they are, where they come from, their implications for health and well-being, and the ways they can be addressed most effectively. In this chapter, we examine three roots of spiritual struggles: significant purpose, the orienting system, and life events and transitions. Throughout, we come back to the story of Gary to see how these factors apply.

HOW SIGNIFICANT PURPOSE
CAN LEAD TO SPIRITUAL STRUGGLES

In the last 35 years of his life, former boxing heavyweight champion of the world Muhammad Ali was ravaged by Parkinson's disease, an illness that attacked many of the qualities that had made him such a distinctive figure, perhaps the most widely recognized figure in the world. The face of the man who never hesitated to call himself "so pretty" was transfigured into a frozen, expressionless mask. The body that had once been able to "float like a butterfly and sting like a bee" trembled and grew increasingly immobile. The voice that had shouted out in protests against the war in Vietnam and expressed a new kind of poetry became mute. Even so, attractiveness, athleticism, volubility, and all the fame they brought were not primary values for Ali, at least not after his conversion to Islam. In an interview given in 1983, Ali said, "I conquered the world, and it didn't give me satisfaction. The boxing, the fame, the publicity, the attention—it didn't satisfy my soul . . . it's all nothing unless you go to heaven. You can have pleasure, but it means nothing unless you please God" (Greene, 1983, p. 139). Ali spent the years of his retirement from the ring and growing disability pursuing what did matter to him—living the life of a faithful Muslim, serving as a model of courage and character for people with disabilities, and doing what he could to share his humanity with the world. Asked how he would like to be remembered, he responded, "I guess I'd settle for being remembered only as a great boxing champion who became a preacher and a champion of his people. And I wouldn't even mind if folks forgot how pretty I was" (Lipsyte, 2016, p. 44). Although we cannot see into his psyche, from all accounts, Ali suffered physically but did not experience great spiritual struggles.

Ali's strength of purpose is a testament to the sentiments expressed in the famous quote from Friedrich Nietzsche: "He who has a *why* to live for can bear with almost any *how*" (cited in Frankl, 1959, p. 97, emphasis added). But the converse of that quote may be just as true; without a fulfilling purpose, people may struggle to find their way in life. Talk of fulfilling purposes takes us into sensitive territory, particularly for mental health professionals. We are generally reluctant to delve too deeply into the values of our clients. Quite rightly, we are taught to respect and affirm the diverse beliefs and values people hold. And yet, there are times when the problems people bring to treatment are entangled with the purposes they are seeking in life. Spiritual struggles can also follow when people strive for limited purposes. So, we cannot avoid the task of evaluating the nature of significance and purpose itself.

Here we introduce a few of the ways in which goals and purposes may be life enriching or life limiting, decreasing or increasing the individual's vulnerability to spiritual struggles. We pay particular attention to the links among spirituality, the purposes people seek out of life, and spiritual struggles.

Strength of Purpose

Muhammad Ali's story suggests that being guided by a strong sense of purpose may help spare people from spiritual struggles, even in very distressing situations. Analyses from two large-scale studies underscore this point. In one study of undergraduates from three universities (Exline, Pargament, & Grubbs, 2014), students who reported that they had a stronger purpose in life were significantly less likely to report spiritual struggles overall. Similarly, a second study of young adult survivors of hematopoietic cell transplant revealed lower levels of spiritual struggles among those who reported signs of stronger purpose, including meaningful life goals, worthwhileness of life, and viewing life as a gift (King, Fitchett, Murphy, Pargament, Martin, et al., 2017).

Ali's story also suggests that having a *sacred* purpose in life may be especially likely to help people avoid spiritual struggles. Why might that be? As we noted in the prior chapter, sacred pursuits seem to have a special place in the individual's goals and strivings, lending a strong sense of direction and purpose to life as a whole, and generating a host of powerful spiritual emotions. Not all sacred purposes are necessarily life enriching, but those that are may reduce the likelihood of spiritual struggles. Conversely, seeking purposes that are more life limiting, sacred and nonsacred, may fail to provide the same advantages of more enriching strivings, and create fertile ground for spiritual struggles. Below we consider a few examples.

Inauthentic Purpose

Some purposes lack authenticity; they are imposed rather than the product of personal reflection, discernment, and choice. Circumstances, social pressures, institutions, and culture can eliminate some dreams and make others virtually impossible to realize. In what has been called the Greatest Generation, those who came of age in the time of the Depression and World War II, many had their hopes and aspirations dashed by terrible financial hardships, the war, or the barriers created by sexism and racism. A number of this generation were able to find new strivings that could be infused with sacred value, such as devoting themselves to raising children who might be able to reach goals their parents could not. Others, however, could never resolve the ache that accompanied the loss of their dreams, dreams that felt irreplaceable. The story is not altogether different today when all-too-many individuals are being blocked from realizing their life choices as a result of barriers erected by a changing world economy and marketplace. In more subtle ways, many people end up drifting into unfulfilling life paths—determined by family, society, or culture—without conscious thought about whether that path is right for them, or recognition where these paths are taking them (Palmer, 2004). In many of these cases, their dreams are not authentically theirs (Wilt, Grubbs, Exline, & Pargament, 2021). The result may be spiritual struggles in many forms: anger at God, conflict with others, the sense that something of ultimate value is missing, and a feeling of being a fraud and a moral failure. The words of Hasidic rabbi Susya are relevant here. Shortly before his death he said, "When I get to heaven they will not ask me, 'why were you not Moses?' Instead, they will ask, 'Why were you not Susya? Why did you not become what only you could become?'" (Yalom, 1980, p. 278).

Elevating Preliminary to Ultimate Concerns

In his book *The Road to Character,* David Brooks (2015) cites some interesting statistics that suggest that a major shift has occurred over the last 50 years in terms of fundamental values and purposes in the United States. From 1966 to 1990, according to the annual survey of college freshmen conducted by the University of California, Los Angeles (UCLA) Higher Education Research Institute, the percentage of students who said they were highly motivated to develop a meaningful philosophy of life declined from 80 to less than 50%. The percentage of freshmen who agreed that becoming rich was an important life goal over the same time period increased from 42 to 74%. Similarly, Google scans of digitized books for key words from 1960 to 2008 revealed a significant increase in the language of self-related words and phrases, such as *I come first, standout,* and *self love* (Twenge, Campbell, & Gentile, 2012).

Tillich (1957) once defined idolatry as the elevation of preliminary over ultimate concerns. By placing primacy on partial and finite issues rather than transcendent concerns, he maintained, people are engaged in a kind of false worship. Brooks (2015) asserts that Western culture as a whole has been engaging in just this kind of misdirected pursuit of significance as it shifts from the traditional values of "little me" to the modern values of "big me." The little me virtues of humility, vocation, self-mastery, dignity, and love, he believes, are being supplanted by big me devotion to pleasure, materialism, celebrity, and self.

All purposes are not created equal, as Brooks (2015) points out. From narcissism to hedonism to consumerism, the big me values are simply less able to carry the weight and fulfill the functions of the sacred than significant purposes that are more deeply rooted in a spiritual framework of meaning (Jones, 1991). As a result, the pursuit of preliminary rather than ultimate concerns may be more likely to generate struggles of value, purpose, and meaning. Perhaps this explains the findings of Ake and Horen (2003), who studied a group of Christian women who had experienced domestic violence. The researchers found that those with a more extrinsic religious orientation, an approach to religion motivated by personal and social gain rather than larger spiritual goals, were more likely to experience spiritual struggles. Certainly, people look to their faith to satisfy many motives: personal, social, and spiritual. But when preliminary ends become the driving force for religious involvement, the stage may be set for spiritual struggles.

Grubbs, Exline, Pargament, Volk, and Lindberg (2017) conducted another investigation that speaks to the struggles that may arise when people organize their lives around addiction. In a 1-year longitudinal study of samples of college students and adult web users, they found that those who reported greater perceived addiction to Internet pornography were more likely to develop spiritual struggles over the course of the year, after controlling for other variables, including their baseline level of struggles. Another study of college students focusing on a more virtuous little me purpose—humility—provided a contrasting result. Students who reported higher levels of humility experienced lower levels of divine struggle (Grubbs & Exline, 2014).

Narrowness and Disunity of Purpose

In some sense, we can think of idolatry as a lack of depth of purpose. A life exclusively devoted to self, pleasure, or material success seems rather shallow, at least by traditional standards. The key here, however, lies in the exclusiveness of the devotion. The very same significant goals take on a different meaning when they become part of a broader set of life purposes that includes devotion to family, friends, and community. Few could find fault with the satisfactions tied to getting a raise at work, going on a vacation, dressing up for a special night on the town, or having a drink with friends, as long as these activities don't become the sole reason for living. Selfism, hedonism, and materialism can lead to spiritual struggles because they are narrow and disconnected from balancing virtues in life. We speak more to this point when we address wholeness in Chapter 6.

However, the same point could apply to spiritual goals that are narrowly defined and pursued to the exclusion of other purposes in life. For example, psychiatrist James Griffith (2010) highlights how sincere efforts to live by the teachings of a religious tradition can become stifling and destructive if they do not allow room for personal expression or they insist on submission to abusive family members or religious leaders. Emmons and Schnitker (2013) have also suggested that problems can arise when people seek out avoidant spiritual strivings, such as "avoiding God's displeasure" and, in the process, overlook more positively oriented spiritual goals, such as "getting closer to God." Griffith points out that avoidant goals in general are linked with poorer subjective well-being and physical health. Thus, the devotion to any one singular narrow pursuit may be problematic.

Ultimately, narrowness and disunity of purpose can lead to spiritual struggles within the individual, between the individual and others, and with the divine. The challenge for practitioners is to help people achieve a broader purpose in life and overcome the polarization that can arise between purposes (self vs. others, self vs. God, others vs. God, higher vs. lower goals, little me vs. big me, ultimate vs. ordinary) to reach a greater unity of purpose.

Significance, Struggles, and the Story of Gary

Gary's story illustrates several of the ways that life-limiting purpose can result in spiritual struggles. Ostensibly, Gary came to college with a strong purpose: the desire to lead a Christian life and be a source of pride to his father, church, and God. But in some sense, Gary's sacred pursuits may have been limited to begin with. His story raises questions about the authenticity of his quest. To what extent had his purpose been imposed on him by his strong-willed father and religious community, and to what extent had he reflected on and come to truly "own" the direction of his life? Gary's purpose in life also appeared to be narrow. In the way he presented himself to his therapist, Gary seemed more driven by steering clear of what he didn't want—avoid displeasing his father, church, and God—rather than what he might want, such as growing in his faith and closeness to God. Moreover, the dominance of his spiritual striving left little room for the other goals so important in the college years: forming mature friendships; developing romantic relationships; and learning how to balance work, relationships, and play. Without other sources of significance, Gary was vulnerable to what was to come, not only an anxiety disorder but a crisis of meaning, a crisis of morality, and a crisis of faith.

We now shift to focus on a second important root of spiritual struggles.

HOW THE ORIENTING SYSTEM CAN LEAD TO SPIRITUAL STRUGGLES

Spiritual struggles are, in part, rooted in limitations within the orienting system. Of course, everyone's orienting system is in some respects limited. Here, we turn to some of the emotional, cognitive, behavioral, social, and spiritual elements of the orienting system that could increase or decrease an individual's vulnerability to spiritual struggles.

Emotion Regulation

Following a lecture on spiritual struggles, one of our undergraduate students dealing with bipolar illness sent this heart-wrenching e-mail:

> "I'm suffering, really suffering. My illness is tearing me down, and I'm angry at God for not rescuing me, I mean really setting me free from my mental bondage. I have been dealing with these issues for ten years now and I am only 24 years old. I don't understand why he keeps lifting me up, just to let me come crashing down again."

People are oriented to life in part by their capacity to regulate their emotions in ways that are appropriate to the demands of situations, the social context, and their life goals (Baumeister & Bushman, 2008). This ability helps people manage both day-to-day challenges and the larger problems in living. Those who struggle to regulate their emotions are also prone to struggles in the spiritual realm, as we can hear in the words of the undergraduate above. A number of studies have shown that people who report greater inability to tolerate emotional distress, neuroticism, and psychiatric disability are more likely to experience spiritual struggles (e.g., Abu-Raiya, Pargament, Krause, & Ironson, 2015; McConnell et al., 2006; Wilt, Grubbs, Pargament, & Exline, 2017). For example, Breuninger et al. (2019) reported that military veterans with a psychiatric diagnosis showed higher levels of divine, doubt, and ultimate meaning struggles than those without a diagnosis.

Most of this research has been cross-sectional in design and, as a result, we cannot know for certain whether (1) the higher levels of emotional dysregulation and distress are stimulating spiritual struggles, (2) the higher levels of spiritual struggles are creating greater emotional distress and dysregulation, or (3) both processes are operating simultaneously. Pargament (2009) labeled these three possible explanations secondary spiritual struggles, primary spiritual struggles, and complex spiritual struggles, respectively. As we see in the next chapter, several studies provide support for a primary spiritual struggles model. However, in support of a secondary struggles model, a few longitudinal studies suggest that spiritual struggles can also grow out of emotional distress and dysregulation. For example, Reynolds, Mrug, Hensler, Guion, and Madan-Swain (2014) measured spiritual struggles and adjustment 2 years apart in a sample of adolescents with cystic fibrosis or diabetes. They found that depression predicted increases in spiritual struggles over the 2-year period for both medical groups. In another 6-month follow-up study of African Americans who had lost a loved one to homicide, people who reported more severe grief reactions (i.e., complicated grief) experienced a higher level of spiritual struggle over time (Neimeyer & Burke, 2011).

In short, people who find it hard to manage their own emotions may also find it more difficult to sustain themselves spiritually, especially when faced with serious challenges. Conversely, those who experience more positive emotions, particularly spiritually related emotions, such as awe and uplift, may be relatively protected from spiritual struggles. Of course, these emotions do not exist in a vacuum. They are closely tied to basic beliefs and assumptions people hold about the world that can make contributions of their own to spiritual struggles.

Core Beliefs

In the search for significance, people are oriented by core beliefs that lend direction, stability, and security to the quest. Psychologist Ronnie Janoff-Bulman (1992) captured this idea in her description of assumptive worlds: "At the core of our internal world, we hold basic views of ourselves and our external world that represent our orientation to the push and pull of the cosmos. . . . Our basic assumptions are guides for our day-to-day thoughts and behaviors" (p. 4). She delineated three fundamental assumptions: (1) the belief that the world, both people and events, are basically benevolent; (2) the belief that there is a meaningful connection between who the person is and what happens to him or her; and (3) the belief in one's own basic self-worth, goodness, and decency. Janoff-Bulman cites considerable research highlighting the frequency with which people hold these core beliefs, even to the point of overestimating the true benevolence of the world and personal competencies, and underestimating the likelihood of negative events. Although they may be in part "positive illusions," Janoff-Bulman maintains that these core assumptions help people approach their lives with an underlying sense of optimism and trust. We would also expect that, as a group, these fundamental beliefs offer some protection for the encounter with spiritual struggles.

Research on the links between concepts of self-worth and spiritual struggles provide some support for this point. In a study of four samples, Grubbs, Wilt, Stauner, Exline, and Pargament (2016) found that people who reported higher levels of self-esteem and greater self-compassion experienced fewer spiritual struggles generally, particularly in the realm of divine struggles. Higher levels of self-esteem were also associated with fewer spiritual struggles in women living with cervical cancer in Ghana (Adom-Fynn, Asamoah, Quainoo, Tetteh, & Acquah, 2019/2020).

It must be added, however, that not all core assumptions are necessarily benevolent and helpful. For example, in a classic series of studies, Martin Seligman (1975) demonstrated how repeated failures to escape painful situations and achieve desired outcomes can lead to a sense of learned helplessness, marked by a deep conviction in one's own powerlessness, the futility of trying in life, and as a result, a greater likelihood of disillusionment and depression. Cognitive-behavioral therapy (CBT) helps people identify and correct fundamental assumptions about life that are maladaptive, such as the beliefs that it is easier to avoid than face problems in life, that it will be catastrophic if things don't turn out the way we hope, and that it is important to be competent at everything and loved by everyone (Beck, 2011).

In the spiritual realm, people can develop beliefs that become problematic when they are either overgeneralized or overly narrow in scope. The belief in a loving God can turn into a belief that God will protect the person from all pain and suffering. The belief in a just God can become a belief that God will ensure that people always get what they deserve. The belief in an all-powerful God can meld into a belief that God will solve the individual's problems without any effort on his or her part. Although these overgeneralized beliefs might sound outlandish, the assumptions we make about God, like other core beliefs, can be held at an implicit, unconscious level, as well as at a more explicit level of awareness (Hall & Fujikawa, 2013). People may be largely unaware of what Carrie Doehring (2015) has described as their "embedded theologies." In this vein, it is not altogether rare to find clients surprised to be feeling that they are being punished by a God for their misdeeds when they consciously disavow or are even repelled by the idea of a God who works in this way.

Although some beliefs about God may be overly generalized, others may be overly narrow. J. B. Phillips (1997) illustrated some of these narrow beliefs in his book *Your God Is Too Small*. These include the God of Absolute Perfection, who insists on flawless performance, and the God of the Heavenly Bosom, who offers limitless nurturance and comfort without ever asking for anything in return. To this list we might add the Jealous God, who provides love and compassion only to those who fall beneath a particular religious umbrella. These gods are problematic because they are insufficient to the task of helping people deal with the full range of life experiences. The God of Absolute Perfection leaves individuals nowhere to turn when they fall short of their goals. The God of the Heavenly Bosom may fail to offer a convincing explanation for an encounter with pain and suffering. The Jealous God fosters tension and conflict with those who lie outside the protection of the divine. Whether overgeneralized or overly narrow, these types of spiritual beliefs are likely to leave the individual more vulnerable to spiritual struggles, especially when people experience problems that underscore the limits of their worldview. We examine some emerging research on the links between spiritually related core beliefs and specific types of spiritual struggle in some later chapters.

Behavioral Practices

People are oriented in their search for significance not only by core beliefs but also by regular life practices. These habits of living can provide stability to the life journey and a sense of confidence that the person does indeed have the strength, resources, and track record of success to handle the challenges that are likely to come up. Mental health practitioners are quite familiar with the fact that many of the most common psychological problems people bring to treatment are accompanied by a breakdown in life routines. And one of the simplest and most helpful recommendations practitioners offer their clients is to "stay in rhythm" by following well-established habits and practices of eating, sleeping, exercising, and talking to family and friends, even if one's heart is just not in it.

Perhaps not surprisingly then, research has shown that people who engage in healthy practices of these kinds are less likely to experience spiritual struggles (Pargament, Wong, Pomerleau, & Krause, 2016). Similarly, people who are more conscientious and self-disciplined in their actions report lower levels of spiritual struggles (Grubbs et al., 2016; Wilt et al., 2016).

Having a variety of practices and coping tools to draw upon can also help people anticipate and deal with a full range of life experiences, heading some challenges "off at the pass" before they become sources of struggle. Spiritual resources can be particularly valuable in this regard. In a longitudinal study of patients with advanced chronic heart failure, those who reported more daily spiritual experiences, such as asking for God's help and finding strength through religion or spirituality, described less spiritual strain 3 months later (Park, Lim,

Newlon, Suresh, & Bliss, 2014). These regular spiritual coping practices may be especially helpful in the context of major stressors, such as heart failure, that are in many respects uncontrollable and not fully responsive to problem-focused strategies.

Of course, not all practices are necessarily healthy. Alcohol and drug misuse, denial, repression, acting out, displacement, and overconscientiousness are a few of the addictive and less mature defensive patterns of responding that may provide some immediate stress relief, but increase the chances of later spiritual struggles (Peteet, 2004).

Relational Connectedness

No one searches for significance in total isolation. We are accompanied by others along the way who can help orient us—supporting, encouraging, suggesting shortcuts, pointing out obstacles that lie ahead. We may also be accompanied by others who at times make the journey even more onerous by giving us wrong directions, nay-saying, and discouraging us when we face challenges. Social connections, at their best, orient and sustain us in our pursuit of purpose in life. At their worst, they make a difficult road all the more difficult. The quality of our connections with others is another important root of spiritual struggles.

In her autobiographical account, Debbie Feldman (2012) makes just this point. Raised as a member of a strict orthodox Jewish movement (Hasidism), Feldman felt set apart from her family and community from her earliest years. She had been abandoned by her mother as a child and was disengaged from her father, who was mentally ill and a source of embarrassment to the community. Although Debbie did have a close relationship with her grandmother, she was alienated from others in her family and the larger community that, she felt, frowned upon her because of her parents and her own tendency to speak her mind. Her sense of profound relational alienation led to powerful spiritual struggles at multiple levels: with God, with her family and community, and within herself. Here is one aspect of her internal struggle:

> On the outside, I keep kosher and dress modestly and pretend to care deeply about being a devout Hasidic woman. On the inside, I yearn to break free of every mold, to tear down every barrier ever erected to stop me from seeing, from knowing, from experiencing. . . . My life is an exercise in secrets, the biggest secret being my true self. . . . I am so tired of being ashamed of my true self. (pp. 233, 239)

Unable to resolve these spiritual struggles within Hasidism, Debbie eventually left her religious community.

Empirical studies indicate that Feldman's experience is not unique. Researchers have tied spiritual struggles as a whole and in various forms to several signs of social alienation, including loneliness (Abu-Raiya, Pargament, Krause, et al.,

2015), poorer social support (Ramirez et al., 2012), a disposition not to forgive others (Anderson-Mooney, Webb, Mvududu, & Charbonneau, 2015), not being in a committed relationship (Exline, Pargament, & Grubbs, 2014), and being part of a less spiritually supportive college campus (Bryant, 2011).

These findings extend to the spiritual realm. Like a parent, God can be understood as a relational figure. And, like that with a parent, the relationship with God may be secure or insecure (Kirkpatrick, 2005; Rizzuto, 1979). Several studies have shown that higher levels of spiritual struggle are more common among people who see God in negative terms (e.g., cruel, distant, negative) or describe their relationship with God as insecure, unstable, or fearful (Ano & Pargament, 2013; Cooper, Bruce, Harmon, & Boccaccini, 2009; Exline, Pargament, & Grubbs, 2014; Sandage & Crabtree, 2012). Conversely, those who see God as a more caring, secure figure (e.g., "protector," "beloved") report less spiritual struggle (Abu-Raiya, Pargament, Exline, et al., 2015; Bryant & Astin, 2008). Of course, these findings apply only to people who see God as a being one can relate to. Even so, in Western cultures, many people continue to view God in this fashion (Granqvist & Kirkpatrick, 2013).

Similar findings have emerged from studies of those alienated at societal and cultural levels. Spiritual struggles are more commonplace within more socially marginalized groups in the United States, such as those with lower education and income (Exline, Pargament, & Grubbs, 2014); people who self-identify as bisexual, gay, or lesbian versus heterosexual (Exline, Pargament, & Grubbs, 2014), Hindus and Muslims versus Catholics, Protestants, and Jews (Stauner, Exline, & Pargament, 2015); and non-white versus whites (King, Fitchett, Murphy, Pargament, Martin, et al., 2017). Interestingly, women and men do not reliably differ from each other in their frequency of spiritual struggles (e.g., Magyar-Russell et al., 2014; Ramirez et al., 2012). This general pattern of findings may reflect the simple fact that socially marginalized groups are more likely to encounter major life stressors that shake their most basic beliefs and practices. Consistent with this idea, a study of a national sample revealed that the significant relationship between lower educational status and spiritual struggles was explained by three mediating factors: greater financial strain, exposure to the stresses of living in rundown neighborhoods, and resulting anger (Krause, Pargament, & Ironson, 2017). As a whole, this body of research shows how spiritual struggles are partly rooted in the ground of our social and spiritual connections.

Spiritual Factors

In the sections above, we have looked at ways spiritual elements of the orienting system may lead to spiritual struggles. What general conclusions can be drawn, if any? Who is more vulnerable to spiritual struggles—those who are less spiritual or those who are more spiritual? A case could be made for both possibilities.

Conceivably, people who are less religious and spiritual lack the strong foundation of beliefs, practices, experiences, and connections that protect them from thorny spiritual issues that may arise. In contrast, those who are more religious and spiritual could be less susceptible to spiritual struggles by virtue of their stronger spiritual framework. There is some support for this idea. We saw that individuals who have more daily spiritual experiences and feel more securely nested in a relationship with God and spiritual community are less likely to encounter spiritual struggles. Higher levels of religiousness and spirituality may also provide some degree of protection against spiritual struggle. In this vein, Maltby et al. (2010) found lower levels of spiritual struggle among people who reported a more intrinsic religious orientation. Similarly, Exline, Pargament, Grubbs, and Yali (2014) noted that people who scored higher on a measure of general religiousness were less likely to experience struggles of ultimate meaning.

On the other hand, we might expect that spiritual struggles go hand in hand with religious and spiritual life. Because of the greater value people who are spiritual place on matters of faith, they may experience more turmoil when their spirituality is challenged, unlike the less spiritually inclined who may feel less at stake even when religious and spiritual problems come up. There is some support for this point of view, too. People who feel religion is more salient to them and engage more in religious activities reported more struggles with the demonic and moral struggles in particular (Exline, Wilt, Stauner, Harriott, & Saritoprak, 2017). In a 1-year longitudinal study of college students, Joshua Wilt and his colleagues found that undergraduates who described their religious beliefs as more important to them were more likely to experience spiritual struggles over the following year (Wilt, Hall, Pargament, & Exline, 2017). The chances of developing greater spiritual struggles over the year were especially high among students at a Christian university in comparison to students attending a public secular and private secular university.

As we saw above, certain specific types of spirituality may also increase the likelihood of spiritual struggles, including overly general or narrow beliefs about God and an insecure relationship with a religious community or sacred figures. One general spiritual orientation—quest—appears to be especially predictive of spiritual struggles. Quest, as Batson and colleagues (1993) describe it, is an ongoing approach to life that emphasizes "open-ended questioning" rather than "clear-cut, pat answers" (p. 166) in the search for truth and meaning. Batson et al. emphasize that the individual who approaches life this way recognizes that the final truths about the deepest questions may never be known. Even so, "the questions are deemed important, and however tentative and subject to change, answers are sought" (p. 166). Batson et al. offer Siddhartha Gautama, Mahatma Gandhi, and Malcolm X as examples of the quest orientation.

Embedded in a quest orientation is a willingness to explore the deepest meanings of existence and grapple with life's greatest mysteries. However, this path may not be for the fainthearted; the life of quest is almost certain to be accompanied by periods of spiritual struggle. Empirical studies have in fact shown strong ties between a quest orientation and spiritual struggles (Bryant & Astin, 2008; Kojetin, McIntosh, Bridges, & Spilka, 1987). Similarly, people who are exposed to challenging new ideas and people of diverse religious backgrounds, such as students entering college, encounter more spiritual struggles over time (Bryant, 2011; Small & Bowman, 2011). Spiritual struggles then may be part of the price to be paid for an open, questioning approach to matters of faith. Conversely, people who may be less spiritually flexible, less open to questioning, and less open to learning about diverse religious beliefs and practices may be spared to a greater extent from spiritual struggles. In a study of Palestinian Muslim college students living in Israel, those who endorsed more fundamentalist beliefs (e.g., "everything in the Sacred Writing is absolutely true without question") and fewer universalist beliefs ("Heaven is open to people of all world religions") experienced fewer spiritual struggles (Abu-Raiya, Pargament, Exline, et al., 2015).

Does it follow that we should discourage people from asking questions and exposing themselves to new ideas and new people? Of course not. These findings simply underscore how spiritual struggles can be a natural by-product of at least some spiritual journeys. In later chapters, we note that even though a more questioning, open, and flexible approach to spirituality may increase the likelihood of spiritual struggles, once these struggles are encountered, the same questing approach may prove to be quite helpful. A less flexible approach to spirituality, on the other hand, may become more problematic when people do come face-to-face with spiritual struggles.

So, returning to the question of what can we conclude about the relationship between spirituality and spiritual struggles, there is no simple answer. Instead, the answer may depend on the kind of spirituality we are considering, and perhaps the specific form of spiritual struggle. Though the research is still in its early stages, it seems clear that certain spiritual beliefs, practices, experiences, and orientations may help protect people from an encounter with spiritual struggles, while others seem to pave the way for times of spiritual trial.

The Orienting System, Spiritual Struggles, and the Story of Gary

Returning to the story of Gary, we can see a number of ways in which his spiritual struggles at college may have been rooted in aspects of his orienting system. Emotionally, Gary had always felt nervous, especially in social situations, and he seemed to lack confidence and skill in managing his uncomfortable feelings. Instead, he dealt with his emotions by becoming overly conscientious and almost exclusively focused on academic success. Lacking experience and expertise in finding the balance between work and relaxation, he veered from overcontrol to out of control when he became completely drunk on one of the first occasions of socializing with friends. His unrelenting pursuit of perfection at school was also founded on a core set of beliefs in an unforgiving God who insisted on absolute perfection, leaving him no room for mistakes. It seems inevitable that Gary would fall short of his impossibly high standards, and when he did, he had nowhere to turn. Abandoned by his mother as a young child, unable to find support from his overly demanding father, and lacking a secure connection with God, Gary felt terribly isolated and stuck in a spiritual struggle. His spiritual struggles then were rooted in a combination of elements of his orienting system to life: emotional, cognitive, behavioral, relational, and spiritual. Underlying many of these limitations was Gary's lack of psychological mindedness—he had had little experience in reflecting on himself, his relationships, and the larger world.

We turn now to the third important root of spiritual struggles.

HOW LIFE EVENTS CAN LEAD TO SPIRITUAL STRUGGLES

Spiritual values, beliefs, and practices are not immune to the effects of life events. They, too, are vulnerable to the stressors, transitions, and traumas of life. Here are some of the spiritual struggles voiced by a young adolescent following the death of her mother:

> I remember being very confused and very angry with God and not understanding how this could happen. . . . I talked to him like, "What did I do wrong?" Why would God take her away from us. . . . You could think "God, God, God" and that all of this [is] a part of his plan, but then you sort of like—why this painful kind of thing? . . . That's when I started to question my faith. (Zuckerman, 2012, p. 49)

Empirical studies clearly show that this example is not unusual. As we will see shortly, stressful life experiences of many kinds, individual and cumulative, can lead to spiritual struggles. Before we discuss this literature, however, it is important to put these findings into a larger context. Spiritual struggles often do follow disruptive life events. Even so, the link between the two is not so strong as to suggest that life's trials and tribulations inevitably result in struggles in the spiritual realm. For example, in one study of over 1,400 survivors of hematopoietic cell transplant, 73% reported that they did not have any religious or spiritual struggles (King, Fitchett, Murphy, Pargament, Martin, et al., 2017). And in a study of responses to Hurricane Hermine (Exline, Stauner, Fincham, & May, 2017), the undergraduate participants, on average, reported almost no anger toward God; those who saw God playing some role in the hurricane were more likely to view God as helpful, protective, or comforting. Clearly, many people are able to come to terms with major life crises without spiritual struggles. Zuckerman (2012) writes cogently to this point:

The reality is that most deeply religious men and women who are committed to the Lord, at some point, face tough life circumstances—such as a failed marriage or financial difficulties. Most experience the failure of prayer. Many experience the untimely death of a loved one. And for most religious men and women, these unfortunate phenomena do not shatter their faith. (p. 55)

Nevertheless, a significant percentage of people do encounter profound spiritual struggles as a result of their crises. If some do and others do not, then the key question is what determines whether stressful life events lead to spiritual struggles?

The answer to this question depends on the implications of life stressors for what people hold significant and their orienting system or, to put it more simply, their destinations and pathways in life. More specifically, theory, research, and practice come together to suggest that people are especially vulnerable to spiritual struggles following an encounter with life events that (1) touch matters of deepest significance, and (2) overwhelm the individual's orienting system.

Life Events, Significance, and Spiritual Struggles

In one episode in the classic movie *Forrest Gump,* Forrest is sent to the Vietnam War where he meets Lt. Dan, an officer descended from a long and illustrious line of military ancestors who had sacrificed their lives in combat. In the midst of a battle, Lt. Dan suffers a terrible wound to his legs. Forrest picks up Lt. Dan and carries him to safety, clearly saving his life. Rather than react with gratitude, however, Lt. Dan responds with rage. On the face of it, Lt. Dan's reaction seems incomprehensible. What the viewer understands though is that Forrest had prevented Lt. Dan from realizing his ultimate goal in life: to sacrifice himself on the field of battle as had his forbearers. Lt. Dan's experience brings to mind a quote from the philosopher Epictetus (1888), almost 2,000 years ago: "[People] are disturbed not by the things which happen, but by the opinions about things. . . . When then we are impeded or disturbed or grieved let us never blame others, but ourselves, that is, our opinions" (p. 3). In the opinion of Lt. Dan, Forrest had prevented him from accomplishing a lifelong goal of heroic self-sacrifice.

The words of Epictetus (1888) and the experience of Lt. Dan fit well with more recent stress and coping theory. In their seminal work, Richard Lazarus and Susan Folkman (1984) demonstrated that how we are affected by major life events depends a great deal on how we appraise them. Particularly important, they noted, are primary appraisals—that is, evaluations of the impact of an event for the individual's significant goals and values. Events that touch matters of greatest spiritual significance likely have even greater power in peoples' lives because, as we described earlier in the chapter, our sacred strivings often become overarching, organizing forces in life that guide and direct much of our behavior and help support and sustain us over the long haul. Situations that threaten, damage, or violate sacred pursuits can then become fundamentally disturbing and destabilizing. They create a loss of spiritual direction and a need to recover or redefine a sense of significance. Spiritual struggles are a natural expression of those disturbing times in life when we are shaken to the core.

A number of studies on spiritual struggle provide support for this idea. Some of the strongest evidence comes from research on the effects of family-related conflicts. These conflicts often cut to the heart of the individual's most sacred values and beliefs: that the individual is important enough to be loved; that trust can be placed in figures of authority; that there is a loving, protective God. Child abuse, in particular, be it emotional, physical, or sexual, often leaves the individual with a tremendous sense of spiritual loss and violation, creating fertile soil for spiritual struggles (Doehring, 1993; Pargament, Murray-Swank, & Mahoney, 2008). Several studies reveal that children who experience abuse are more likely to show signs of spiritual struggle later in their lives (e.g., McCormick, Carroll, Sims, & Currier, 2017; Walker, Reid, O'Neill, & Brown, 2009). For example, in a study of 1,000 Czech respondents, religious and nonreligious, those who experienced more childhood trauma reported higher levels of all six types of spiritual struggles as adults (Janů, Malinakova, Kosarkova, & Tavel, 2020). One survivor of rape as an adolescent wrote a letter to God voicing her feelings of disappointment and abandonment:

> Dear God, I don't understand how you can do this? I believed in you; I trusted you. "Why have you forsaken me?" I try to tell myself to have faith, to believe, to remember Jesus on the cross. But, I can't keep feeling this pain. Why is there such pain and tragedy? I feel as though you never answer me. I feel abandoned by you.. (Murray-Swank & Waelde, 2013, p. 335)

Abuse perpetrated by clergy creates particular vulnerability to spiritual struggles. In one study of adult Catholics in the United States, Rosetti (1995) compared survivors who had been abused by clergy as children with those who had been abused by someone who was not a clergy person, and those who had not been sexually abused. Both groups of adults who had been sexually abused as children reported more difficulty trusting priests and God than those who had not experienced childhood sexual abuse. However, among the three groups, adults who had been sexually abused by priests were the most likely to report signs of spiritual struggle. It is the spiritual nature of the abuse that lends it such extraordinary power. "This guy had my soul in his hand," a victim of clergy sexual abuse said. "It was devastating to know that someone would step out of the powers of spiritual liberty to take over someone else's soul. . . . I still have anger about a lot of that and I think more of the anger is about the spiritual loss than anything to do with the sexual abuse" (Fater & Mullaney, 2000, p. 290).

Although clergy sexual abuse is undoubtedly singular in many respects, other religiously based stressors can trigger appraisals of spiritual loss and desecration. Many lesbian, gay, bisexual, and transgender (LGBT) individuals describe a variety of negative religious experiences that violate their fundamental beliefs about God and religious communities, and that lead to spiritual struggles (Wood & Conley, 2014). These include experiences of spiritual neglect, spiritual bullying, and sexual microaggressions in which LGBT are denigrated or invalidated by religious individuals and communities for their "otherness." More frequent encounters with events such as these may help explain why LGBT individuals report higher levels of spiritual struggles than their heterosexual counterparts (Exline, Pargament, & Grubbs, 2014).

Seemingly secular events can also be viewed and appraised through a spiritual lens. As we discussed in the previous chapter, aspects of life, such as marriage, parenting, work, health, the environment, and social justice, can all be imbued with qualities often associated with divinity. Life events that violate, threaten, or damage these sacred objects (e.g., divorce, unemployment, illness, pollution, racial discrimination) can then take on added power and make spiritual struggles more likely. In fact, studies (Krumrei, Mahoney, & Pargament, 2011; Magyar-Russell et al., 2013; Pargament, Magyar, Benore, & Mahoney, 2005) have shown that people who appraised various life stressors as more of a spiritual loss and desecration also reported higher levels of spiritual struggle.

Before concluding this section, it is important to add that other events and times of life can elicit spiritual struggles not because they represent a spiritual loss or violation but because they reveal a need for greater significance and meaning in life. For example, studies have shown that spiritual struggles appear to become less commonplace as people age (Pargament, Wong, Pomerleau, et al., 2016; Stauner et al., 2015). The time of emerging and young adulthood may be particularly ripe for spiritual struggles. In analyses with a nationally representative sample, those ages 18–25 reported the highest level of spiritual struggles of all age groups (Krause, Pargament, Hill, Wong, & Ironson, 2017; Stauner et al., 2015). From a developmental perspective, this makes good sense, for the period of emerging adulthood is a challenging time of differentiation from families of origin and formation of one's own significant strivings, identity, and orientation to life. And, we might add, aging may also produce greater wisdom that protects people from struggles (Krause, Pargament, Hill, et al., 2017). Thus, spiritual struggles may be a natural outgrowth of these developmental trends and transitions.

Life Events, the Orienting System, and Spiritual Struggles

People are also especially vulnerable to life events that point to the limited ability of their orienting systems to understand and deal with these situations (Pargament, 1997). Once again, it must be stressed that people generally have a great deal of resilience to difficult problems in life—through their beliefs, practices, history of experience, coping resources, and networks of support they are able to resolve many of these problems before they rise to the level of spiritual struggles. Often, the individual is able to assimilate the challenging situation into his or her orienting system and, as a result, his or her guiding framework is sustained and conserved. None of us is totally invulnerable, however. We are most susceptible to spiritual struggles when we encounter events that overwhelm our orienting systems.

People can find themselves overwhelmed when they face an accumulation of stressful experiences—none in and of itself might lead to spiritual struggles, but the sum total of these events can undermine individuals' resources. Here are the words of a war veteran who suffered the death of five members of his family in 5 months: "I've always been the person in the family that people could depend on. I could always fix the problem and solve the problem. And when all of them started dying, I realized that I couldn't fix it . . . I became really overwhelmed and it really crushed me and I couldn't fix it" (Teng, Stanley, Fletcher, Pargament, & Exline, 2015). What followed for him was an intense spiritual struggle: "Why" he asks God, "would you empty my life like that? I don't have anybody to do nothing for . . . I'm really really really struggling to process that now. I still struggle with it constantly." Several studies have shown that the likelihood of spiritual struggles increases as people accumulate greater numbers of stressful life experiences. In a study of three college samples and one adult sample, the accumulation of life stressors was associated with all six forms of spiritual struggles as assessed by the Religious and Spiritual Struggles (RSS) Scale (Stauner, Exline, Pargament, Wilt, & Grubbs, 2019). A longitudinal study of college students reported that those who had more stressful experiences were more likely to face spiritual struggles a year or more later (Wortmann, Park, & Edmondson, 2011).

As a side note, it is important to recognize how recent life stressors can take on added power when they trigger earlier unresolved traumatic experiences. Baider and Sarell (1983) present the example of an older man whose diagnosis of lung cancer brought up earlier, unresolved feelings of anger toward God that had grown out of his experience in the Holocaust.

Of course, some single events can be powerful enough on their own to overwhelm the individual's orienting system, resulting in spiritual struggles. They are, as Sharon Parks (2000) puts it, "shipwrecks" that upend the individual's world. One grandfather describes this kind of upheaval and struggle following the loss of his baby granddaughter in childbirth:

> God, you don't even give her a chance to come into the world and see what it is about. . . . What did she do. . . . Is it a punishment; what is it? I mean why would you create a beautiful creation and not give it a chance to see what you created; to allow it to have a part in what you created? I just, I can't fathom that. (Teng et al., 2015)

The experience of combat, too, can throw the individual's world off-kilter. In a study of returning military veterans from Iraq and Afghanistan, soldiers who faced higher levels of combat exposure also described higher levels of spiritual struggle (Park, Smith, et al., 2017). Ai, Tice, Huang, and Ishisaka (2005) conducted a study of Muslim war refugees from Kosovo and Bosnia, and found that those who encountered more war-related trauma experienced more spiritual struggles.

We have noted how stressful experiences can lead to spiritual struggles by overwhelming the individual's orienting system. How do life stressors, in fact, overwhelm people? It's worth considering this question in a bit more detail. We suggest three ways this effect occurs. First, life stressors can push people beyond the capacity of their orienting systems to guide them toward their destinations. Events can push friends, family, and helping systems beyond their ability to provide needed support. Events can push people beyond the resources that keep their lives on an even keel: a regular paycheck, problem-solving skills, emotion regulation abilities, healthy habits, optimism, and a sense of trust in the world. And events can push people beyond their core spiritual beliefs, revealing the limits of their framework for understanding stress and suffering.

Second, stressful life events can become overwhelming when they directly threaten, damage, or violate the fundamental assumptions that underlie the orienting system. Life stressors can lead to basic questions about many of the central beliefs people live by: that life is fair, that life is controllable, that life is predictable, that God answers our prayers, and that we have the resources to handle the challenges that we face. In her theory of trauma and meaning, Crystal Park (2016) makes a similar point using the language of meaning systems and meaning-making. She describes how traumatic situations can create discrepancies between the events and the individual's global meaning system and goals. For example, a physical assault may be hard to square with a core belief in the trustworthiness of others and the goal of physical safety and security. The end result is distress, psychological and spiritual, and meaning-making efforts to reduce it. In support of these ideas, empirical studies have found links between spiritual struggles and events that throw fundamental assumptions into question (Ano & Pargament, 2013). For example, cancer patients who appraised their illness as a violation of their beliefs in the fairness of life, and the controllability of situations by themselves, God, or the medical profession, were more likely to experience anger at God (Exline, Park, Smyth, & Carey, 2011). In a related vein, spiritual struggles are more likely to follow when people experience misfortune that takes them by surprise, such as the COVID-19 pandemic (Yildirim, Arslan, & Alkahtani, 2021), an unexpected hospital admission (Fitchett, Winter-Pfändler, & Pargament, 2013), or when their prayers have gone unanswered (Maunu & Stein, 2010).

Third, stressful life experiences can overwhelm the orienting system by targeting particular areas of vulnerability, vulnerabilities that vary from person to person. In ordinary times, these points of fragility in the orienting system may be less consequential, but in the midst of stressful circumstances, they limit the person's ability to maintain stability, essentially making tough times even tougher. Trevino, Pargament, Krause, Ironson, and Hill (2019) conducted one of the first studies of what happens when stressful life events and vulnerability factors in the orienting system collide. Working with a national sample, they identified several orienting system variables that increased the likelihood of spiritual struggles as people encountered increasing numbers of major life stressors. Higher levels of trait anger, death anxiety, social isolation, smoking, and insecure attachment to God were all related to higher levels of spiritual struggles, and these effects were stronger among those who had been exposed to a larger number of stressors.

If fragile points in the orienting system can increase the susceptibility to spiritual struggles, might points of strength in the orienting system protect people from these same conflicts? As yet, researchers have only just begun to address this question. San Roman et al. (2019) studied a sample of church-affiliated members who were indirectly affected by a mass shooting. They found that the effects of the shooting on spiritual struggles were buffered by support from God, religious leaders, and religious peers. A few other studies have offered contrasting results. The effects of stressful life events on spiritual struggles were not buffered by higher levels of general religiousness in one study (Stauner, Exline, Pargament, et al., 2019), nor by resources including self-esteem, optimism, and emotional support in another (Trevino et al., 2019). Further research is needed to identify other factors (e.g., various spiritual coping methods, forgiveness, gratitude) that might help cushion the effects of major life events on spiritual struggles.

Life Events and the Story of Gary

Even though Gary was still an emerging adult, he had already encountered more than his fair share of major life stressors. Some of these events had occurred in his earlier years: abandonment by his mother as a toddler, the demands of an authoritarian father, and bullying and harassment by classmates as an adolescent. Others were more recent: the shock of getting a D on a test in mechanical engineering, and his episode of drunkenness and questionable sexual activity.

A poor grade and a night of excess in college are not inherently stressful. After all, many students experience these events with little distress, spiritual or otherwise. The power of these events lay instead in their capacity to fundamentally disrupt both the destination and pathway that defined Gary's distinctive life journey. To Gary's mind, the combination of a poor academic performance and moral lapse posed a serious threat to his dreams of academic success, making his father, church, and God proud, and living a life of Christian virtue. The same stressors revealed vulnerable areas of Gary's orienting system: his belief that he had no room to make mistakes, his social inexperience, and his difficulty in regulating negative emotions. At a deeper level, these stressors may have brought up old unresolved fears of abandonment that had been etched into Gary's psyche when his mother left the family and when he felt ostracized by his classmates as an adolescent. With these limitations in his orienting system, Gary was ill equipped to sustain himself through this stressful period on his own.

CONCLUSIONS

We have covered a lot of ground in our attempt to answer the question "Where do spiritual struggles come from?" (See Table 3.1 for a summary.) Research in this area is still in its early stages and there is much to learn. Nevertheless, the findings suggest that spiritual struggles grow out of three key interrelated factors: the individual's significant goals and purposes in life, the character of the individual's orienting system, and the life events the individual encounters in his or her life journey. We have seen that spiritual struggles are, in part, an outgrowth of limitations in what the person seeks out of life and how he or she pursues these ends. For some, spiritual struggles are part and parcel of a preferred way of life, one that involves an open-ended search for answers to ultimate questions.

We have avoided speaking of spiritual struggles as a sign of weakness or pathology. Spiritual struggles are a normative part of development, coming to

TABLE 3.1. The Roots of Spiritual Struggle

Significant purpose

  Inauthentic purpose
  Elevation of preliminary concerns to ultimate concerns
  Narrowness and disunity of purpose

Orienting system

  Emotion dysregulation
  Negative worldviews
  Overgeneralized and overly narrow beliefs
  Breakdown in life routines
  Unhealthy behavioral practices
  Limited set of coping tools and resources
  Social disconnection
  Insecure spiritual attachment
  Quest orientation
  Limited reflectiveness

Life events

  Cumulative life stressors
  Events that threaten, damage, or violate significant purposes
  Emerging adulthood
  Events that overwhelm the orienting system
  Events that target areas of vulnerability in the orienting system

the foreground in emerging adulthood and in response to major life stressors. Moreover, spiritual struggles have value. Without some degree of struggle, the individual would be stuck in a rigid spirituality, unable to change or grow. Spiritual struggles may signal the need for a reorientation to life and change in life direction. This point applies to everyone, for everyone's approach to life is limited in some respects. As we will see in subsequent chapters, through the process of spiritual struggles, people have opportunities to move toward greater wholeness and growth in their search for significance.

With a clearer understanding of the roots of spiritual struggle in hand, we can now shift to a more practical set of questions: Do spiritual struggles in fact matter? Do they affect our development, our health, our well-being? In the next two chapters, we take up these questions. We will see that spiritual struggles are often pivotal times in life that can lead toward distress, brokenness, and decline; toward well-being, wholeness, and growth; and, for some, toward both growth and decline.

CHAPTER 4

Do Spiritual Struggles Lead to Decline?

THE PAINFUL SIDE

Susan, a 28-year-old mother of two young children, has come to your office complaining of nervousness, depression, headaches, tiredness, and light-headedness. Her physician had not found any underlying physical reason for her complaints, and Susan had not improved following brief CBT with her employee assistance program (EAP) counselor. She did not want to take any psychotropic medications.

You learn that Susan comes from a close, working-class, church-centered family. She had grown up in a small conservative congregation that believed in the healing power of prayer, a belief reinforced by the fact that she and the members of her immediate family had never experienced a major health problem. Her husband is also Christian, but does not share her beliefs in healing through prayer.

About 2 years ago, Susan developed a bad cold with a deep and persistent cough, and high fever. She refused her husband's pleas to get medical help and, instead, following her mother's advice, prayed to God for a healing. Her condition continued to deteriorate until she collapsed and was admitted to the emergency room after her husband called 911. In the hospital, she was treated for pneumonia. The doctors told her that she could have died if she had waited much longer for medical treatment. Susan left the hospital weakened physically and emotionally.

In the course of treatment, it becomes clear that Susan's symptoms of depression, anxiety, and vague physical complaints grew out of her spiritual struggles. Susan had always tried to live according to the teachings of her church, but now she was being flooded with painful questions: Had her illness been the result of a weakness in her faith life? Had she unknowingly turned away from God? Was God punishing her for her transgressions, and was the punishment a "wake-up call" to get right with God? How could she deal with the conflicting spiritual advice from her mother and her husband, which left her feeling like a "Ping-Pong ball" hit back and forth in a game over which she had no control? What Susan feared most was the idea of getting sick again. What would she do? Even worse, what if one of her children got sick? Would she pray for a healing or seek medical help? Susan had no answers. She felt worn down by her spiritual struggles and by the emotional turmoil they were creating for her.

Susan's case is not unusual. In this chapter, we delve into a growing and now significant body of research on the relationship between spiritual struggles and signs of distress, disorientation, and serious problems. These findings challenge any idea that spirituality is invariably helpful. This is not to discount the large amount of evidence that spiritual and religious expressions are often beneficial to people in terms of their health, well-being, and even longevity (Koenig, King, & Carson, 2012; Oman, 2018). The point we make is that some forms of spirituality, spiritual struggles in particular, have different implications for health and well-being. We review evidence of robust ties between spiritual struggles and markers of pain, distress, and decline. The results of these studies should not be altogether surprising; after all, spiritual struggles involve tensions and conflicts about matters of deepest, sacred value within ourselves, with others, and with the supernatural. True, these struggles focus on the spiritual domain, but spirituality is not disconnected from other parts of our lives—we are biopsychosocial spiritual beings, and tensions and conflicts within one dimension are likely to ripple out and affect other life domains. In fact, the evidence suggests they do. This is more, however, than an interesting scientific finding. There is a very important practical lesson to be drawn from this accumulating evidence base: spiritual struggles have to be taken seriously in clinical work.

THE LINKS BETWEEN SPIRITUAL STRUGGLES AND DISTRESS, DISORIENTATION, AND DECLINE

Empirical studies of the relationship between spiritual struggles and various measures of psychological, social, physical, and spiritual distress have increased rapidly over the past 25 years. Literally hundreds of empirical studies have now examined these linkages. One way of summarizing this growing body of research is through meta-analysis. A meta-analysis is a method for combining the results of multiple studies to arrive at a potentially stronger and more reliable estimate of the relationship between variables than any one study can provide. In 2003, Smith, McCullough, and Poll conducted a meta-analysis of the links between spiritual struggles and depressive symptoms across 147 independent research studies. Smith and colleagues found a small but statistically significant relationship between higher levels of spiritual struggles and more depressive symptoms. In 2005, Ano and Vasconcelles completed a meta-analysis of 49 studies on the ties between spiritual struggles and a variety of measures of psychological adjustment. They found a modest but significant statistical relationship between more spiritual struggles and poorer psychological adjustment. Over 2,000 contradictory results from other studies would have been needed to disconfirm this result. Reynolds, Mrug, Wolfe, Schwebel, and Wallander (2016) conducted a more focused meta-analysis of 14 studies among youth coping with chronic illness. Spiritual struggles were associated with more internalizing problems, lower quality of life, and poorer physical health. Most recently, Bockrath et al. (2021) completed a meta-analysis of 32 longitudinal studies of the relationship between spiritual struggles and negative psychological adjustment, and found that spiritual struggles predicted declines in adjustment over time. Some studies have reported nonsignificant relationships between measures of spiritual struggles and maladjustment. However, these latter studies appear to be exceptions to the rule. Overall, meta-analytic findings, gleaned from hundreds of studies of spiritual struggles, point to the same general conclusion: *Spiritual struggles are consistently associated with a variety of indicators of distress and disorientation.*

But . . . Some Critical Questions

The answers that come from research investigations always lead to more questions. That's simply the way science moves forward. In the case of these meta-analytic findings, a few critical questions arise.

The first is a chicken-and-egg question. Evidence of an association between spiritual struggles and poorer adjustment begs a key issue, one that holds important practical implications: Which comes first, spiritual struggles or signs of distress and disorientation? As noted in the previous chapter, there are three possible answers (Pargament, 2009). Conceivably, spiritual struggles could be the end result or secondary to the experience of distress. We cited a few studies that provide support for the *secondary spiritual struggles model* in which higher levels of psychological distress predicted increased levels of spiritual struggles over time (e.g., Neimeyer & Burke, 2011; Reynolds et al., 2014). On the other hand, spiritual struggles could be primary to distress—that is, spiritual struggles may lead to greater distress and disorientation. As we will see shortly, we can also find support for the *primary spiritual struggles model*. Of course, both secondary and primary spiritual struggle models may apply in a *complex spiritual struggles model*. Just like chickens lay eggs and eggs hatch into chickens, spiritual struggles can lead to distress and distress can lead to spiritual struggles.

A second important question is whether the relationship reported between spiritual struggles and distress is simply inaccurate. Perhaps this association is confounded or distorted by other variables. For instance, people who struggle spiritually may be more negative in general and this overall tendency to be "gloom-and-doom" oriented may be the culprit in predicting distress rather than spiritual struggles. Or perhaps those who struggle with their spirituality have a generally higher or lower level of religious commitment and it is this overall degree of religiousness rather than spiritual struggles per se that actually predicts distress. To rule out the possibility of confounding in research studies, it is important to control for these variables when possible. As we will see, a number of studies in this area have done just that.

Spiritual Struggles, Distress, and Disorientation

Let's now take a closer look at some of these findings. We begin by examining the ties between spiritual struggles and signs of distress and disorientation within the general population and then within clinical samples and people exposed to major stressors. By distress and disorientation we are referring to markers of unease, dissatisfaction, anxiety, depression, lower well-being, and general malaise. We then shift our attention to studies that go beyond indicators of distress and disorientation to show that spiritual struggles may signal even more serious problems and decline. Although most of these studies have been conducted on predominantly Christian samples in the United States, we will see that the findings extend to a variety of religious and spiritual groups, as well as people from other cultures. Note that because this literature is now so large, we cannot review every study that has been conducted on the topic. Instead, we are thorough but not exhaustive. Also note that our focus in this chapter is on spiritual struggles as a whole, as assessed most commonly by the negative subscale of the Brief RCOPE (Pargament, Feuille, & Burdzy, 2011), the Religious Strain Scale (Exline et al., 2000), and the RSS Scale (Exline, Pargament, Grubbs, & Yali, 2014). We examine more specific struggles later in this book.

General Population Studies

We have described spiritual struggles as a normal though potentially distressing and disorienting part of the search for significance. Generally speaking, spiritual struggles disrupt the stories people live by and hope to live out. They challenge the plot line in our narratives, our cast of characters, our own role in the story, and the way we expect it to unfold. The story line can become confused and disorganized. No wonder then that spiritual struggles may become a source of distress and disorientation. If this perspective is accurate, then we should find a significant tie between spiritual struggles and signs of distress and disorientation not only among people seeking help for their personal problems, such as the case of Susan, but also among people in the general population.

A number of studies of this kind have shown that those who experience spiritual struggles are more likely to report signs of distress and disorientation (e.g., Bjorck & Thurman, 2007; Bryant & Astin, 2008; Ellison & Lee, 2010). For example, in one study of a representative sample of adults in the United States, higher scores on five subscales of the RSS Scale were associated with higher levels of depression and anxiety, and lower levels of life satisfaction and happiness (Abu-Raiya, Pargament, Krause, et al., 2015). These findings controlled for demographic indicators and measures of neuroticism, social isolation, and religious commitment, so the results could not be explained by any general tendency of spiritual strugglers to be more negative, alienated, religious, or nonreligious. In another study of a national sample in the United States, individuals who reported a more troubled relation with God, negative interactions in religious settings, and religious doubts also indicated higher levels of psychological distress, even after controlling for the effects of demographic variables and religious involvement (Ellison & Lee, 2010). This pattern of findings held true for almost all of the demographic subgroups. Also noteworthy is research by Wilt, Grubbs, Pargament, et al. (2017), who measured cumulative spiritual struggles in a large sample of community-dwelling adults and college students, finding that those who had accumulated greater spiritual struggles over their lifetime reported lower well-being. Finally, a study of five different adult samples from the United States made use of advanced statistical methods and replicated a key finding from many other studies: Spiritual struggles were associated with greater distress, in the form of greater depression, anxiety, and perceived stress (Stauner, Exline, Grubbs, et al., 2016). Even though spiritual struggles were associated with both religiousness and distress, they were distinguishable from these latter constructs.

In one notable large-scale, follow-up national study of undergraduates in the United States, college juniors who experienced more spiritual struggles also reported feeling more overwhelmed and depressed, even after adjusting for their levels of self-esteem, feeling depressed, and feeling overwhelmed when they had been freshmen (Bryant & Astin, 2008). Because of its longitudinal design, this study provides stronger evidence in support of a primary spiritual struggles model in which spiritual struggles lead to distress. Similarly, in their work with an African American sample, Park, Holt, Le, Christie, and Williams (2018) found that a brief measure of spiritual struggles predicted greater depression and negative affect 2.5 years later after controlling for baseline levels of well-being.

Investigators have also begun to examine the connection between spiritual struggles and distress among other religious groups and within other cultural contexts. Researcher Hisham Abu-Raiya has directed a number of investigations in this area. For example, he and his colleagues found that Palestinian Muslim college students who struggled more spiritually showed more depression and generalized anxiety and less life satisfaction (Abu-Raiya, Pargament, Exline, et al., 2015). Among Jewish Israeli students who completed a Hebrew version of the RSS, spiritual struggles were associated with more depression and anxiety and less life satisfaction (Abu-Raiya, Pargament, Weissberger, et al., 2016). In another investigation of Jews in New Jersey and New York, Rosmarin, Pargament, and

Flannelly (2009) reported that higher levels of spiritual struggle were linked with lower levels of mental and physical health. Working with a sample of Roman Catholic students in Poland, Zarzycka (2019) found that spiritual struggles were associated with greater depression, lower life satisfaction, and poorer general health. These effects were mediated by less of a tendency to forgive others following spiritual struggles. Nalini Tarakeshwar and her collaborators developed a measure of Hindu religious coping, including a subscale that assessed anger toward God, feeling punished by God, and religious passivity (Tarakeshwar et al., 2003). She gathered a sample of Hindus in the United States and found that higher scores on this subscale were associated with less life satisfaction, less marital satisfaction, and more depressed mood. Similarly, in a sample of Sikh immigrants, the largest group of South Asians in the United States, higher levels of spiritual struggles were associated with higher levels of depression (Roberts, Mann, & Montgomery, 2016).

One recent study is especially noteworthy. It involved two large samples of college students and adult Internet respondents, including atheists as well as theists. Although the atheists reported significantly fewer spiritual struggles overall than a comparative group of theists, atheists who manifested more spiritual struggles also reported higher levels of depression and anxiety, and lower levels of life satisfaction and meaning in life (Sedlar et al., 2018). These findings highlight a key point: Spiritual struggles are relevant to the mental health of atheists, as well as religiously involved people. We should add here that in many of the studies involving the general population, the average level of spiritual struggles is relatively low. Even spiritual struggles of lower intensity, however, are often tied to significant distress and disorientation.

In short, studies of spiritual struggles among people with diverse orientations to religion and within diverse cultural contexts are just emerging. Even so, it appears that the link between spiritual struggles and psychological distress may well apply to the general population of people from a variety of religious and social backgrounds.

Clinical and Stressed Population Studies

To what extent do the findings from the general population apply to people facing medical problems, psychological problems, and other major life stressors? Because their resources may be more strained and they may feel less equipped to handle their challenges, clinical and stressed populations may be particularly vulnerable to the effects of spiritual struggles. This appears to be the case.

Medical Population Studies. In research with a national sample, McConnell and colleagues (2006) found significant ties between spiritual struggles and greater depression, anxiety, and other psychological problems; notably, these effects were significantly stronger among people who had experienced an illness or injury in the past year. Other studies of a variety of medical populations have shown similar results (e.g., Damen et al., in press; Fitchett et al., 2004; Lee, Nezu, & Nezu, 2014; Sherman, Simonton, Latiff, Spohn, & Tricot, 2005; Tarakeshwar et al., 2006). For example, Lee et al. focused on individuals with HIV/AIDS and found that people who reported higher levels of spiritual struggles also manifested more depressive symptoms and a lower quality of life, after controlling for a variety of clinical and demographic factors.

Several investigations of patients with medical problems made use of longitudinal designs that provide stronger support for a primary spiritual struggles model. In a study of outpatients in various stages of HIV/AIDS, spiritual struggles were associated with declines in overall quality of life and increases in depression over a period of 12–18 months after controlling for initial levels of these variables (Trevino et al., 2010). Sherman, Plante, Simonton, Latif, and Anaissie (2009) followed patients with multiple myeloma undergoing autologous stem cell transplantation. Higher levels of spiritual struggle prior to the transplantation were predictive of greater depression and anxiety, and poorer emotional well-being after the procedure, controlling for baseline levels of these measures of distress. Similarly, higher levels of spiritual struggles among older adults who were medically ill and hospitalized for a number of serious conditions (e.g., cancer, cardiac, gastrointestinal) were associated with declines in quality of life and increases in depression over the following 2 years, controlling for a variety of demographic, medical, and mental health variables at baseline (Pargament, Koenig, Tarakeshwar, & Hahn, 2004). Spiritual struggles seem to have negative implications for people at the other end of the age spectrum as well. In two studies of children and adolescents with asthma, higher levels of spiritual struggles were linked with increases in anxiety 1 month posthospital discharge (Benore, Pargament, & Pendleton, 2008) and increases in depression (Cotton et al., 2013), after adjusting for initial levels of anxiety and depression, respectively.

A few studies have also examined the connection between spiritual struggles and distress among people with medical problems in other cultures, with similar results. Ramirez et al. (2012) worked with patients from Brazil with end-stage renal disease and reported that spiritual struggles were associated with greater depression and anxiety and poorer health-related quality of life in a variety of forms, even after controlling for various clinical risk factors. In a study of Muslim patients with cancer and a control sample in Pakistan, higher levels of spiritual struggles were tied to significantly greater depression, anxiety, and fear of death among patients with cancer and among the controls (with the exception of fear of death; Khan, Sultana, & Watson, 2009). Pedersen, Pedersen, Pargament, and Zachariae (2013) studied 111 Danish patients with lung disease and found that spiritual struggles were associated with poorer quality of life; this finding is especially notable since it comes from one of the most secularized countries in Europe.

All in all, the results of these studies, including some well-designed longitudinal studies, show a clear link between spiritual struggles and signs of distress and disorientation among medical populations facing a variety of illnesses in different social contexts.

Studies of People with Psychological Problems. Studies of people with psychological problems also show that spiritual struggles are significantly linked to signs of distress and disorientation. Working with patients with a psychiatric diagnosis in a partial hospitalization program, Rosmarin, Bigda-Peyton, Öngur, Pargament, and Björgvinsson (2013) reported that spiritual struggles were tied to greater depression, anxiety, and lower levels of well-being prior to treatment. In their study of veterans diagnosed with PTSD, Witvliet, Phipps, Feldman, and Beckham (2004) found that higher levels of spiritual struggles were related to more anxiety and depression. Similarly, in a study of patients with serious psychiatric disabilities, spiritual struggles were tied to greater psychological distress and lower life satisfaction (Warren, Van Eck, Townley, & Kloos, 2015). Robertson, Magyar-Russell, and Piedmont (2020) conducted a noteworthy study of men on a Sex Offense Registry and found that higher levels of struggles with God and with a faith community were associated with greater depression, anxiety, shame, and hopelessness. Another 2-week longitudinal study of orthodox Jews dealing with worry and stress also found support for a primary rather than a secondary spiritual struggles model, with spiritual struggles predicting changes in depression rather than the reverse (Pirutinsky, Rosmarin, Pargament, & Midlarsky, 2011).

Only a few studies of the spiritual struggles–distress connection have been conducted among people with psychological problems from diverse cultures and religious traditions. Stroppa and Moreira-Almeida (2013) studied Brazilian outpatients with a bipolar diagnosis and found that more spiritual struggles were associated with poorer quality of life. In research with Dutch patients and parishioners with mental health issues, higher levels of spiritual struggle were tied to greater anxiety and less existential well-being (van Uden, Pieper, & Zondag, 2014). A study of Iranian patients with psychiatric diagnoses showed that spiritual struggles were associated with poorer adherence to medications (Movahedizadeh, Sheikhi, Shahsavari, & Chen, 2019).

Given the historical antipathy of many leaders of the mental health field (e.g., Freud, Ellis, Skinner) to religion and spirituality, it is important to stress that the findings we have presented here do not support the sweeping claims about the detrimental role of religion in mental health voiced by these leading figures. The research we have presented has focused solely on spiritual struggles rather than other expressions of spirituality and religion—in fact, many studies have shown that faith in a variety of its forms can serve as an important resource for people with serious psychological problems (e.g., Mohr, 2013). Nevertheless, the general pattern of findings we reviewed in this section points to a significant connection between spiritual struggles, distress, and disorientation among people with psychological problems, as well as physical health problems.

Studies of People Dealing with Major Life Stressors. Several investigators have looked at the relationship between spiritual struggles, distress, and disorientation among people facing major life stressors. Here, too, the results reveal a connection among these variables. In one study of sexual assault victims (Ahrens, Abeling, Ahmad, & Hinman, 2010), higher levels of spiritual struggles were tied to greater depression, and in another study of Christian survivors of domestic violence (Ake & Horen, 2003), spiritual struggles were associated with greater psychological distress. Among young adults whose parents had divorced, those who recalled greater spiritual struggles around the marital breakup reported more current depression, feelings of loss and abandonment, intrusive thoughts, and self-blame (Warner, Mahoney, & Krumrei, 2009). Spiritual struggles among family caregivers to loved ones with dementia were also generally associated with greater depressive symptoms and caregiver burden (Wong & Pargament, 2019).

Studies in other contexts have yielded similar results. Berzengi, Berzenji, Kadim, Mustafa, and Jobson (2017) conducted an investigation of two Muslim samples exposed to trauma in London and the Middle East, and demonstrated a tie between spiritual struggles and greater depression in both groups. Abu-Raiya, Sasson, Paalchy, Mozes, and Tourgeman (2017) worked with Christian, Jewish, Muslim, and Druze women who had survived intimate partner violence in Israel and reported that higher levels of spiritual struggles were associated with greater depression. Among adults in Saudi Arabia dealing with the COVID-19 pandemic, spiritual struggles were tied to depression, anxiety, and stress (Yildirim et al., 2021). In one of the few empirical studies of Buddhists, Falb and Pargament (2013) identified a sample of Buddhist hospice caregivers and found that spiritual struggles, particularly feelings of being a "bad Buddhist," were associated with greater depression and less of a sense of meaning and peace.

These cross-sectional findings have been supplemented by several longitudinal studies that provide more direct support for the primary role of spiritual struggles in fostering distress and disorientation among people encountering major life stressors (see Bockrath et al., 2021, for a meta-analysis). For example, Chan and Rhodes (2013) examined the long-term effects of spiritual struggles on psychological distress among low-income female survivors of Hurricane Katrina 4 years later. After controlling for initial levels of distress, spiritual struggles were predictive of greater psychological distress. In a study of divorced individuals, those who reported more spiritual struggles experienced more depressed symptoms 1 year later, after adjusting for initial levels of depression (Krumrei, Mahoney, & Pargament, 2011). Some investigations have yielded inconsistent or nonsignificant findings (see Koenig, 2018a, for a review). For example, a 2-year longitudinal study of parents of children with cystic fibrosis found that, although spiritual struggles were correlated with higher levels of depression over time, spiritual struggles at baseline did not predict shifts toward more depression (Szcześniak, Zou, Stamper, & Grossoehme, 2017). The authors note that this pattern of results is more consistent with a secondary or complex model of spiritual struggles.

More controlled research in this area is rare, but a study by Lee, Roberts, and Gibbons (2013) was an exception to this rule. The researchers had college students, who were grieving the loss of a family member, friend, or acquaintance, engage in a grief induction exercise through an interview in which participants were asked to talk about their loss, their relationship with the deceased, their fondest members of the person, and their feelings since the death. The researchers measured the intensity of participants' feelings of grief before, immediately after, 1 minute after, and 5 minutes after the grief induction. Higher levels of spiritual struggle were predictive of greater grief intensity and a longer time to recover from their grief following the loss interview. These findings illustrate how spiritual struggles may foster emotional dysregulation after a death.

Overall, the research shows modest but consistent connections between spiritual struggles and signs of distress and disorientation. The findings are robust. They apply to the general population, to diverse clinical samples, and to people facing a diverse array of life stressors, including death, war, sexual assault, domestic violence, and natural disasters. Although most of the research focuses largely on Christians in the United States, several researchers have expanded these studies to other religious groups and cultures, and arrived at similar conclusions.

So far, we have focused on the implications of spiritual struggles for markers of distress and disorientation, such as anxiety and depression. However, it is important to recognize that, on average, the levels of anxiety and depression in these studies did not rise much beyond mild to moderate levels. An important question remains: Do spiritual struggles have potentially more serious implications for an individual's health and well-being? We turn now to that literature.

Spiritual Struggles, Serious Problems, and Decline

Recalling our model of spirituality (see Chapter 2), spiritual struggles could be tied to more serious psychological and physical decline. What do the data show?

Studies of Serious Psychological Problems

Relatively few studies have examined the implications of spiritual struggles for serious psychopathology (see Pargament & Exline, 2021, for a review). Earlier, we noted an exception to this rule in a study by McConnell et al. (2006), who found that spiritual struggles were significantly associated with symptoms indicative of several types of serious psychological problems that went beyond anxiety and depression to encompass paranoid ideation, obsession–compulsion, somatization, and phobic anxiety. In another study, notable because it measured psychopathology not by self-report but by informant's ratings, McGee, Myers, Carlson, Funai, and Barclay (2013) found that reports of spiritual struggles by patients with mild Alzheimer's disease were tied to informant's ratings of greater frequency and severity of neuropsychiatric symptoms, including delusions, hallucinations, agitation, disinhibition, and nighttime disturbances. A third study of orthodox Jewish adolescent girls showed spiritual struggles to be significantly associated with higher levels of disordered-eating pathology (Latzer et al., 2015). In all three of these studies, however, data were collected at only one point in time (i.e., cross-sectional in design), and as a result, questions about whether spiritual struggles are primary or secondary to psychopathology were left unanswered.

Studies of PTSD. One type of serious psychological problem has received more attention: PTSD. PTSD occurs in response to a trauma and is marked by disruptive symptoms that include reexperiencing and trying to avoid the trauma, feeling on edge, problems with memory, trouble sleeping, angry outbursts, negative thoughts about oneself and the world, alienation from others, a lack of motivation, and difficulty working. Can spiritual struggles produce this level of life disruption among those who have experienced a traumatic experience?

Several researchers have demonstrated higher levels of symptoms of PTSD among people who experience more spiritual struggles. These findings have emerged in studies of military veterans in the United States (Park, Smith, et al., 2017; Witvliet et al., 2004), Croatian war veterans (Mihaljević, Aukst-Margetić, Vuksan-Ćusa, Koić, & Milošević, 2012), Muslims exposed to trauma in London and the Middle East (Berzengi et al., 2017), caregivers dealing with their child's hematopoietic stem cell transplant (Chardon, Brammer, Madan-Swain, Kazak, & Pai, 2021), and survivors of the Oklahoma City bombing (Pargament, Smith, et al., 1998).

Longitudinal studies of college freshmen facing traumatic and nontraumatic life events (Wortmann et al., 2011) and U.S. military veterans (Currier et al., 2015) provide support for a primary spiritual struggles model in which spiritual struggles increase the likelihood of PTSD symptoms. For example, in an investigation of U.S. military veterans in a 60- to 90-day residential treatment program for combat-related PTSD, spiritual struggles at baseline were predictive of poorer outcomes of PTSD over the course of the program (Currier et al., 2015). These researchers also tested for a secondary spiritual struggles model by examining whether higher levels of PTSD at the beginning of treatment predicted changes in spiritual struggles over time. They did not. In contrast, Harris et al. (2012) found support for a complex model of spiritual struggles. They conducted a 1-year follow-up study of a sample of church members who had been coping with a range of acute and chronic stressors: physical and sexual assault or abuse, war, natural disasters, accidents, a diagnosis of a serious illness, or an unexpected death. They found that spiritual struggles mediated the relationship between posttraumatic stress symptoms at baseline and 1 year later. In other words, posttraumatic stress symptoms at baseline predicted higher levels of spiritual struggles, and spiritual struggles, in turn, predicted higher levels of posttraumatic symptoms 1 year later. Thus, these studies point to a connection between spiritual struggles and symptoms of PTSD, with the weight of the evidence suggesting that spiritual struggles set the stage for PTSD symptoms.

Studies of Suicidality. One important set of studies documents an increased risk among spiritual strugglers for suicidal ideation and attempts. Some research has focused on military veterans, a particularly relevant population given the fact that suicide is a major cause of death in this group in the United States (Currier, Smith, & Kuhlman, 2017). Strikingly, in 2012 and 2013, deaths as a result of suicide in the military were more common than deaths through combat (cited in Currier et al., 2017). In the Currier et al. study, veterans from the Iraq and/or Afghanistan wars completed a comprehensive measure of suicidality, including questions about lifetime suicidal ideation and/or prior attempts, the frequency of suicidal ideation over the past 12 months, suicidal threats, and the likelihood of suicide attempts in the future. Higher levels of spiritual struggles were strongly tied to greater suicidality. For every 1-point increase in the spiritual struggles measure, the veterans were 1.44 times more likely to have discussed a plan to commit suicide with a desire to die, and 1.51 times more likely to attempt suicide in the future. Spiritual struggles were uniquely associated with suicidality—in fact, suicidality was not predicted by any of the other variables in the study, including the number of deployments, combat-related exposure, moral injury experiences, depression, and PTSD symptoms.

Few studies have examined the relationship between spiritual struggles and suicidality in other cultures. One exception to this rule comes from a large-scale study of 11 Muslim countries. The researchers reported that higher levels of spiritual struggles were associated with more suicide attempts—interestingly, struggles were not related to suicidal ideation (Eskin et al., 2020).

People with psychological and physical health problems are also at risk for suicidality, and studies have identified spiritual struggles as a significant predictor of suicidality for this group (Paika et al., 2017; Rosmarin et al., 2013; Trevino, Balboni, Zollfrank, Balboni, & Prigerson, 2014). For example, Trevino et al. worked with 724 patients with advanced cancer and found that higher levels of spiritual struggles were associated with more frequent suicidal ideation, even after controlling for a number of other potentially confounding variables, including the stage of diagnosis, physical quality of life, religiousness and spirituality, and secular and religious social support. In another study of Greek patients with diabetes, chronic obstructive pulmonary disease (COPD), and rheumatic diseases, higher levels of spiritual struggle were associated with greater suicidality, depressive symptoms severity, and negative illness perceptions (Paika et al., 2017). In one of the few prospective studies in this area, Rosmarin et al. investigated patients in a psychiatric treatment program with current or past psychosis, and reported that spiritual struggles prior to treatment were strongly predictive of subsequent greater frequency and intensity of suicidal ideation. They concluded that "spiritual struggle potentially represents a significant safety concern for psychotic patients" (p. 185).

Additional longitudinal studies are needed to determine whether spiritual struggles lead to greater suicidality, as in the primary spiritual struggles model, or vice versa. Recall, however, that longitudinal studies have shown a connection between spiritual struggles and increased levels of depression, anxiety, and PTSD symptomatology over time, problems that increase the risk for suicidality. These findings would be consistent with the assertion that spiritual struggles can trigger higher levels of suicidality. In any case, mental health professionals should be alert to the potentially serious implications of spiritual struggles for suicidality among their clients.

Studies of Physical Symptomatology. Several studies have considered the ramifications of spiritual struggles for physical health. Cross-sectional studies have shown a link between spiritual struggles and indices of poorer physical health, including more HIV symptoms (Trevino et al., 2010), lower self-rated physical health among Muslims (Abu-Raiya, Pargament, Mahoney, & Stein, 2008), and poorer medication adherence among Iranians with epilepsy (Lin, Saffari, Koenig, & Pakpour, 2018).

Spiritual struggles have also been consistently tied to greater pain-related symptoms. More specifically, high levels of spiritual struggles were associated with greater pain, fatigue, and physical symptomatology among people who had stem cell transplants for multiple myeloma (Sherman et al., 2005); greater pain, physical role limitations, and poorer self-rated physical health among Jews (Rosmarin et al., 2009); and greater catastrophization and interference of pain with behavioral and emotional functioning (mediated by depression) among veterans with chronic pain (Harris et al., 2018).

A few longitudinal studies have addressed the question of whether spiritual struggles are primary or secondary to physical symptomatology. Fitchett, Rybarczyk, DeMarco, and Nicholas (1999) followed a group of 98 patients in medical rehabilitation from hospital admission to 4-months postadmission, and found that higher levels of spiritual struggles at admission were predictive of poorer functional status at follow-up, even after controlling for their initial functional status (e.g., ability to self-care). Similar results were reported by Pargament et al. (2004) in their longitudinal follow-up to the study of older adult patients who were medically ill and hospitalized. Spiritual struggles were related to declines in functional status after controlling for initial functional status, mental health, and physical health. Park, Wortmann, and Edmondson (2011) followed a group of patients with end-stage congestive heart failure over a 3-month period. Higher levels of spiritual struggle at baseline were associated with more nights of hospitalization and, marginally, greater physical impairment 3 months later. These studies, as a group, support a primary spiritual struggles model.

Studies of Mortality. Perhaps the most compelling support for a primary model of spiritual struggles comes from a study by Pargament, Koenig, Tarakeshwar, and Hahn (2001). Over the course of their 2-year study, 176 of their initial sample of 596 older adult patients who were medically ill died. The researchers found that higher levels of spiritual struggles at baseline were predictive of greater risk of mortality even after the effects of demographic variables, mental health variables, and physical health status at baseline were controlled. Numerous studies have shown that more frequent attendance at religious congregations is strongly related to a lower risk of mortality (e.g., Shanshan, Stampfer, Williams, & VanderWeele, 2016). The Pargament et al. study of spiritual struggles was, as far as we know, the first to identify one form of spirituality that may work in the opposite direction, increasing rather than reducing the likelihood of mortality. This finding was more recently replicated in a study of 177 HIV patients in the midstage of their disease (Ironson, Kremer, & Lucette, 2016). After controlling for a variety of medical and demographic variables, higher levels of spiritual struggles, as measured by qualitative content analysis of interviews, predicted increased rates of mortality over 17 years.

Why might people who experience more spiritual struggles be more likely to die sooner? (In this instance, only a primary spiritual struggle model makes sense since the idea of a secondary struggle—dying resulting in a spiritual struggle—would be hard to fathom.) At this early stage in the research on this topic, we can only speculate on some possible answers to this question.

Perhaps people who engage in more spiritual struggles take poorer care of their health. Park, Edmondson, Hale-Smith, and Blank (2009) tested this possibility in a study of young to middle-age adults with cancer. They found that those who struggled more spiritually were less likely to adhere to their doctor's advice and to their medications. They also tended to engage in more days of drinking alcohol. Another study of a nationally representative sample of adults showed that higher levels of spiritual struggles were tied to an elevated risk of problem drinking, especially among young adults (Krause, Pargament, Ironson, & Hill, 2018). In a longitudinal study of entering college students, Faigin, Pargament, and Abu-Raiya (2014) hypothesized that addictive behavior represents a response to the anguish and sense of emptiness that accompanies spiritual struggles. To test this idea, they had students report their frequency of engaging in 17 types of addictive behaviors at two points in their freshman year. As predicted, those who experienced more spiritual struggles on entry into college were more likely to develop 11 of the 17 addictive behaviors 5 weeks later, including gambling, drug use, smoking, and excessive undereating.

A second related explanation for the spiritual struggles–mortality connection is that spiritual strugglers may be more likely to experience a sense of hopelessness, helplessness, and other negative emotions that, in turn, interfere with the motivation to engage in good health practices and persist in the face of challenging circumstances. The consistent ties between spiritual struggles, depression, and suicidality would fit with this explanation, as would the finding by Park et al. (2009) that the relationship between spiritual struggles with poorer medical adherence and more drinking among cancer patients was mediated by the emotions of guilt and shame.

A final explanation is more biological in nature. Spiritual struggles may increase the risk of dying earlier (and physical illness more generally) as a result of their impact on the biological paths that lead to disease progression. A few studies have begun to examine this possibility. Trevino and colleagues (2014) focused on whether spiritual struggles predict changes in a cluster of differentiation 4 (CD4) counts and viral load over time among people with HIV/AIDS. CD4 T lymphocytes provide an indication of how well the immune system is working and the degree to which the disease is progressing. Viral load measures the amount of HIV viral particles in the individual's bloodstream. The researchers reported that people with low to moderate levels of spiritual struggles showed some improvement in their CD4 levels over time, while those with higher levels of spiritual struggles showed declines in CD4 levels, after controlling for baseline CD4, positive religious coping, and demographic variables. No effects were found for viral load. However, Ironson, Stuezzle, Fletcher, and Ironson (2006) did find that patients with HIV who saw God as more punishing and judgmental showed faster disease progression over a 4-year period, according to both CD4 counts and viral load, adjusting for antiretroviral medications. Focusing on a sample of 235 patients with cardiac disease about to undergo surgery, Ai, Seymour, Tice, Kronful, and Bolling (2009) examined the relationships between spiritual struggles and interleukin-6 (IL-6), a cytokine. Cytokines are involved in the immune-inflammatory response and healing of wounds. However, when cytokine levels are elevated chronically, they can lead to inflammation in the arteries, which contributes, in turn, to cardiac disease. IL-6, in particular, has been linked to cardiac disease, as well as cardiac surgical morbidity and mortality. Ai et al. reported that even after controlling for a variety of physical health and mental health variables, patients who experienced more spiritual struggles had higher IL-6 levels. Finally, Tobin and Slatcher (2016) studied a large national sample of adults in the United States over a 10-year period and found that the unhealthy relationship between lower levels of religious participation and the stress hormone of cortisol was explained by higher levels of spiritual struggles. These findings are intriguing and point to the need for further research on the biological pathways—psychoendocrine, psychoneuroimmune, epigenetic—that could lead from spiritual struggles to physical deterioration and decline.

Signs of Social Problems

Before concluding this section, we should also note that a few studies have begun to examine the implications of spiritual struggles for signs of social problems. In one study of survivors of the 1995 Oklahoma City bombing, higher levels of spiritual struggles were associated with greater callousness toward others (Pargament, Zinnbauer, et al., 1998). Another study of veterans dealing with PTSD and their partners reported that spiritual struggles were associated with more negative communication between veterans and their partners according to both groups (Harris et al., 2017). Negative communication mediated the ties between spiritual struggles and lower relationship satisfaction for veterans but not for their partners. In an investigation of Muslim patients from Pakistan with cancer, spiritual struggles were tied to higher levels of hostility (Khan et al., 2009). Perhaps the strongest evidence for a link between spiritual struggle and social problems comes from a disturbing study of Rwandan perpetrators of genocide who completed a measure of spiritual struggles and appetitive aggression—that is, aggression driven not by its practical value but by the satisfaction or pleasure it produces (Schaal, Heim, & Elbert, 2014). An illustrative question from this measure is "Once you got used to being cruel, did you want to be crueler and crueler?" (p. 935). The researchers note abundant evidence of the role religion and spirituality play in inhibiting violence, and find in their study that positive religious coping was tied to less appetitive aggression. Spiritual struggles, however, worked in the opposite direction with higher levels of spiritual struggles associated with reports of greater appetitive aggression. Whether the aggression is a cause and/or consequence of spiritual struggles could not be determined in this cross-sectional study.

The growing body of research we just reviewed suggests that the implications of spiritual struggles go beyond distress and disorientation. The weight of the evidence appears to link spiritual struggles in a modest but consistent fashion to signs of more serious problems, deterioration, and decline, including psychopathology, posttraumatic stress symptoms, suicidality, physical health problems, potentially greater risk of mortality, and social problems.

And what about religious and spiritual involvement? As yet, relatively few studies have focused on the implications of spiritual struggle for the religious and spiritual life of the individual. We would expect that spiritual struggles increase the likelihood of dissatisfaction and perhaps disengagement from spiritual and religious activity and identification. A few studies suggest this may be the case. In one investigation, spiritual struggles were tied to spiritual dissatisfaction and decline (Cole, Hopkins, Tisak, Steel, & Carter, 2008). Another study among American orthodox Jews linked spiritual struggles with the coronavirus to negative impact on religious observance and faith in God (Pirutinsky, Cherniak, & Rosmarin, 2020). And in a study of college students, spiritual struggles were more common among those who had disengaged from organized religion or moved to a nonreligious identity in comparison to students who held more stable religious identities (Exline, Van Tongeren, et al., 2020). It is important to add here that religious and spiritual disengagement could be perceived as distressing by some and as a positive change by others. We have more to say on this point in the next chapter.

SPIRITUAL STRUGGLES AS A PATHWAY FROM STRESSFUL LIFE EVENTS AND A LIMITED ORIENTING SYSTEM TO DISTRESS, DISORIENTATION, AND DECLINE

In the previous chapter, we examined the roots of spiritual struggles. In this chapter, we focus on the painful consequences of spiritual struggles—namely, distress, disorientation, and potentially more serious problems. How do we pull this growing body of literature together? In our model of spirituality (see Chapter 2, Figure 2.1), we suggest that stressful life events, a limited orienting system, and problems of purpose or significance may essentially "work through" spiritual struggles to create problems. To put it another way, spiritual struggles may help to explain why stressful life events, weaknesses in the orienting system, and problems of purpose increase the individual's vulnerability to subsequent problems in living. Several studies have, in fact, tested this model by examining whether spiritual struggles mediate the relationships between (1) life events and signs of distress, disorientation, and serious problems; and (2) limitations in the orienting system and signs of distress, disorientation, and serious problems. No studies, as yet, have examined whether spiritual struggles might mediate a relationship between problems of purpose and distress and disorientation.

Spiritual Struggles as a Pathway between Stressful Life Events and Signs of Distress, Disorientation, and Serious Problems

Spiritual struggles represent an important transitional place that can be found in between the experience of a major life event and subsequent distress and disorientation. In line with this view, a few cross-sectional studies produce results consistent with a model that stressful life events work through spiritual struggles to produce poorer outcomes. Bradley, Schwartz, and Kaslow (2005) conducted a study of low-income African American women with a history of intimate partner violence and child abuse. Women who had encountered greater violence and abuse reported more PTSD symptoms, but when spiritual struggles were entered into the equation, the relationship between abuse and PTSD symptoms was significantly reduced. This pattern of findings suggests that spiritual struggles help to account for the link between the severity of abuse and PTSD symptoms. Similarly, McCleary-Gaddy and Miller (2019) studied a sample of African Americans and found that the effects of their experiences with prejudice on psychological distress were fully explained by spiritual struggles. Working with a sample of older Polish patients with cancer, Krok, Brudek, and Steuden (2019) found that spiritual struggles helped explain the link between more negative appraisals of the illness and lower psychological well-being. Chen, Bechara, Worthington, Davis, and Csikszentmihalyi (2019) studied groups of Colombian survivors of lengthy war conflict and a landslide, and reported that spiritual struggles mediated the relationship among trauma symptoms, the virtues of forgiveness and hope, and psychological well-being. Finally, Pomerleau et al. (2020) examined data from a national sample of adults in the United States and also found support for a mediational model in which spiritual struggles helped to explain, in part, the relationship between experiencing a greater number of stressful life events with greater distress and lower well-being.

Stronger support for the possibility that stressful life events produce some of their harmful effects by triggering spiritual struggles comes from a small set of longitudinal investigations. In one study of divorced people from the community, Krumrei et al. (2011) found that spiritual struggles mediated the relationship between appraisals of the divorce as a sacred loss or violation and depression 1 year later. Magyar-Russell et al. (2013) followed a group of patients in medical rehabilitation from admission to 6- to 8-weeks postdischarge and also reported that spiritual struggles helped to explain the relationship between appraisals of the stressor as a sacred loss or desecration, and depression and anxiety at postdischarge. Finally, in a study of college students exposed to traumatic and nontraumatic events in their first year, Wortmann et al. (2011) reported that spiritual struggle partially mediated the link between the experience of trauma and PTSD symptoms at the end of the academic year, after controlling for initial PTSD symptomatology. The authors conclude that spiritual struggles represent a "potential mechanism in the development and maintenance of PTSD symptoms" (p. 447).

As a group, these studies offer support for a new explanation that helps account for the negative effects of stressful life events on mental and physical health: Negative life experiences trigger struggles in the spiritual domain that lead to distress, disorientation, and decline. More practically, these findings should alert clinicians to the spiritual power of major life stressors—that is, their capacity to elicit spiritual struggles and, in turn, the capacity of these struggles to elicit psychological and physical problems.

Spiritual Struggles as a Pathway between Limitations of the Orienting System and Signs of Distress, Disorientation, and Serious Problems

Spiritual struggles may also help to explain why limitations of the orienting system—maladaptive core beliefs, social isolation, emotional dysregulation—can cause distress and decline. Only a few studies have focused on this possibility, but the results have been interesting. In a study of patients with cardiac disease before and after surgery, Ai and colleagues (2009) found that a combination of spiritual struggles and IL-6 mediated the relationship between a reliance on anger and anxiety as a way of coping before surgery and postoperative hostility. Another pair of studies examined spiritual struggles as a mediator of the effects of aspects of the spiritual orienting system on indicators of distress. Working with Christian women who were experiencing domestic violence, Ake and Horen, (2003) found higher levels of trauma symptoms among those who had a more extrinsic religious orientation, an orientation marked by the use of religion to meet social and personal needs rather than religious ones. The relationship between extrinsic religiousness and trauma symptoms was partially mediated through spiritual struggles. Using a large sample of college students and an adult web sample, Wilt et al. (2016) found that spiritual struggles—divine struggles in particular—mediated the relationship between beliefs about God's role in suffering and higher distress and lower well-being. As expected, spiritual struggles mediated the effects of a less benevolent theodicy (God causes suffering) on greater distress and lower well-being. Harder to understand, however, was the finding that spiritual struggles also mediated the effects of a more benevolent theodicy (suffering is part of God's benevolent plan) on greater distress and lower well-being. Finally, one rather complex study considered how spiritual struggles mediate the relationship between both stressful life events and orienting system variables and symptoms of physical health problems (Krause, Pargament, & Ironson, 2017). Working with a nationally representative sample of U.S. adults, the researchers found support for a causal chain in which (1) lower education level leads to (2) chronic economic problems that contribute to (3) living in rundown neighborhoods that triggers (4) greater anger, leading in turn to (5) spiritual struggles, and then ultimately (6) more symptoms of physical illness.

Overall, these findings provide relatively strong support for the idea that stressful life events contribute to distress and serious problems in part by triggering spiritual struggles. Further research is needed to determine whether spiritual struggles play a similar role in linking limitations within the orienting system and problems of significant purpose to significant problems in life.

CONCLUSIONS, QUESTIONS, AND IMPLICATIONS

We have reviewed what has become an impressive and still growing literature on the relationship between spiritual struggles with indicators of distress, disorientation, and serious problems. In this section, we summarize the key take-home points from this literature, raise questions that require further study, and consider the implications of these findings for clinical practice.

Conclusions

We can draw several conclusions from our review of this growing literature.

1. *There is a robust relationship between spiritual struggles and signs of distress and disorientation.* This relationship has been demonstrated within diverse groups: the general population; people facing physical health problems, mental health problems, and major life stressors; and demographically diverse groups. Although the large majority of this research has been conducted among predominantly Christian samples in the United States, several studies have shown similar results within people from other cultures and other religious traditions (e.g., Jewish, Muslim, Hindu), as well as atheists. Moreover, even relatively low levels of spiritual struggles can be tied to distress and disorientation.

2. *Spiritual struggles are associated with more serious problems.* The implications of spiritual struggles for adjustment go beyond signs of distress and disorientation to include symptoms of psychiatric disorders and PTSD, suicidality, symptoms of physical illness, a weakened immune system, perhaps greater risk of mortality, and social problems.

3. *The connection between spiritual struggles, distress, and serious problems cannot be explained away by potentially confounding variables.* The relationship remains even after controlling for variables, such as personality, demographic factors, general levels of religiousness, positive spiritual coping, or any tendency among spiritual strugglers to be generally more negative about themselves and their lives.

4. *Spiritual struggles can be both a cause and effect of psychological and physical health problems.* Consistent with a primary spiritual struggles model, a number of longitudinal studies and one meta-analysis (Bockrath et al., 2021) of these findings demonstrate that higher levels of spiritual struggles are predictive of declines in mental health. A smaller number of studies have shown similar results with respect to physical health. On the other hand, in keeping with a secondary spiritual struggles model, some longitudinal studies have shown that psychological distress and, to some extent, physical health problems can lead to spiritual struggles. And it is important to note a recent test of all three

models of spiritual struggles—primary, secondary, complex—in a longitudinal study of people with chronic illness (Cowden et al., in press). Spiritual struggles were found to be predictive of increased psychological distress over two points in time, and psychological distress predicted increased spiritual struggles over these time points. This study and the pattern of findings overall suggests that a complex model of spiritual struggles may be the most accurate of all. In other words, the best response to the chicken-and-egg question of what comes first, spiritual struggles or psychological and physical problems, may be "all of the above"—spiritual struggles can result in problems and problems can trigger spiritual struggles.

5. *Spiritual struggles do not inevitably lead to distress and decline.* Even though the relationship between spiritual struggles and distress, disorientation, and decline has been consistently shown across many studies, the statistical magnitude of this relationship is generally modest. What this means is that many people who struggle spiritually do not necessarily experience distress and serious problems.

6. *Spiritual struggles help to explain why stressful life events and limitations in the individual's orienting system can produce distress and serious problems.* Several studies show that spiritual struggles mediate the relationship between stressful life events and subsequent problems. A few studies have also suggested that spiritual struggles mediate the connection between limitations within the orienting system and maladjustment. These findings support a model in which life events and orienting system variables "work through" spiritual struggles to generate distress and problems. Further research is needed to determine whether problems of purpose and significance also work through spiritual struggles to produce distress and decline.

Questions

A number of questions arise from the findings we have reviewed here. Perhaps the most basic of these is a "why" question: Why is the connection between spiritual struggles, distress, disorientation, and decline so robust? Drawing on our perspective on spiritual struggles, we can suggest a few possible reasons. First, because spiritual struggles touch our deepest values and our basic orientation to life, they have an inherent capacity to produce pain and disruption at all levels: emotional, cognitive, behavioral, social, biological, and spiritual. Second, coming to terms with spiritual struggles can deplete our resources or reveal the limitations in our resources, making it difficult to sustain ourselves. Further "close-up" studies that follow people over time as they go through spiritual struggles are needed to test these ideas.

A second key question is how far-reaching are these findings? Further studies of spiritual struggles are needed among groups that have not received much attention, such as Buddhists, atheists, native and indigenous peoples, and those from African and Asian cultures. Additional studies should also consider how spiritual struggles affect social, biological, religious, and spiritual outcomes. And even though a number of longitudinal studies have been conducted on spiritual struggles, participants have generally been followed up over relatively short periods of time. This leaves us with an important unanswered question: How long-lasting are the effects of spiritual struggles? Because struggles can touch people so deeply, it may take a great deal of time to marshal the resources to sustain and conserve oneself or, if necessary, transform one's most basic orientation and purposes in life.

As noted above, the relatively modest size of the connection between spiritual struggles with signs of distress, disorientation, and serious problems indicates that spiritual struggles do not invariably lead to painful outcomes. This raises a third set of relevant questions: Why is it that some spiritual strugglers run into trouble while others do not? What factors potentially cushion the negative effects of spiritual struggles? What factors potentially make matters worse? We take up these vital questions in Chapter 6.

Finally, it is important to ask whether the ties between spiritual struggles and signs of trouble are the full story. Is the best we can hope for that an encounter with spiritual struggles will not lead to pain, disorientation, and decline? Many writers have likened spirituality to a life-giving process that moves from "dream sleep to awakening, illusion to realization, darkness to enlightenment, imprisonment to liberation, fragmentation to wholeness, separation to oneness, being in exile to coming home, seed to flowering tree, being on a journey to arriving, and death to rebirth" (Decker, 1993, p. 36). Is this simply rich poetic language or is there in fact a brighter side than the one we have explored in this chapter? Is there a potential for growth and transformation through spiritual struggles? We examine this question in the next chapter.

Implications for Clinical Practice

We have emphasized that spiritual struggles are often not a sign of pathology but rather a natural part of life. This doesn't mean, however, that they are not potentially painful or problematic. Like other experiences and times of life—adolescence, pregnancy, childbirth, aging—spiritual struggles are accompanied by risks. We cannot assume that spiritual struggles are inevitably resolved with minimal (if any) pain. Spiritual struggles really matter. The data are clear: People can and do suffer psychological and physical distress and decline as a result of their spiritual struggles. These are sobering findings. They bring to mind the concern Paul Tillich (1957) expressed over a half-century ago: "It may well be that with the vanishing of the god the believer breaks down without being able to reestablish his centered self by a new content of his ultimate concern" (p. 18).

It follows that many people may need help in understanding and coming to terms with their spiritual struggles. In some cases, spiritual struggles might be resolved by helping people deal with what could be more basic psychological problems. We have noted studies that support a secondary spiritual struggles model in which struggles are the end result of social, situational, and psychological factors. Attending to these more basic problems, in some instances, might resolve the spiritual struggles as well. We have also seen though that spiritual struggles can play a more primary role, creating significant distress and problems of their own. On these occasions, spiritual struggles are likely to require direct attention.

Unfortunately, however, spiritual struggles may be hidden from view when people seek help. One Vietnam War veteran with PTSD spoke to this point: "The physical wounds are not the most significant wounds of war. The wounds of the soul, the spiritual wounds, the emotional wounds—they are far deeper, though less obvious" (Thomas, 2004, p. 138). Here, we have reviewed findings that begin to shed light on this "less obvious" aspect of spirituality, one that may well be a vital mechanism for change. For example, if you recall, we started this chapter with the case of Susan, who came to therapy with symptoms of depression, anxiety, vague somatic concerns, and suicidality following an illness that was almost fatal for her. On the face of it, Susan's problems were simple and straightforward, provoked by her confrontation with mortality. And on the face of it, the solution would be straightforward as well: simply help Susan process her traumatic encounter with a frightening physical health event. This approach, however, might not be effective, for it would overlook the central role Susan's spiritual struggles played in her unfolding story. Susan's stressful life experience was especially problematic *because* it triggered spiritual struggles and these struggles were, in turn, the most direct source of her presenting mental health problems. Progress in treatment then would likely rest on helping Susan talk about her spiritual struggles. We believe that spiritual struggles represent an important target of conversation and mechanism for potential change in many other cases, as well. In chapters to come, we explore the ways practitioners can help people address spiritual struggles in treatment.

CHAPTER 5

Do Spiritual Struggles Lead to Growth?

THE BRIGHTER SIDE

"If I hadn't struggled with a lot of stuff, I never would've come to [a] more
   sincere faith and really questioned some of my beliefs and where I stand."

"I'm kind of becoming more outspoken because I do have ideas, I have things
   to say, and I guess that's part of me feeling more spiritual and feeling
   more whole and trying to figure out who I am."

"Things die in the wintertime; they come back in the spring."
                              —ROCKENBACH, WALKER, AND LUZADER (2012, p. 68)

These are the voices of college students reflecting on the impact of their spiritual struggles—from the struggle to reconcile belief in a loving God with tragedy, to the challenges of coming out as a gay man to friends and family, to the struggle of staying true to one's religious faith. Each of their stories is marked by accounts of great distress, confusion, and disorientation, but there is more to their stories than pain. In their accounts, we also hear words of strength, confidence, positive transformation, and renewal. Painful though their spiritual struggles were, the students feel that they have undergone powerful, life-changing shifts in their sense of significance and their orientation to themselves, the world, and the sacred. In reflecting on their spiritual struggles, the students speak the language of growth. It is, as Rockenbach and colleagues (2012) concluded, the "bright side" of spiritual struggle (p. 69).

Given the rather dark picture of spiritual struggles that emerged in the previous chapter, it may come as a relief to shift gears and focus on this brighter side. Of course, the notion that spiritual struggles can lead to growth may not be any big surprise. After all, one of the core narratives in the United States is built on the theme that people can grow through their most difficult times (McAdams,

2013), as we hear in many old sayings: "Suffering builds character. . . . " "No pain, no gain. . . . " "What doesn't kill me makes me stronger. . . . " "God writes straight with crooked lines. . . . " "Broken bones heal stronger." Therapists are also steeped in this narrative; by conveying a sense of hope and possibility to clients who come to psychotherapy often feeling the very opposite, therapists try to lift clients' spirits and foster commitment to counseling and growth.

And yet, uplifting and inspirational as this narrative is, before we conclude that spiritual struggles in fact lead to growth, we need to ask some hard questions: Are stories of growth through spiritual struggles commonplace or are they unusual? Do reports of growth reflect actual change or are they simply refrains of the cultural narrative that pain leads to gain? Similarly, are the "old sayings" grounded in reality? Does suffering really build character? Are people inevitably strengthened by their greatest trials, including spiritual struggles? Or are the old sayings and stories of growth through struggle simply fanciful illusions that help us cope with pain or simply avoid our fears that suffering may not have a happy ending?

We take a careful look at these questions in this chapter, drawing on theory, research, and clinical accounts. Our findings challenge the notion that spiritual struggles inevitably lead to growth. Claims of "growth guaranteed" through spiritual struggle are simply false. What spiritual struggles do offer is *potential*—the potential for growth and positive transformation.

A brief word on definitions: Although the term *growth* has been defined in a variety of ways (Jayawickreme & Blackie, 2014; Linley & Joseph, 2004; Tedeschi & Calhoun, 1995), we speak about growth in this chapter to refer not only to resilience and recovery of health and mental health after a spiritual struggle but also to positive, potentially transformational changes in the individual's larger purpose in life and orientation to him- or herself, the world, and the sacred. We begin by considering some classic religious and psychological writings on growth and its links to spiritual struggle.

RELIGIOUS PERSPECTIVES ON SPIRITUAL STRUGGLES AND GROWTH

The potential value of spiritual struggle for growth is affirmed in the writings of several religious traditions. In one of the foundational stories within the Hebrew Bible, prior to his fateful confrontation with his brother Esau, Jacob wrestles with the angel in the dark. Although he is scarred through that struggle, he is also transformed, taking on the new name of Israel (meaning "wrestles with God") and becoming the third patriarch of the Hebrew people. Jews are also told to lay the most central commandments "upon your heart." Why? A Hasidic tale contains an answer: "It is because as we are, our hearts are closed, and we cannot place the holy words in our hearts. So we place them on top of our hearts. And there they stay until, one day, the heart breaks, and the words fall in" (Palmer, 2004, p. 181). Pain, suffering, and struggle then can become gateways to greater wisdom. They are, Karff (1979) says, opportunities for teachable moments.

Christianity imbues spiritual struggles with higher purpose. As Exline, Hall, Pargament, and Harriott (2017) note, within the Bible, human trials are depicted as ways that God purifies people, like a vine being pruned (John 15:2), silver being refined (Isaiah 48:10), or clay being shaped by the potter's hands (Jeremiah 18:1-6). Through these difficult times, Christians are taught that they can experience growth through greater endurance (James 1:2-4); the ability to provide solace to others (2 Corinthians 1:4); and the fruits of the Holy Spirit that include love, joy, peace, patience, gentleness, and self-control (Galatians 5:22-23a). Weakness then can become a source of strength and even embraced as Paul describes: "Therefore I will boast all the more gladly about my weaknesses, so that Christ's power may rest on me. That is why, for Christ's sake, I delight in weaknesses, in insults, in hardships, in persecutions, in difficulties. For when I am weak, then I am strong" (2 Corinthians 12:10). More contemporary Protestant theologian Paul Tillich (1948) describes periods of suffering and struggle as opportunities to experience grace: "Grace strikes us when we are in great pain and restlessness. . . . Sometimes at that moment a wave of light breaks into our darkness, and it is as though a voice were saying, 'You are accepted' " (p. 163).

Within Buddhism, the shattering of illusions is seen as a desirable, even necessary, step along the road to enlightenment. The orienting systems of Zen Buddhists, for instance, are challenged by seemingly nonsensical koans or riddles, such as "What is your original face before your parents were born?" and "Two hands clap and there is a sound; What is the sound of one hand clapping?" It is the ensuing struggle and disorientation that may elicit a deeper understanding of life. Commenting on Zen Buddhism and growth, Campbell, Brunell, and Foster (2004) write:

> A self that experiences the richness and fullness of life with a sense of awe and appreciation may reflect the deconstruction rather than reconstruction of the self. . . . The self may be jarred out of its cocoon and given the opportunity to see the world more as it is—no reconstruction necessary or desirable. (p. 25)

Within Islam, and especially within the Sufi tradition, the concept of *spiritual jihad* refers to a battle between the higher and lower parts of the self, in which the aim is to cultivate virtue and thereby draw closer to God (see Saritoprak & Exline, 2021; Saritoprak, Exline, & Abu-Raiya, 2020, for a review). In two samples of U.S. Muslims (Saritoprak, Exline, & Stauner, 2018), a spiritual jihad mindset in response to moral struggles was associated with more positive religious coping and more spiritual and posttraumatic growth. In one of the two samples, the spiritual jihad mindset was also associated with greater self-reports of virtuous behaviors along with lower levels of depression and anxiety.

PSYCHOLOGICAL PERSPECTIVES
ON SPIRITUAL STRUGGLES AND GROWTH

Many theories of psychological and spiritual development mirror the religions of the world in the value they place on struggle in general and spiritual struggle in particular as a precursor to growth. Earlier, we described Erikson's (1998) view that people are forged by the way they come to terms with the psychosocial crises they face at every phase of life. In his classic theory of cognitive development, Jean Piaget (1954) described how intellectual growth is the direct result of the child's encounter with the tension and frustration that occurs when he or she cannot assimilate new experiences into old ways of thinking and experiencing the world. A young child given a small rubber ball may initially try to eat it, thinking that small objects are to be chewed. When the rubber proves to be inedible, the child may grimace, give a shout, or throw or drop the ball, and when the latter takes place, learning results. Aha, some objects are more fun to throw than eat—they bounce! However, the key point to take from Piaget here is that frustration is essential to the creation of a new way of viewing the world.

Psychologist of emotion W. Gerrod Parrott (2014) has also spoken to the ways in which negative emotions may foster adjustment, growth, and development. Certainly, problems arise when people are unable to regulate their emotions. Anger, sadness, guilt, shame, and anxiety can cause tremendous problems when they are dysregulated, leading to disorders (often called emotional disorders), such as depression, intermittent explosive disorder, and generalized anxiety disorder. Even so, painful as they may be, these emotions also have adaptive value. Fear can mobilize escape when it is essential to survival. Anger can signal to others an unwillingness to tolerate mistreatment of the self or others. Embarrassment can lead to efforts to restore social standing. One fascinating study speaks to this point. Borowiecki (2017) studied the relationship between negative emotions and the creative output of three famous composers: Mozart, Liszt, and Beethoven. Specifically, the voluminous correspondence of these composers was analyzed for the frequency of negative emotional terms, such as *hurt, grief, nervous,* and *sad.* He then examined whether periods of greater negative emotionality were followed by the creation of more important classical compositions in the next year. Negative emotions, particularly sadness, were indeed succeeded by more creative musical output. Parrott (2014) concludes that negative emotions are intrinsic to a life of value, a life well lived: "To engage passionately with all aspects of life gives rise to negative emotions that will be meaningful because they are connected to commitments and goals that are treasured" (pp. 292–293).

Several theorists have written about the growth-inducing potential of stressful life experiences, including the most major of traumas. For example, Parks (2000) maintains that out of turbulent times of transition, "shipwreck" college students can grow in their understanding of the world. "The gladness on the other side of shipwreck arises from an embracing, complex kind of knowing that is experienced as a more trustworthy understanding of reality" (p. 30). Similarly, Pearce (2020) writes that, like the cactus that blooms only in the dark, some people require a period of loss and darkness to fully blossom and grow. Tedeschi and Calhoun (2004) coined the term *posttraumatic growth* to describe the positive benefits that can result from the experience of major life changes. No doubt, having one's schema for making sense of the world shaken may be quite distressing, but this disruption sets the stage for growth and transformation. Tedeschi and Calhoun go on to make an important point: "Growth . . . does not occur as a direct result of trauma. It is the individual's struggle with the new reality in the aftermath of trauma that is crucial in determining the extent to which posttraumatic growth occurs" (p. 5). From the perspective of the model of struggles we present in this book, we would agree that growth is not a direct result of trauma. However, we would add that whether spiritual struggles lead to growth depends not only on the struggle itself but also on the way people come to terms with it. This is a point we take up in greater detail in the following chapter.

The psychologists we reviewed so far describe how struggles of many kinds can lead to positive, transformational change. A smaller number of theorists have zeroed in on the implications of *spiritual* struggle for growth. Most famously, James Fowler (1981) has described faith in terms of a series of developmental stages that unfold in parallel to the stages of cognitive, moral, and personality development as the result of new environmental demands and challenges that call for new ways of knowing and behaving in the world. He writes, "Growth and development in faith also result from life crises, challenges and the kinds of disruptions that theologians call revelation. Each of these brings disequilibrium and requires changes in our ways of seeing and being in faith" (pp. 100–101). Through the experience of these disruptions, Fowler asserts, the individual is able to move toward a faith of greater reflectiveness, depth, and universality.

The possibility of growth is also embedded in the model of spiritual struggles we have presented in this book. We have noted that spiritual struggles may reveal the limits of both the significant purposes we pursue and the orienting system that guides us toward these destinations. Chittister (2003) offers a powerful description of how spiritual struggles confront us with our human limitations: "We know things now that we never knew before. We know how meager is our imagination, how limited our vision. We know how small we can really be. . . . Nothing else unmasks us to the same degree" (p. 85). Though disorienting, this discovery can set the stage for fundamental transformation in both the purposes we seek and in the pathways we take to reach our goals. Chittister goes on to capture the growth and transformation in self and spirit that can occur through spiritual struggles: "The whole purpose of wrestling with God is to be transformed into the self that we are meant to become, to step out of the confines of our false securities and allow our creating God to go on creating in us" (p. 98). At its best, spiritual struggle "gives life depth and vision, insight and understanding. It not only transforms us, it makes us transforming as well. . . . It teaches us our place in the universe. It teaches us how little we really need in life to be happy. It teaches us that every day life starts over again" (pp. 82, 85).

Writings from religious and psychological perspectives converge then to paint a hopeful picture of spiritual struggles; though they may be a source of pain and suffering, they also offer the potential for powerful life-altering change.

NARRATIVE ACCOUNTS
OF SPIRITUAL STRUGGLES AND GROWTH

As compelling as much of this literature is, questions remain about the degree to which it applies to people facing struggles in the world. Is this literature merely inspirational or do people actually experience growth through their spiritual struggles? One way to answer this question is by examining the stories of people who have struggled spiritually.

Foundational Stories from the World's Great Religious Traditions

Stories of growth through spiritual struggles are central to the world's great religious traditions. In his seminal book *The Hero with a Thousand Faces,* Joseph Campbell (2008) described how the leaders of these traditions—Osirus, Buddha, Moses, Muhammad, Jesus—all took the "hero's journey," in which they were called to leave their ordinary existence, underwent a time of testing and struggle with external or internal forces, and returned home as victors, transformed into world redeemers, saints, or reconciled with their communities.

Let's focus on some of these key stories here. The story of Moses, the most central narrative of Judaism, is filled with spiritual struggles. Moses struggles within himself and with God about his own reluctance to become the leader of the Hebrew people; he struggles with the pharaoh of Egypt, who refuses to release the Israelites from slavery; and he struggles with the Hebrew people, who rebel at times against Moses and God. But these struggles ultimately lead to a social transformation: the Exodus and delivery of the Israelites from enslavement to freedom.

Likewise, the Passion of Christ, describing the days leading up to the crucifixion of Jesus, is marked by spiritual struggles with the high priests of the temple, the Roman governor Pontius Pilate, Jesus's disciples, and Jesus's questions about God himself on the cross. Yet, these struggles are only a prelude to the culmination of this narrative so central to Christianity: the resurrection of Jesus from the dead, a transfiguration that allows Christians to experience a new way of life.

Perhaps the most important narrative within Buddhism is the story of Gautama Siddhartha beneath the Bodhi tree. There he sat for 7 days, and there he encountered the demon, Mara, who tried to lead Siddhartha away from his spiritual quest by distracting him through fearful images and tempting visions of beautiful women. Siddhartha's ability to master his internal spiritual struggles sets the stage for his transformation into a Buddha, a fully awakened being, and his decision to share his enlightenment with others.

And where would Confucianism be without the struggles Confucius experienced in the context of the moral decline of Chinese society in the 6th century B.C.E.? How could we imagine Islam without Muhammad's struggle with polytheism and the ruling elites of Mecca? What would Mormonism be without the story of struggle with prejudice and persecution leading to the dramatic escape of a people across the American continent to found a new Zion? It is critical to add that none of these stories ends with spiritual struggles. Instead, these periods of tremendous tension, strain, suffering, and conflict become vehicles that lead to positive transformation, be it freedom, rebirth, a new awakening, enlightenment, a new code of morality and virtue, or unification. Powerful and compelling though they are, these stories are not ultimately about spiritual struggles; they are about growth and transformation through spiritual struggles.

Are these stories a thing of the past? Do people describe growth through spiritual struggles today? Many do. We turn now to more current narrative accounts of growth through spiritual struggles.

Current Stories of Spiritual Struggles and Growth

In the stories below, people describe important shifts in both their guiding purposes and in their orientation to life, including their relationships with themselves, others, the world, and the sacred.

Growth in Ultimate Purpose and Significance

In some accounts of spiritual struggles people experience a change in their ultimate purpose or significance. The shift is toward the pursuit of something sacred, although the nature of that sacred transformation varies. Some describe a new religious purpose that comes to them suddenly, akin to a religious conversion. Commenting on what she has learned from her own spiritual struggles, one college student says:

> People reach a point [in their spiritual journeys] where they feel that nothing else is happening. They just feel like . . . they're burned out and they're dead. . . . And then all of a sudden there's a new spark of life and a new passion—a new goal to achieve. (Rockenbach et al., 2012, p. 68)

Be it a sudden or a gradual process, people seek a reason for living when confronted by their spiritual struggles with the limitations of themselves and their former lives. In one of their richly descriptive interviews of women with HIV/AIDS, Siegel and Schrimshaw (2000) share the words of one person who finds a faith "to hold on to" through her spiritual struggle:

Well, first I went through this anger thing. God wasn't on my side, and God didn't care about me, and why should I pray to him anymore? He could have saved me from getting this [HIV]. And then what happened was I realized that if I don't turn to God, if I don't have some kind of hope and some kind of faith, then what do I have left to hold onto? So I ran back to [the church], and what happened was I got deeper into my faith . . . and what happened was everything in life that I thought was important became so unimportant. (p. 1548)

Another man dealing with brain cancer and religious doubts talks about a shift in focus in which he has to "move out of the way" to make room for God in his life (Piderman, Egginton, et al., 2017):

There are times where I questioned why God did certain things, and now when I get to my prayers, I thank God for being who He is and how He is and you know, where He is. I had to move out of the way. . . . It's not all about me, you know. Much of what it takes is just simply having faith and belief that these things [having cancer and seizures] were done for us, and moving out of the way and letting God do it. But it's . . . hard to move out of the way, as we think we can do it [ourselves, but] . . . we can't. (p. 23)

Still another woman struggling with the disapproval of members of her church following a drug-related accident involving her fiancée, recounts how she gave up the goal of pleasing others and became more focused on pleasing God (de Castella & Simmonds, 2013): "now . . . it's not about anybody else because it's about me personally bettering myself . . . other people don't discourage me, or I don't look at what they're doing because I need to be right with God and not anybody else" (p. 543).

People also report an alteration from the lack of an overarching significance in their lives to more generative goals that involve caring for others and making the world a better place. One Puerto Rican woman with symptomatic HIV spoke to this change (Siegel & Schrimshaw, 2000):

Well when I found out [about my HIV status], I didn't have any career or nothing. No goals or nothing. You know, it's now when I have goals . . . I'm an activist for HIV now. I like doing that, and I also like helping people in recovery. You know, get their life together. . . . A goal of mine is to one day, um, get my GED . . . work for [an AIDS organization] and be an HIV coordinator. Then get my condo and all that. So, my goals have changed tremendously. (p. 1551)

In certain instances, we can hear a subtler, but nonetheless profound, change in values following difficult life experiences and spiritual struggles. This is a shift from more superficial material matters to a focus on the sacredness that can be found in everyday life. One woman with AIDS comments on her change in this direction (Siegel & Schrimshaw, 2000):

> I value life more now. I value moments and memories, and you know, what is good about life. Things, material things don't mean like anything anymore. Never never before did I ever notice the sky like I notice the sky now. You know and the clouds. I savor a sunset when I see a nice sunset. Life is different now. You see things more clearly. (p. 1549)

An early psychologist of religion, George Coe (1916) once wrote that "Possibly the chief thing in religion, considered functionally, is the progressive discovery and reorganization of values" (p. 65). The narrative accounts above suggest that Coe is right in his judgment: at least some individuals experience a fundamental shift in their guiding purpose in life as a result of their spiritual struggles. The character of the transformation involves a change from more extrinsic, self-centered, or superficial values to more internally held, sacred-centered, and generative pursuits. Other narratives of spiritual strugglers describe growth not only in the ultimate purposes people seek in life but also in the pathways they take to reach their destinations.

Growth in the Orienting System

In the stories of growth and transformation following spiritual struggles, we can hear three commonly described positive changes in the orienting system: new-found personal resources, a shift in the person's stance toward the world, and an altered relationship to religious and spiritual involvement.

Perhaps the most common of all transformations reported by people who struggle spiritually involves the development of strength of character. Through their struggles, people describe a shift toward greater independence and self-confidence. Rockenbach and colleagues (2012) capture these changes in their qualitative analysis of in-depth interviews of college students who experienced spiritual struggles. One student says that as a result of her time of struggle: "It's almost like I've found my own place and don't necessarily need to cling to other people as much." Another comments, "Each time I face a new situation it brings me back to a point where I am more centered, because I have faced it and I have overcome it. And I can accept it for what it is and know . . . I can work through it." A student summed up her experience succinctly: "It's made me a stronger person" (p. 68).

Another positive change often heard in the narratives of people who struggle spiritually involves a new way of relating to the world, including other people, the future, and stress and struggle. As a result of their struggles, people in narrative studies describe growth in their sense of closeness to others. Listen to the experience of one woman who had encountered spiritual struggles following a hemorrhage after childbirth and subsequent treatment for melanoma: "Other people have things happen in their lives and sort of when you hear all these different things that people have experienced . . . sort of forms a jigsaw puzzle and you get an understanding of them, that we are all in this together" (de Castella & Simmonds, 2013, p. 552). Another survivor of physical and sexual abuse by her father spoke of becoming less judgmental and more loving of others: "I'm not the same person I was . . . black and white view has gone out the door . . . it's letting go of . . . moralistic thinking. . . . You're not judging anyone's sin. . . . It's loving the person" (p. 550). Others talk about how their spiritual struggles have led them to a more hopeful, positive view of the future. Reflecting on his own struggles, one college student captured this sense of hope: "I feel stripped down sometimes. I feel like I have nothing left, but I know that I'm going to grow back again . . . and it's gonna be more beautiful than ever" (Rockenbach et al., 2012, p. 68). And some describe the development of a new perspective on periods of struggle in life, one that brings to mind the writings of Viktor Frankl (1959), who spoke of the fundamental freedom to choose one's attitude toward adversity. Following her experience in a psychoeducational group for students experiencing spiritual struggles, one participant put it this way:

> I've become a lot more positive about my struggles. I had a lot of rash emotions coming into this experience. . . . [Now] I look at my struggles as more of a positive. It is a learning and growing experience. I've matured in my view of the struggle—it doesn't have to be resolved right now. . . . Now it's not so much a struggle as an evolution. (Dworsky et al., 2013, p. 309)

One more theme common to the stories of positive change following spiritual struggles is important to note: growth in the individual's relationship to religion and spirituality. People often describe a deepening in their understanding of God. This may involve a new capacity to reconcile their struggle and suffering with their belief in a caring God. In response to her struggles with God around the severe emotional, physical, and sexual abuse she had suffered, a woman said:

> I had to go through this process of understanding why God had allowed me to go through all that suffering because it was the most hellish thing ever, to be so abused. You know your whole integrity is just taken away . . . and then being able to somehow reconcile that with a God who loves me and then a God who's my best friend. (de Castella & Simmonds, 2013, p. 545)

Another person talked about a shift to a more intimate relationship with God after a period of religious doubts in response to a life-threatening illness: "I have an ongoing day-to-day, minute-by-minute relationship with God. So it's not something that happens in church on a Sunday morning, and that, that is really sustaining and supportive for me and comforting for me to have that kind of relationship" (de Castella & Simmonds, 2013, p. 548).

The change experienced by yet another struggling individual involved a greater ability to see God in the midst of darkness: "God is like [a] redbird . . . sitting on these branches of a tree that has no leaves in front of a gray sky. It's like that light in the darkness, that reminder that there is something greater; there is something bigger than all of us" (Rockenbach et al., 2012, p. 6).

Other people describe a shift in the character of their faith as a result of their times of pain and spiritual struggle. This change may take the form of an intensified faith. One of the participants in Piderman, Egginton, et al.'s (2017) study of patients with brain cancer said:

> If I did not grow my faith during this period of time and [was] dealing with my illness as the person I was before, I would have been torn into pieces from the inside. I would have ended up in depression. I would have ended up in anger. I would have had a different personality than what I think I should be. I just like me now. (p. 24)

In some cases, the change in faith is more an alteration in kind than intensity. One woman dealing with religious doubts reported a change from a literal interpretation of Scriptures to a new appreciation for the mystery that lies at the heart of spirituality. She said, "Having experienced that growth . . . allowed me to kind of step out of bounds and trust something that I normally wouldn't have trusted and kind of believe a little more abstractly, not so literally" (Rockenbach et al., 2012, p. 6).

Finally, a number of stories depict changes in the individual's relationship with his or her religious congregation. In some cases, the shift is toward deeper institutional involvement, as we hear in the words of one woman who had experienced a struggle with her church after an experience of rape:

> I have a much, much deeper understanding of why I go to church. . . . I understand . . . what I receive from attending the mass. And what I gain from attending the mass and having all that understanding . . . strengthens my spirituality, which means that I'm able to live my life daily in a new way. (de Castello & Simmonds, 2013, p. 547)

In other instances, institutional involvement is de-emphasized in favor of a personal connection with the sacred. One woman struggling with a brain tumor said:

> After the experience there was a . . . real profound change. There was . . . greater depth and breadth to my faith. . . . I see spirituality as . . . a personal relationship with the Lord, and I see . . . religion as more of an institutionalized sort of thing. (de Castello & Simmonds, 2013, pp. 547–548)

It is also important to recognize cases in which people report growth and transformation through religious disaffiliation. In his extensive interview study of 87 religious apostates, Philip Zuckerman (2012) challenges the notion that people who leave their congregations and faith following a time of struggle necessarily encounter emotional pain and loss. Some, he notes, experience a growing sense of relief and freedom. Read the words of former Catholic atheist philosopher Andre Comte-Sponville:

> It felt like a liberation—everything suddenly seemed simpler, lighter, stronger and more open. It was as if I had left childhood behind me, with its fantasies and fears, its closeness and languorousness, and entered the real world at long last—the adult world, the world of action, the world of truth, unhampered by forgiveness or Providence. Such responsibility! Such joy! Yes, I am convinced that my life has been better—more lucid, freer, and more intense—since I became an atheist. (Zuckerman, 2012, p. 32)

Judging from the stories of the ordinary people we have reviewed here, reports of growth through spiritual struggles are not restricted to the world's great religious figures. Many people describe positive change—in some instances, wholesale change—as a result of their encounters with spiritual struggles. Growth is reported in both the destinations people seek in their lives and in the pathways they take to reach these goals. More specifically, growth is said to manifest itself through shifts in ultimate purpose and significance, strength of character, the individual's stance toward the world, and his or her relation to religion and spirituality. On the face of it then, these findings would seem to say that spiritual struggles do in fact lead to growth, at least among some individuals. Skeptics, however, would caution us against jumping to any quick conclusions.

EMPIRICAL STUDIES OF SPIRITUAL STRUGGLES AND GROWTH

Compelling though many of these stories are, they also raise several questions: How well do these stories represent the experiences of most people facing spiritual struggles? Are the accounts we have heard unusual or are they more commonplace? And even more important, are these stories valid? Do people really grow through their struggles? To answer these questions we shift our focus now from stories to empirically based studies of spiritual struggles and growth.

Studies of Prevalence of Growth

In the aftermath of major life stressors, research studies show that many people report positive changes and growth (see Linley & Joseph, 2004). For example, McMillen, Smith, and Fisher (1997) interviewed survivors of three community groups that encountered a traumatic event: a tornado that had led to loss of life and terrible destruction in a northern Florida town, a plane crash into a hotel that killed nine employees, and survivors of a deadly mass shooting in a cafeteria in Texas. Three to 4 months later, the majority of those interviewed reported some type of benefit or positive change as a result of these stressors. Three years later, many people continued to indicate that they perceived benefits as a result of their trauma. In a more recent study of military veterans with signs of PTSD, 50% indicated that they had experienced at least moderate growth as a result of their worst traumatic event (Tsai, El-Gabalawy, Sledge, Southwick, & Pietrzak, 2015). Even in the most dire of situations, these findings seem to say, people can find ways to change and grow in positive directions. Interesting as these findings are, they don't zero in on our particular focus of interest: spiritual struggles. How common are reports of growth following periods of tension, conflict, and strain surrounding the sacred?

Only a few studies have addressed this question directly. Desai and Pargament (2015) worked with college students who were undergoing a struggle with the divine or doubts about their religious beliefs. When asked to select whether they felt they had grown and/or declined as a result of their struggles, almost half (49%) of the participants said they had grown through their struggle, 29% said they had experienced both growth and decline, and 21% indicated neither growth nor decline. It was striking that only 3% felt they had simply declined as a result of their struggle. In another larger-scale study (Exline, Pargament, & Hall, 2014a), college students responded to the Posttraumatic Growth Inventory (PTGI; Tedeschi & Calhoun, 1996) in terms of the degree to which they had experienced growth as a result of their spiritual struggles. A majority indicated moderate to a great degree of agreement with items indicating growth in several areas, such as "My priorities about what is important in life" (53%), "Being able to accept the way things work out" (50%), and "Having compassion for others" (56%).

A few studies have focused more specifically on the extent to which people feel they have grown spiritually following a spiritual struggle. In the Exline et al. (2014a) study noted above, college students also completed the Spiritual Transformation Scale with reference to their spiritual struggles (Cole et al., 2008). Once again, many students agreed that they had experienced moderate to a great deal of spiritual growth as a result of their spiritual struggles on items such as "I have grown spiritually" (52%), "Spirituality has become more important to me" (48%), and "I more often look for a spiritual purpose in my life" (41%). Similar results have emerged from studies of military veterans who saw service in Iraq and Afghanistan (Breuninger et al., 2019; Teng, Stanley, Exline, & Pargament, 2016). For example, in the Teng et al. study, a majority of veterans moderately or strongly agreed with these aftereffects of spiritual struggles: "I have grown spiritually" (52%), "Spirituality has become more important to me" (69%), and "I more often look for a spiritual purpose in my life" (62%). In a follow-up of these veterans 6 months later, an even higher proportion reported moderate or greater levels of spiritual growth from their spiritual struggles.

These results lead to a very clear conclusion: A sizable number of people report at least moderate growth through their spiritual struggles. Thus, the stories of struggle-related growth, both classic and contemporary, do not seem to be unusual. However, it is important not to overstate these findings. A smaller but still sizable number of people also feel they have either not grown at all or grown only to a modest degree following times of struggle. Struggle-related growth may not be rare, but it is not universal either.

Before delving more deeply into empirical studies of spiritual struggles and growth, we take a brief detour now to address some relevant questions and criticisms that have been raised about measures of self-reported growth following difficult life situations.

How Much Faith Should We Put in Self-Reports of Growth?

Several researchers and theorists have voiced concerns about the validity of measures that assess whether people feel they have grown through their times of stress. Although this literature does not generally focus on spiritual struggles or spirituality more broadly, for that matter, it remains relevant to our interest here. The fundamental question is whether the chief method for assessing growth— perceptions of positive change when looking back on oneself following a stressful event—reflects actual growth or something else. What could that "something else" be? Several alternative explanations have been offered. Self-reports of growth could be

- Efforts to bolster self-worth by deprecating who the person was prior to the stressor, and highlighting the progress the individual has made since the hard time (McFarland & Alvaro, 2000).
- Self-deceptive defense mechanisms involving denial and wishful thinking designed to minimize the darkness of the trauma and place it in the brighter light of growth, thereby avoiding the confrontation with real pain and problems (Maercker & Zoellner, 2004).
- Ways of actively coping with stress through positive interpretations that make meaning of the difficult period (Jayawickreme & Blackie, 2014).
- Expressions of a cultural script that leads people to believe that "good things do come from traumatic events" (Linley & Joseph, 2004, p. 19).

Each of these explanations casts doubt on whether self-reports of growth measure the actual changes that may unfold before and after periods of strain and struggle. In support of this critical perspective, a few empirical studies have shown that measures of growth, such as the PTGI, are not consistently related to actual growth and change following a trauma or stressor. For instance, in a longitudinal study, Park and Fenster (2004) found that actual changes in the worldview of college students did not predict their reports of posttraumatic growth. According to another longitudinal study of undergraduates, scores on the PTGI were not generally related to actual changes experienced by students in specific domains of life, though the PTGI was predictive of actual changes across all of the domains as a whole and increases in religious commitment (Frazier et al., 2009). In one study more directly related to spirituality, Trevino, Naik, and Moye (2016) followed a sample of adult military veteran cancer survivors over 18 months postcancer diagnosis and found that more perceived growth was associated with perceived changes in religious or spiritual beliefs but not actual changes in these beliefs.

In short, important questions have been broached about the validity of self-reports of growth. However, significant counterarguments have also been generated in response to these concerns and a body of empirical evidence has emerged that offers some support for the validity of these self-reports. We simply highlight these counterarguments and studies below:

- In contrast to the argument that self-reports of posttraumatic growth are a form of self-deception, these perceptions have been corroborated by the perspectives of significant others, including family members, close friends, and partners (Park, Cohen, & Murch, 1996; Shakespeare-Finch & Enders, 2008).

- Contrary to the argument that self-reports of growth are efforts to protect self-image and avoid distress, measures of posttraumatic growth have not been generally associated with the tendency to present the self in a socially desirable way (Calhoun & Tedeschi, 2004), nor with lower levels of anxiety and distress (Helgeson, Reynolds, & Tomich, 2006). Commenting on their own experiences with bereaved parents, Calhoun and Tedeschi describe how they are struck "by the raw honesty of many of these parents who are unable to muster attempts at impression management in the midst of their grief. We see them as people who are usually looking at themselves and their world with the blinders off. They may be less prone to cognitive bias" (p. 94).

- In contrast to the suggestion that self-reports of growth are dysfunctional defense mechanisms, longitudinal studies have shown that reports of posttraumatic benefits and growth predict better mental health and physical health outcomes, such as less risk of developing PTSD (McMillen et al., 1997), lower risk of heart attacks and better physical health among patients who suffered a heart attack (Affleck, Tennen, Croog, & Levine, 1987), and less psychological distress among family members coping with the loss of a loved one (Davis, Nolen-Hoeksema, & Larson, 1998).

- Contrary to the assertion that self-reports of growth are not associated with actual changes, several studies have linked perceptions of posttraumatic growth to real increases in personal resources and a positive state of mind (Park & Fenster, 2004); more intrinsic goals among patients with cancer (Ransom, Sheldon, & Jacobson, 2008); and greater optimism, positive affect, and social support (Park et al., 1996). In the only study as yet to focus on reports of spiritual growth and actual changes in spirituality, Haugen (2011) found that perceptions of greater spiritual growth following a stressor were associated with several actual religious and spiritual changes, including higher levels of salience, participation, integration, and belief–behavior congruence in the spiritual realm.

How do we reconcile the critiques of self-reports of posttraumatic growth with the counterarguments? Perhaps there is a grain of truth to each point of view. Reports of growth following stressful life experiences may be, in part, efforts to protect oneself from pain, bolster self-image, and cope in ways that make meaning out of a difficult time. These same reports may also be, in part, indicators of real change, noticeable by others, and predictive of other positive changes over time. Thus, perceptions of growth may be both coping efforts and coping results (Maercker & Zollner, 2004). More studies are needed to clarify the ties between reports of growth and actual growth. Challenging as they are to implement, studies that follow people over a longer period of time are also needed because some research as well as clinical experience suggests that it takes time for growth to fully emerge following difficult life situations, perhaps months and years rather than days and weeks (e.g., Helgeson et al., 2006; Richards, Acree, & Folkman, 1999). Reflecting on their interviews with struggling college students, Rockenbach et al. (2012) noted, "The 'bright side' of spiritual struggle did not typically materialize in the moment of the struggle, but through individual efforts to reflect on and make meaning of the struggle in retrospect" (p. 69).

We believe there is sufficient evidence in support of the validity of self-reports of stress-related growth that they should be taken seriously. There is one final reason we believe these reports deserve attention: They are clinically meaningful. People seek out help, often because their life story has been disrupted or no longer makes sense to them. Part of the job of psychotherapy is to help people reconstruct their narrative to one that holds more meaning and promise. Growth following life stressors is a reflection of a story in the process of reconstruction. As Pals and McAdams (2004) put it, "Posttraumatic growth may be best understood as a process of constructing a narrative understanding of how the self has been positively transformed by the traumatic event and then integrating this transformed sense of self into the identity-defining life story" (p. 65). Facilitating stress and struggle-related growth in the process of therapy can then be understood as a key clinical task.

We return now to our central focus: empirical studies of spiritual struggles and growth.

Studies of the Connection between Spiritual Struggles and Reports of Growth

If spiritual struggles do, in fact, lead to growth, then it would be reasonable to expect that those who encounter spiritual struggles to a greater extent will also experience more growth. Several studies have addressed this question, but the results are not crystal clear.

Higher levels of spiritual struggle have been associated with stress-related growth in several investigations. In one set of studies, spiritual struggles were tied to reports of more growth in three samples: college students facing various life stressors, older adults who had been hospitalized for physical illnesses, and people who lived close to the site of the Oklahoma City bombing (Pargament, Smith, et al., 1998). Spiritual struggles were associated with greater spiritual fortitude through adversity in an adult community sample (Van Tongeren, Aten, et al., 2019). In a sample of Swiss churchgoers dealing with stressful life events, spiritual struggles were linked with higher levels of stress-related growth (Winter et al., 2009). Zeligman, Majuta, and Shannonhouse (2020) studied a group of drought survivors from Botswana and found that spiritual struggles were predictive of posttraumatic growth. In a prospective study of college students dealing with the 9/11 terrorist attacks, spiritual struggles shortly after the tragedy predicted more stress-related growth 3 months later (Ai, Tice, Lemieux, & Huang, 2011). Similarly, Gall, Charbonneau, and Florack (2011), working with a sample of patients with breast cancer before they were diagnosed and 24-months post-surgery, found that higher levels of spiritual discontent prior to the diagnosis were predictive of more posttraumatic growth 2 years later.

On the other hand, in some instances, researchers have found that spiritual struggles are tied to significantly *lower* rather than higher levels of growth following life stress and struggle. These include studies of veterans of the Iraq and Afghanistan wars (Park, Smith, et al., 2017), college students over a 3-year period (Bryant & Astin, 2008), parents of children with autism (Tarakeshwar & Pargament, 2001), and Hindu caregivers in India (Thombre, Sherman, & Simonton, 2010). In a longitudinal study of military veterans, higher levels of spiritual struggle were predictive of struggle-related spiritual decline (Wilt, Pargament, Exline, Barrera, & Teng, 2019).

Complicating matters further, several investigations yielded mixed findings, with signs of both pain and gain linked to spiritual struggles. In one study of college students, people who experienced more severe struggles reported significantly more struggle-related secular growth *and* significantly less struggle-related spiritual growth (Desai & Pargament, 2015). Similarly, Mussett (2012) worked with parents of children with Down syndrome and found that those who recalled higher levels of spiritual struggles at the time their child was diagnosed reported both greater posttraumatic growth and greater spiritual decline. Higher levels of spiritual struggles have also been tied to both posttraumatic growth *and* distress (e.g., anxiety, depression, distress) in studies of cancer survivors (Trevino, Archambault, Schuster, Richardson, & Moye, 2012), college undergraduates facing a variety of traumatic events (Gerber, Boals, & Schuettler, 2011), and patients in medical rehabilitation during hospitalization and at discharge (Magyar-Russell et al., 2013).

And it is important to note that no significant ties between spiritual struggles and spiritual and secular growth have been reported in several instances, such as studies of sexual assault survivors (Ahrens et al., 2010), bereaved undergraduates (Lord & Gramling, 2014), survivors of Hurricane Katrina (Chan & Rhodes, 2013), military veterans (Wilt, Pargament, et al., 2019), survivors of cancer (Park & Cho, 2017), and Muslims who lost their children as a result of traffic accidents (Abu-Raiya & Sulleiman, 2020).

How do we make sense of these inconsistent findings? If we average across all of these positive, negative, mixed, and null results, we might conclude that higher levels of spiritual struggles are simply unrelated to reports of more growth. This is just the conclusion Ano and Vasconcelles (2005) reached through their meta-analysis of 16 studies on this topic: Overall, spiritual struggles were unrelated to indicators of positive adjustment, including growth. But to discount all of the positive, negative, and mixed findings might be premature. Perhaps we need richer measures of growth that capture this important process in more subtle and complex ways. Perhaps, as we noted above, it takes more time than these studies have allowed for people to realize significant change through their struggles. Or perhaps these inconsistent findings accurately reflect a more complex reality: that spiritual struggles have the potential to foster and/or impede growth.

CONCLUSIONS

Do spiritual struggles lead to growth? This is the seemingly simple question we raised to start this chapter. As we delved into it more deeply, however, we found that the answer may not be so simple. To review what we learned:

• According to psychological perspectives, spiritual struggles can indeed be a source of growth and positive change.

• Stories from the world's great religious traditions, as well as those of ordinary people today, provide us with many rich descriptive accounts of growth through spiritual struggles.

• Empirical studies suggest the need for a more nuanced answer to the question of whether spiritual struggles lead to growth. Surveys that ask people about their perceived growth show that many feel they have grown through their spiritual struggles. Not everyone, though—we can find others who do not share the same feeling. In addition, higher levels of spiritual struggles are not consistently tied to growth and, in fact, appear to be associated with perceptions of decline in some cases.

A definitive answer to the question of whether spiritual struggles lead to growth awaits further research. We need studies that follow people over a longer period of time to see whether it takes months or even years for growth to emerge following spiritual struggles. We need to think about and measure growth in ways that integrate positivity with the bittersweet, poignant, and melancholy nature of life. We also need to study whether spiritual struggles result in not only perceived change but also actual change in significance and the individual's orientation to life. What does seem safe to conclude at this point is that while spiritual struggles may lead to growth, growth is not an inevitable result of spiritual struggles. The encounter with spiritual struggles offers a possibility, not a guarantee of positive change and transformation.

And how do we reconcile the findings from this chapter on the brighter side of spiritual struggles with the findings on the darker side of struggles from the previous chapter? There we saw that spiritual struggles are robustly associated with signs of distress, disorientation, and decline. This is not to say that everyone who struggles spiritually inevitably declines. Nevertheless, this research underscores how profoundly disruptive spiritual struggles can be to our most fundamental values, beliefs, practices, and relationships. True, growth may eventually emerge out of spiritual struggle but the process itself may be quite painful, even destructive, and not everyone necessarily realizes positive change. To illustrate the point in the context of a major life stressor, Lehman, Wortman, and Williams (1987) conducted a study of parents who had lost a child 4–7 years earlier. While 74% reported at least one positive life change (most often greater self-confidence and enjoying the present) over that time, in comparison to a group of nonbereaved parents, those who had lost a child showed significantly more signs of depression, hostility, phobic anxiety, and greater likelihood of divorce. Eighty percent reported that they could make no meaning out of the loss and 47% indicated that they had been dealing with suicidality and drug abuse. With respect to spiritual struggles more specifically, if growth takes place, it may also evolve out of a context of pain. In surveys of people who struggle spiritually, reports of perceived growth appear to go hand in hand with descriptions of distress and decline for at least some individuals. As we noted earlier, Desai and Pargament (2015) found that 29% of college students who were struggling spiritually indicated that they had *both* grown and declined as a result of their conflicts. Thus, it may be most accurate to speak of spiritual struggles in terms of what Bryant (2011) described as their "interlocking promise and pain" (p. 456).

These findings should caution practitioners against sentimentalizing spiritual struggles. Ours is a "culture of cheerfulness" (cf. Parrott, 2014), replete with the common folk wisdom that suffering builds character, that broken bones heal more strongly, and that out of darkness comes light. This narrative can offer powerful sources of inspiration and hope to those in pain, but it can also be misused when applied to spiritual struggles and other sources of strain, especially when growth becomes a yardstick by which to judge the progress of strugglers. Speaking to these dangers with respect to people who have experienced trauma, Wortman (2004) says:

> Survivors often suffer at the hands of others who expect them to be recovered from their trauma or loss rather quickly. . . . If outsiders believe that growth is prevalent, this can become a new standard that survivors' progress is measured against. Such a standard may lead to negative judgments toward those who do not show personal growth, making them feel like coping failures. (p. 89)

In working with spiritual strugglers then, it is important to acknowledge and appreciate the very real pain as well as the potential for both growth and decline that accompany the experience.

We are left then with a few important practical questions: What determines the trajectory of spiritual struggles? How is it that some people experience positive transformation and growth while others head downhill? Having a spiritual struggle in and of itself, we believe, may be less important for growth and decline than how people come to terms with that struggle. If that is the case, then what are the ingredients that lead to growth and/or decline in the encounter with spiritual struggles?

In the next chapter, we turn to these vital questions, so critical to any practical effort to help people in their times of spiritual struggle.

CHAPTER 6

What Shapes the Outcomes of Spiritual Struggles?

For many people, spiritual struggles signal the loss of their spiritual map or compass. Unable to find their bearings, people who struggle spiritually experience a sense of disorientation in their search for whatever holds significance to them. However, spiritual struggles indicate more than loss and disorientation: they also signal that an effort is underway to reorient, to regain or transform one's life orientation and sense of significance. There is no guarantee of immediate or even long-term success through this reorientation process. As we learned in Chapter 4, spiritual struggles can lead to serious decline—psychological, social, physical, and spiritual. However, we also saw in the prior chapter that some people describe powerful life-changing awakening, transformation, and growth through their spiritual struggles.

Spiritual struggles can be pivotal, even momentous, times in life, with the power to direct the individual's journey in a positive or negative direction. What determines whether spiritual struggles lead to growth, decline, or to some degree both? In this chapter, we focus on this question. As with other important psychological questions, the answer here is not simple; no single value, trait, attitude, or skill holds the key to whether struggles lead to growth or decline. Instead, the trajectory of spiritual struggles depends on the dynamic interplay among a host of factors that define the search for significance: psychological, social, physical, spiritual, situational, and cultural. The extent to which people are whole or broken, we believe, holds an important key to the trajectory of spiritual struggles. Wholeness, as we define it, has to do with how well we put the bits and pieces of our lives together. At our best, we are able to pull these disparate ingredients of our lives into a relatively unified, well-integrated whole. At our worst, we are unable to do so and instead experience brokenness and dis-integration. Research on wholeness is only just beginning to emerge (e.g., Hart, Pargament, Grubbs, Exline, & Wilt, 2020), but we believe thinking about spiritual struggles in the context of wholeness and brokenness will prove quite helpful to practitioners in their day-to-day efforts to foster growth among their clients who are struggling spiritually. We begin this chapter by discussing the meaning of wholeness and brokenness.

Maria's world fell apart when she was only 14 years old. Kidnapped from her family and village in South America, she was taken to a large city and forced into prostitution. After 7 years, she escaped and made her way to the United States. Her "nightmare years" were marked by constant fear, struggle, and disorientation. Why hadn't someone tried to rescue her? What had she done to deserve this pain? Where was God in all of her suffering? Who had she become? How could she continue to live? The questions were overwhelming. To cope, Maria tried to disconnect from the intense pain and confusion surrounding her trauma and struggles, living day-to-day by being there but not really being there.

Maria's therapist learned that Maria's personality had fragmented during her traumatic experience. She had five alters: a rageful persona, a suicidal persona, a grieving persona, an intellectual persona, and a child-like persona. Each alter expressed an important aspect of her identity, but none of the personas was able to communicate directly with the others. The therapist became the point of connection.

Much of the initial work in therapy focused on helping Maria stay safe and alive—no insignificant task given the power of her emotions and the active threat she represented to herself. Gradually, Maria was able to develop greater self-control and the focus of therapy shifted to helping her move to greater wholeness. This was another tremendous challenge, for Maria was disconnected in multiple ways: from her family, her village, her faith, her culture, and from the multiple personas within herself. "I'm just a broken piece of pottery," she often said. Over the course of 20 years of therapy, Maria was able to put some pieces of her life back together. She went to school and became a teacher to visually impaired children. She reached out to other survivors of rape and prostitution and helped form a spiritual center for women who were recovering from sexual abuse and trauma. Though Maria was unable to achieve the degree of integration she had hoped for, she was able to reach a truce among her conflicting personas, and she now experiences some measure of inner peace.

Few people encounter experiences as shattering as those of Maria, but her case offers a dramatic illustration of a dynamic common to human development and common to the work of psychotherapy: the movement from brokenness to greater wholeness in the search for significance. In their own distinctive ways, various models of psychotherapy share an interest in addressing areas of human disconnection and brokenness, and fostering greater integration and wholeness. It may take the form of building greater insight into hidden aspects of oneself (psychoanalysis), fostering more reality-based cognitions and emotional self-regulation (CBT), developing greater self-compassion and acceptance (client-centered therapy), or repairing relational conflicts and rifts through healthier patterns of communication (marital and family therapy).

Religious and spiritual writings, both classical and contemporary, are especially concerned with issues of brokenness and wholeness (see Pargament, Wong, & Exline, 2016). The term *holy* itself derives from the Old English word *hurlig,* meaning wholeness, health, and happiness (New World Encyclopedia, 2008). Fundamental to the world's religious traditions is the notion that people are in some ways broken. As a remedy to this condition, each tradition encourages its adherents to follow a pathway toward greater wholeness. For example, according to the Jewish mystical account of creation, God withdrew from the infinite realm to form a finite vessel and then injected a ray of divine light into this space (Frankel, 2005). However, unable to fully hold this light, the vessel shattered. Thus, brokenness was a defining quality of the universe from its very beginnings. Humans are then called upon to bring wholeness and healing back to a fragmented world through acts of compassion and justice.

According to classical Christian thought, Adam and Eve brought sin and death into the world when they ate from the fruit of the tree that had been divinely forbidden. This transgression resulted in the loss of their unrestricted access to God (Smith, 1958). Through the sacrifice of Jesus Christ on the cross, however, the breach between humankind and the divine was repaired, and redemption was offered to all those who accept Jesus as savior.

Nontheistic religions also recommend pathways to achieve greater wholeness. Within Buddhism, suffering is understood as basic to the human condition, a natural state of imperfection or brokenness. According to the Mahayana tradition, the Buddha provided a solution to suffering through wholesome ways of action that move individuals along the path toward enlightenment, an ideal state of completeness (Bhikkhu, 1985).

Psychologists of religion and spirituality have also stressed the movement from brokenness to wholeness as an essential developmental task. One of the founders of the field, William James (1902), saw the unification of the divided self—the material self, the social self, the spiritual self, and pure ego—as central to the achievement of human functioning at its best. In their seminal book, Kurtz and Ketcham (1992) articulated a "spirituality of imperfection" that rests on the assumption of "the basic and inherent flaws of being human" (p. 2). And yet, they argue, this isn't the full story; people are also motivated to seek out a larger wholeness in spite of the fact that perfection is never fully attainable: "For to be human is to be incomplete, yet yearn for completion; it is to be uncertain, yet long for certainty; to be imperfect, yet long for perfection; to be broken, yet crave wholeness" (p. 19). Approaching the topic of wholeness and brokenness from a somewhat different vantage point, Palmer (2004) maintains that each of us contains an inner wholeness. Internal and external constraints, however, limit our ability to attain this wholeness. The end result is the pain of alienation from other people and from our authentic selves. The developmental challenge then becomes one of overcoming this disconnection by locating and cultivating one's true spirit. In his theory of faith development, Fowler (1981) also proposes a shift over the lifespan toward greater integration and wholeness. He describes the movement from undifferentiated, literal, and socially conventional stages of faith to more individually reflective and ultimately universalizing stages that place the emphasis on inclusive visions of humanity.

In spite of these important contributions, the concepts of wholeness and brokenness are not often well articulated in psychological and spiritual writings. We believe there may be great value in moving these constructs from the background to the foreground of our thinking and practice. In this chapter, we take a step in that direction in the context of spiritual struggles and their end results. More specifically, we turn to some ingredients of wholeness and brokenness as they affect whether the trajectory of spiritual struggles leads to growth or decline. We pay special attention to the spiritual dimension of these ingredients. It may seem counterintuitive that spirituality could be a source of wholeness and growth to people dealing with spiritual struggles, but it is important to keep in mind that spiritual struggles are not equivalent to spiritual disengagement or disconnection. Moreover, struggles may occur in one area of spirituality and leave other aspects of spiritual life unaffected. Thus, our discussion highlights the double-edged nature of spirituality: It may contribute to the ingredients of wholeness and growth, and/or to brokenness and decline. We now consider three interrelated dimensions of wholeness and brokenness in relation to spiritual struggles: breadth and depth, life affirmation, and cohesiveness.

BREADTH AND DEPTH

Greater wholeness is marked in part by the capacity to see and approach life in its fullness. This is, however, no easy task. "Reality," Karff (2015) writes, "is too complex to be caught in the net of one symbolic language system" (p. 284). It requires breadth and depth of language, vision, and skill. What goes into breadth and depth? First, the broader and deeper approach to life rests on access to a variety of living tools and resources that enable people to deal with the full range of life's challenges. A second related element of breadth and depth is the ability to see and accept the darker as well as the lighter sides of life. Third, breadth and depth rest on the recognition that life can be viewed from multiple vantage points, that appearances can indeed be deceiving, and that beneath the surface of human experience lie dimensions that make life deeper, richer, and at times, more complicated. Let's take a closer look at these factors.

Access to a Variety of Resources and Tools for Living

Philosopher Abraham Kaplan (1964) once wrote, "Give a small boy a hammer and he will find that everything he encounters needs pounding" (p. 28). This tendency may apply not only to small children but also to all of us who rely on the implements we have in our toolbox to fix the problems we encounter, whether or not they are best suited to the task at hand. We might think about this very human tendency as an example of the problem of overgeneralization mentioned in Chapter 3—that is, the application of a familiar but narrow set of resources that leaves the individual unprepared to meet the demands raised by his or her evolving challenges. For example, the relentless self-criticism that has helped a military officer rise in the ranks may be of no help when she faces the uncontrollable chaos of combat and can find no compassion or forgiveness for herself. The hugs and kisses, constant presence, and day-to-day guidance from parents that worked so well in raising a young child no longer do the trick when the child enters adolescence and needs a different style of parenting.

The solution to the problem of overrelying on a few instruments is to become equipped with a full range of tools for living—diverse ways of thinking, behaving, feeling, and interrelating—that can be accessed to realize a significant set of purposes. In times of spiritual struggle, it may be especially important to be able to think about problems from different points of view, generate a variety of possible solutions, access a wide repertoire of adaptive skills, experience a multitude of feelings, and seek out a configuration of life-enriching purposes (e.g., Szcześniak, Kroplewski, & Szałachowski, 2020).

Of course, no single person can be the repository of all possible skills, resources, and qualities. We are, after all, only human, and each of us is faced with choices about how to allocate our finite resources and how to define ourselves and our ultimate sources of significance. If we avoid these hard choices and, instead, try to master every tool for living, we are bound to be frustrated. In this vein, Sampson (1977) critiqued the movement toward "self-contained individualism" in the United States, arguing that ultimately those "who hope to be entire unto themselves" are likely to be dissatisfied and disconnected from one another (p. 770). Better, he maintained, to recognize our incompleteness and become part of a larger network in which people help support, sustain, and complete one another. God or other representations of the sacred can be perceived as part of that network for those who are more spiritually minded. Having access to a variety of tools for living doesn't mean the individual must own each of these tools him- or herself. Tools can be borrowed and shared as well.

Without enough instruments in our toolbox (self-crafted, bought, or borrowed), without sufficient breadth in our orientation to life and our reasons for living, we may be crippled in our efforts to resolve challenging situations, including spiritual struggles. Maria, the survivor of sexual trauma who had fragmented into multiple personalities, was unable to function effectively for much of her life because each of her personas lacked the tools and resources to stand on its own for very long: her rageful persona had no access to positive emotions; her grieving persona was devoid of any hope that might have sustained her; and her intellectual persona was unable to draw on potentially guiding emotions.

Goodman, Rubinstein, Alexander, and Luborsky (1991) conducted a study that illustrates the consequences that may follow from a limited set of tools and resources. In their clinical interactions with older women who had lost an adult child, the researchers observed that the older Jewish mothers appeared to be having a particularly difficult time coping with their loss. Interviews and surveys of the women seemed to confirm their clinical observations. Compared to the non-Jewish mothers, the Jewish mothers showed significantly lower levels of well-being and higher levels of depression and loneliness. The Jewish mothers seemed to be more "stuck" in loss and grief. The researchers wondered why this might be the case and came to the conclusion that the difference might have to do with the more exclusive focus of the Jewish mothers on the well-being of their children, a source of significance and meaning supported and encouraged by not only the mothers but also by Jewish culture as a whole. In contrast, the authors noted, the non-Jewish mothers appeared to have a more multifaceted sense of significance. As terribly painful as the loss of their adult child was, they were able to turn to other sources of purpose and satisfaction to sustain themselves in their time of grief. In short, the Jewish mothers were more vulnerable to problems not because of their devotion to their children but because of the exclusiveness of their devotion.

As this example suggests, a lack of breadth can extend to the spiritual realm. Many people center their spirituality on a small number of beliefs and rituals that have been selectively drawn from a much larger religious body of thought and practice (Nielsen, Johnson, & Ellis, 2001). The spiritual narrowness that results can take many specific forms. One example involves a spirituality that confers humanity only upon those who share the same identity, beliefs, practices, and values. In this vein, Hall, Matz, and Wood (2010) conducted a meta-analysis of studies showing that beliefs in the exclusive truth of one's own religion are tied to higher levels of right-wing authoritarianism that are linked, in turn, to more prejudice toward outgroups, including sexual minorities, African Americans, Jews, and Muslims. Narrowness can also take the form of regular religious practices that fail to touch the heart or encourage a sense of sacredness. Krause, Pargament, Hill, and Ironson (2020) conducted a study relevant to this point. They asked participants from a large-scale community study to identify themselves as either religious and spiritual, religious but not spiritual, not religious but spiritual, or not religious and not spiritual. They found that, in comparison to the other three groups, the religious but not spiritual group was at much greater risk for poorer self-rated health, depression, and alcohol use in response to lifetime trauma. The religious but not spiritual group may have been more vulnerable to problems because their religious involvement was not accompanied by a sense of spiritual connection.

The individual's social network can also be constricted in its capacity to offer support in spiritual strugglers. In a study of hospitalized patients who indicated spiritual struggles, Ellis, Thomlinson, Gemmill, and Harris (2013) found that only one-third received some kind of spiritual or psychological care from family members, congregation members, spiritual leader, or chaplain. Commenting on this breakdown in social support, Marty (1983) writes:

> [Many potential caregivers] simply run out of the ability to be spontaneous about identifying with someone else, to take into themselves the agony of nerves exposed, the plotlessness of pain that never stops. They have their own coffee pots to put on, their own paychecks to draw, their own bright moments to celebrate. (p. 128)

Each of these signs of spiritual narrowness may hamper the person's ability to resolve and grow from spiritual struggles. One particular challenge to achieving a life of breadth deserves some extra attention.

The Ability to See and Accept the Darker Side of Life

None of us goes through life unscathed. Pain, suffering, imperfection, frailty, and struggle are all part of the human condition. Even with access to the best of health care, the scrupulous avoidance of all bad habits, and the comfort of living in a secure nest of the most loving relationships, the reality is we will still age; encounter accidents, loss, and illness; and eventually die. Most recently, we have come face-to-face with this reality in the form of the COVID-19 pandemic. What makes these dark, existential truths especially problematic, many writers agree, is the unwillingness to face them. That reluctance can be encouraged by social institutions, families, and friends. Religious traditions can play a part in fostering the avoidance of the dark side of life. "The verdict is unanimous," Barbara Brown Taylor (2014) writes, "Darkness in the Bible . . . is bad news. In the first testament, light stands for life and darkness for death. . . . In the second testament, light stands for knowledge and darkness for ignorance" (p. 43). Taylor notes that her exposure to what she called "the full solar version" of faith taught her to steer clear of the dark places: the smoky nightclubs, the dark bedrooms, the hidden back alleys, the dim jail cells.

By avoiding the dark side, however, many people may be left with one particularly common form of spiritual narrowness, a bright and sunny spiritual orientation that cannot address the challenges raised by times of upheaval, turmoil, and loss. For example, those who see God as a "heavenly bosom" (cf. Phillips, 1997)—a being who assures that they will never encounter undeserved suffering—may end up surprised, unprepared, and unsupported when they do face terrible loss. That spiritual orientation may extend to religious networks of support that can offer only expressions of a "summer spirituality" (cf. Marty, 1983) to those going through their "wintry" seasons of life. As a result, Beck (2007) notes, "Winter experience is marginalized and left without a voice" (p. 75). In this vein, psychologist and theologian Carrie Doehring (personal communication, April 12, 2014) described a vigil service she attended for the 12 people killed in the 2012 Aurora Theater shooting. Many of the religious leaders offered prayers invoking the theme of resurrection and encouraging the survivors to move toward healing. Only a few of the leaders, however, offered what was also needed by survivors: a period of lament in which they could give voice to their suffering and reflect on the precariousness and darkness that are also part of life. Even further, expressions of spiritual struggle can be met with more explicitly critical reactions. In a study of adults who had negative feelings toward God following a life stressor, among those who had shared their feelings with others, about half reported some kind of unsupportive response, such as statements that it is wrong to feel negatively toward God or statements that made them feel guilty, judged, or ashamed (Exline & Grubbs, 2011). These kinds of critical responses were associated with greater odds that people would try to suppress their struggles with the divine, along with greater difficulty resolving their anger toward God, a greater chance of exiting the relationship with God, and higher levels of substance use.

The inability to accept pain and struggle comes at a cost. According to acceptance and commitment therapy (ACT), avoiding unpleasant experience consumes needed energy and prevents the individual from developing the confidence and skills that lead to the realization of personal goals (Hayes, Strosahl, & Wilson, 2016). Avoidance can become a habit resulting in an increasingly constricted and fear-based existence. This is the conclusion Trappist monk Thomas Merton (1948) reached as a result of his struggles in witnessing the death of his much-loved father:

> Indeed, the truth that many people never understand, until it is too late, is that the more you try to avoid suffering, the more you suffer, because smaller and more insignificant things begin to torture you, in proportion to your fear of being hurt. The one who does most to avoid suffering is, in the end, the one who suffers the most. (p. 91)

The costs of the avoidance of suffering and struggles can extend to the spiritual realm. Once again we can turn to William James (1902), who commented on the limits of a "healthy-minded" perspective that does not acknowledge the darker side of life:

> There is no doubt that a healthy-mindedness is inadequate as a philosophical doctrine, because the evil facts which it refuses positively to account for are a genuine portion of reality; and they may after all be the best key to life's significance, and possibly the only openers of our eyes to the deepest levels of truth. (p. 160)

Taylor (2014) speaks to the same point in more explicitly religious terms. Although the religious traditions often depict darkness in terms of sin and ignorance, that is not the full picture. Darkness is also a place where people can encounter God: Abraham was promised more descendants than the stars in the night. Paul experienced conversion after he lost his sight. By turning away from darkness, Taylor concludes, people run away from an opportunity to encounter God.

Empirical research has pointed to the psychological, social, and physical costs of the avoidance of negative inner experiences (see Ruiz, 2010, for a review). These findings appear to apply to the experience of spiritual struggles as well. Working with a sample of adults, Dworsky, Pargament, Wong, and Exline (2016) found that higher levels of experiential avoidance of spiritual struggles were associated with greater depression, anxiety, somatic symptoms, and difficulty regulating emotions. These effects were even stronger for people who reported higher levels of spiritual struggles.

Struggles and suffering may be inevitable, but the added pain that comes from efforts to avoid these experiences is not. According to one quote often attributed to psychiatrist R. D. Laing: "There is a great deal of pain in life and perhaps the only pain that can be avoided is the pain that comes from trying to avoid pain" (Binau, 2007, p. 29). The mental health challenge is finding a way to "avoid the avoidance" by gently accepting life's heartaches as part of being human without becoming overwhelmed by the experience of darkness, for that experience is also a key to wholeness (Frankel, 2005). Taylor (2014) comes to a similar conclusion in her book *Learning to Walk in the Dark*: "I have learned things in the dark that I could never have learned in the light, things that have saved my life over and over again, so that there is really only one logical conclusion. I need darkness as much as I need light" (p. 5).

The Ability to See Beneath the Surface

We live in a multilayered world made up of strata that we do not fully apprehend. On the crust of the planet, we walk while paying no mind to the dynamic forces operating miles beneath our feet in the Earth's mantle, outer core, and inner core. On water, we drift, often unaware of the rich life teeming beneath the tides and turbulence at the surface. In the air, we process a marvelous world of sight and sound while remaining blind and deaf to the continuously unfolding waves of light and sound that fall outside of our perceptual range. We live in a psychological world of thought and feeling not fully aware of the motivations and yearnings that lie within our unconscious selves. And yet, we also have the capacity to see more deeply, to look beneath the surface, and experience life in more of its fullness, richness, and complexity. This capacity may be especially important in periods of struggle.

What does it mean to see beneath the surface? It means that things are not necessarily what they appear to be, that there may be a greater reality underlying our usual sense of reality (Yaden et al., 2017). When we see beneath the surface, we take issue with popular phrases, such as "That's all there is to it" or "It is what it is." Instead, a closer look reveals that sometimes there's more to "it" than meets the eye—sometimes it *isn't* what it is.

Seeing beneath the surface means looking beyond the foreground of a picture to view it in depth. The remarkable cellist Yo-Yo Ma (2016) illustrates this point in an interview in which he describes the richness that can be experienced in something as seemingly simple as the interval between two notes of music:

> Well, how do you get from A to B? Is it a smooth transfer? . . . Or do you have to mentally and effortfully reach to go from one note to another? Could the next note be part of the first note? Or could the next note be a different universe? Have you just crossed into some amazing boundary, and suddenly the second note is a revelation?

Yo-Yo Ma continually explores the deeper possibilities and potentials that lie beneath the most basic of musical expressions.

Seeing beneath the surface rests on the skill of taking a step back and reflecting on the thoughts, feelings, and experiences of oneself and others with appreciation for their depth. Reflectiveness or "mentalization," as Jon Allen (2013) describes it, is the capacity to know one's own mind; the mind of others; the larger world; one's past, present, and future; and, for some, a transcendent reality. Reflectiveness involves not only rational processing, analysis, and reasoning but also simple awareness, mindfulness, and intuitiveness. To be able to reflect provides a safeguard against getting overly caught up in experience and rushing to overly simple solutions—it is essential to regulating emotions, thoughts, behaviors, and relationships. More generally, reflectiveness is one of the keys to creating a significant life purpose and to enacting and, at times, correcting the plan that allows people to realize their dreams. Unable to reflect, it is easy to get lost in the search for significance, for the individual is essentially flying blindly, incapable of reading all of the indicators on the instrument panel that offer essential guidance. It follows that a lack of reflectiveness increases the chances of serious problems among spiritual strugglers. People who are more psychologically minded, on the other hand, may be better able to put their spiritual struggles into a larger growth-enhancing perspective.

Seeing beneath the surface also means sensitivity to the world of multiple perspectives and meanings—to recognize that chicken soup may be good for you but not so good from the chicken's point of view, as Frankel (2005) put it. Many theories of growth and development emphasize the importance of the progression from simple to more complex differentiated ways of viewing the world and oneself (e.g., Calhoun & Tedeschi, 2004; Loevinger, 1976). This deepening and broadening of perspectives emerges as a key theme in a set of qualitative studies of Israelis who described the spiritual change they experienced outside of religious institutions (Russo-Netzer & Mayseless, 2014). One 44-year-old woman said:

> I feel that I have learned on this path that I am not one being but that there are all sorts of voices, all sorts of parts of me, that I can contain them all, and one of them is me . . . it's an expansion of consciousness, of my acceptance of myself and everything, expansion of my experience, of my ability to experience different experiences, different people . . . it's like your vision opens up. You can see more, you experience more, accept more, and contain more. (p. 28)

Spirituality and the Ability to See Beneath the Surface

The ability to see beneath the surface receives special emphasis within the religious and spiritual world; there we find no shortage of references to spirituality as a way of "seeing" (Wong & Pargament, 2017). In many renderings, the Buddha is shown having a third eye between his brows. Other religious traditions, such as Taoism, Hinduism, and New Age spirituality, also make mention of a third or "divine" eye. Alan Watts (2004) once said that "Zen is spiritual ophthalmology." And the language of sight and vision are prominent within Islam and Sufi mysticism in particular (Nicholson, 1914).

One of the major functions of all religious institutions is to help its people see more deeply. Indeed, the very act of thinking about God may promote deeper self-reflection according to an investigation conducted by Michael Kitchens (2015). In a set of four experimental studies, he primed participants to think about God by having them recall the Ten Commandments or rate various adjectives according to the degree to which they described God. They then completed measures that indicated how well they reflected on their inner thoughts and feelings. In all four studies, compared to those who were primed to think about topics other than God (e.g., friends), participants who were thinking about God reported significantly higher levels of internal reflection. Interestingly, these findings applied to both believers and nonbelievers in God, suggesting that thinking about the divine promotes deeper reflection on personal beliefs and values regardless of personal faith commitments.

Prominent theologians have stressed the importance of being able to go beyond surface appearances and see the world with greater depth, including its mysteries and unknowns. To focus only on the surface is to miss the essence of spirituality. In this vein, Tillich (1957) strongly warned against the dangers of religious literalism. As finite beings, he said, we cannot fully grasp the sacred. Symbols are necessary to reach out to the infinite because they point to something beyond themselves. However, symbols can only hint at what that "something" may be. To treat symbols literally then, Tillich argues, "deprives God of his ultimacy, and, religiously speaking, of his majesty. It draws closer to the level of that which is not ultimate and conditional. . . . Faith, if it takes its symbols literally, becomes idolatrous" (p. 52).

Perhaps most basically, seeing beneath the surface in the spiritual realm involves an ability to perceive the sacred. People can find the sacred in many aspects of life: work, nature, strivings, marriage, sexuality, parenting, close relationships, virtues, special moments in time, and life as a whole (Pargament & Mahoney, 2005; Pomerleau, Pargament, & Mahoney, 2016; Wong & Pargament, 2017). Seen through a sacred lens, life takes on greater dimensionality and depth, as we can hear in the way Chief Seattle of the Squamish Tribe (Smith, 1887) perceives nature:

> Every part of this soil is sacred in the estimation of my people. Every hillside, every valley, every plain and grove, has been hallowed by some sad or happy event in days long vanished. Even the rocks, which seem to be dumb and dead as they swelter in the sun along the silent shore, thrill with memories of stirring events connected with the lives of my people.

As these words suggest, the perception of sacredness elicits deep spiritual emotions—gratitude, awe, uplift, elevation, joy—that can soothe, comfort, and empower. In Chapter 2, we described how the process of seeing more deeply situates life within a larger spiritual context that can be a source of greater meaning and purpose, an identity that links past and future, and enduring connections among people who share in their understanding of the sacred. In support of this point, a recent meta-analysis of 40 studies showed that sanctification of a diverse array of life domains was associated with more positive psychological adjustment and less negative maladjustment (Mahoney, Wong, Pomerleau, & Pargament, 2021).

People who perceive the sacred in their lives may also be better equipped to sustain themselves in times of spiritual struggle. In a national study, Abu-Raiya, Pargament, and Krause (2016) found that people who see life as sacred were better protected from the detrimental effects of spiritual struggles on unhappiness and depression. Wilt, Pargament, and Exline, (2018) focused on the potentially beneficial role of sacred moments in life—that is, moments that are felt to be transcendent, boundless in space and time, and bearers of ultimate truth. The researchers asked a sample of adults to describe a particular spiritual struggle they were experiencing, and then followed up with these participants at five time points over 6 months to assess various outcomes of the struggle. Those who experienced sacred moments more frequently across time generally reported better outcomes of their spiritual struggles, including better struggle resolution, more spiritual growth, and less spiritual decline.

The Depth of Spiritual Commitment

The ability to see the sacred in life may also help people in periods of strain and struggle, in part, by deepening their spiritual commitments. These deeper levels of spiritual commitment, in turn, have been associated with greater well-being in the face of spiritual struggles. For example, among college students who were experiencing spiritual struggles, those who integrated religion and spirituality more fully into their daily lives were more likely to report spiritual growth as a result of their struggles (Desai & Pargament, 2015), less spiritual decline, and more general struggles-related growth (Hart et al., 2020). Similarly, U.S. military veterans who attached higher importance to their religious beliefs reported more spiritual growth through their spiritual struggle at both baseline and 6-month follow-up (Wilt, Pargament, et al., 2019). Among a national sample in the United States, higher levels of religious commitment reduced the strength of the connection of spiritual struggles with depression and unhappiness (Abu-Raiya, Pargament, & Krause, 2016). However, a few other studies have yielded contradictory findings (Ahles, Mezulis, & Hudson, 2016; Ellison, Fang, Flannelly, & Steckler, 2013; Park et al., 2011).

If religious commitment generally helps people work through their spiritual struggles, how do we square this conclusion with some of the findings presented in Chapter 3 showing that higher levels of religious commitment may increase the likelihood of developing spiritual struggles? Recall the study of college undergraduates in which those who described their religious beliefs as more important to them, particularly undergraduates at a Christian university, were more likely to experience spiritual struggles over the following year (Wilt, Hall, et al., 2017). The answer may be that there is truth to both sets of findings. People with a deep spiritual commitment may be more prone to developing spiritual struggles because they are more often engaged in the challenge of integrating the events of their lives, large and small, into their core spiritual values, beliefs, and commitments. Spiritual struggles in this sense go hand in hand with spiritual development for many faithful people. On the other hand, once spiritual struggles have emerged, those with a deeper spiritual commitment may have a stronger set of resources to help them come to terms with their struggles.

Of course, not everyone sees with spiritual depth or manifests a deep spiritual commitment, including those who identify as religious or spiritual. Some use their faith as a form of "spiritual bypass" to avoid or protect themselves from confronting life's deeper meanings, complexities, and paradoxes (Cashwell, Bentley, & Yarborough, 2007). Many others have given little thought to deeper spiritual issues or find it hard to develop or hold on to a spiritual vision in a larger culture that encourages the pursuit of more tangible, material rewards. This may leave them among those with a spirituality Gallup and Lindsay (1999, p. 45) described as "only three inches deep" (p. 45) or living in what Kushner (1989) described even more starkly as "a flat, monochromatic world, a world without color or texture" (p. 205). Without a depth of spirituality to draw from, people may also find it difficult to sustain themselves and grow through times of spiritual struggle.

We turn now to a second ingredient of wholeness.

LIFE AFFIRMATION

Recall the story of Maria. Although her personality had fragmented into several alters—rageful, suicidal, grieving, intellectual, child-like—they had one thing in common: none was able to offer any compassion for herself or hope for her future. Weighed down by the tremendous shame she felt, Maria had been unable to share her story with others and receive the support they might have provided. Spiritual support was also out of the question when she first came to therapy. After all, how could she seek help from a God so intimately wrapped up in her spiritual struggles, so devoid of caring? In short, Maria was unable to find any affirmation in her life, a deficit that made it virtually impossible for her to move forward from her trauma and spiritual struggles. One of the main reasons she persisted in therapy over the years was that her therapist offered her that vital ingredient of compassion and hope she was unable to generate for herself. Therapy also helped her recover a sense of affirmation from others and from the sacred.

Life affirmation (cf. Doehring, 2015) speaks to the degree to which the individual's life is infused with compassion, hope, and support. By affirmation, we are referring to a host of qualities—strength, resources, virtues, competence, capability, benevolence, gratitude, patience, kindness—that color the individual's life orientation and goals. Life affirmation does not mean that suffering, pain, and struggle are minimized or ignored. That would lead only to the myopia that creates problems of its own, as we just noted. Although an affirming perspective does not discount the reality of the darker side of life, it insists that darkness does not have the only word or final say on life; hope in a better tomorrow remains. Doehring (2019) provides a personal and poignant illustration in the way she found some level of healing in the wake of the suicide of her much-loved 27-year-old son, a loss that had triggered deep spiritual struggles. The experience of affirmation, she found, the "embodied sense of being held within a relational web of love," was an essential part of her movement to greater wholeness (p. 241). Affirmation is, in short, another key to wholeness. Without some degree of life affirmation, it is difficult to sustain oneself, especially when spiritual struggles arise.

Support for the power of affirmation can be found in a growing body of theory and research that has focused on those qualities that make for "the good life" or what we call a life of wholeness. This area of study, "positive psychology," rests on the assumptions that life at its best is more than the absence of distress and disorder, that the positive in life is as authentic as the negative, and that building strengths may be as important as addressing weaknesses in helping people through hard times. Better mental health and physical health (even longer life in some instances) have been tied to a host of indicators of positivity: social support, purpose, optimism, courage, empathy, joy, humility, gratitude, forgiveness, love, and compassion, to name just a few (see Snyder, Lopez, Edwards, & Margues, 2021, for reviews).

Some of the most important work in this area comes from psychologist and author Barbara Fredrickson, who proposed that positive emotions contribute to well-being and success by broadening the individual's repertoire of thoughts and actions, which lead over time to a deepening of resources. She noted, for instance, that emotions of joy in children create a desire for play that stimulates creativity, intellectual resources, social skills, and brain development (Fredrickson, 1998). She and her colleagues also demonstrated the important role of positive emotions in "undoing" the detrimental effects of negative emotions. For example, in one study, participants underwent a task that would strike fear in the hearts of most people: delivering a speech under a great deal of time pressure (Fredrickson, Mancuso, Braningan, & Tugade, 2000). Following that experience, participants watched one of four films, two designed to elicit positive emotions (contentment and amusement), one designed to trigger sadness, and one used as a neutral film. The researchers then compared the speed of cardiovascular recovery among the four groups. The films that elicited positive emotions led to faster cardiovascular recovery than the sad or neutral films.

Several studies suggest that an affirming approach to life can be similarly helpful to people dealing with spiritual struggles. In a study of Polish adults, the negative effects of spiritual struggles on life satisfaction were reduced in part by higher levels of self-esteem (Szcześniak & Timoszyk-Tomczak, 2020). Among college students struggling spiritually, those who reported more optimism and greater compassion for others indicated more spiritual growth and general growth as a result of their struggles (Hart et al., 2020). Similarly, military veterans who found more social support from others and meaning in their spiritual struggles reported greater spiritual growth (Wilt, Pargament, et al., 2019). Within a national sample, higher levels of hope (and religiously based hope in particular) reduced the strength of the ties between spiritual struggles with depression and unhappiness (Abu-Raiya, Pargament, & Krause, 2016).

In contrast, people who lack compassion toward themselves or others are more prone to a variety of repercussions. Consider the contempt one woman with eating disorders directed toward herself: "I wanted to kill the me underneath. That fact haunted my days and nights" (Hornbacher, 1999, p. 205). Research indicates that people who show more signs of negativity (e.g., pessimism, shame, and guilt) following spiritual struggles report less existential well-being (Kvande, Klöckner, Moksnes, & Espnes, 2015), greater distress (Warren et al., 2015), and are more likely to disregard medical recommendations and use alcohol (Park et al., 2009).

Religious and Spiritual Sources of Affirmation

Historically, religious systems of thought and practice have been particularly prominent sources of life affirmation. Few traditions deny the existence of evil, pain, or suffering, but virtually all place darker forces in a larger, ultimately benevolent context, be it the promise of salvation for Christians, the hope that a broken world can be repaired within Judaism, the attainment of enlightenment in Buddhism and liberation in Hinduism, or the possibility of eternal life within Islam. In spite of the many troubles we find in our world and in ourselves, these traditions maintain that "life is a precious gift, not a dirty trick" (Karff, 1979, p. 143), and that there is something to hope for.

In modern times, many people continue to draw on the resources of religion and spirituality in difficult periods (see Gall & Guirguis-Younger, 2013). Following the September 11, 2001, attack on the World Trade Center and Pentagon, 90% of people reportedly turned to religion for solace and support according to a national survey in the United States (Schuster et al., 2001). In fact, among some groups, such as older adults and African Americans, many say that they look first to their faith in a crisis, even before seeking out help from family, friends, or the health system (e.g., Segall & Wykle, 1988–1989). Religious people in particular make more frequent and effective use of cognitive reappraisals of stressful situations (Vishkin et al., 2016).

Part of the power of religion and spirituality may lie in their ability to assist people searching for a number of significant purposes, such as mastery and control, meaning, emotional comfort, intimacy with others, life transformation, and/or closeness to God (Pargament, 1997). Pargament, Koenig, and Perez (2000) identified a variety of positive spiritual coping resources designed to serve these functions. These include efforts to find comfort and care from God; reframing of negative situations in a more benevolent spiritual light; seeking out spiritual support from family, friends, and clergy; collaborating with God to solve problems; and looking for divine help in finding forgiveness. A number of studies have linked this cluster of positive spiritual coping methods to greater well-being, mental health, and growth (e.g., Ano & Vasconcelles, 2005; Smith et al., 2003; Van Tongeren et al., 2018). For example, in one meta-analysis of over 100 studies that examined various predictors of posttraumatic growth, such as optimism and social support, Prati and Pietrantoni (2009) found that positive spiritual coping emerged as the strongest predictor.

Only a small number of studies have zeroed in on the role of positive spiritual coping with spiritual struggles, but they have generated similar findings. Reynolds et al. (2014) worked with a sample of adolescents with cystic fibrosis over 2 years. They found that spiritual struggles were tied to more positive spiritual coping over time, which predicted, in turn, lower levels of depression. Similarly, more use of positive spiritual coping was associated with various indicators of struggle-related growth among military veterans (Wilt, Pargament, et al., 2019) and college students (Desai & Pargament, 2015). In another study of minority older adults, positive religious coping buffered the effects of spiritual struggles on anxiety and depression (O'Brien et al., 2019).

Let's consider a few specific forms of benevolent spirituality in more detail.

Benevolent Spiritual Reframing

Many religious traditions encourage their adherents to view stressful experiences in a positive spiritual light. From a spiritual vantage point, problems in living can be seen as the will of God, an opportunity to experience closeness with the divine, or a pathway to growth more generally. One of the most well-known examples within Christian scriptures comes from Paul. Struggling with a thorn in his flesh (which could be interpreted as physical, emotional, or spiritual pain), Paul cries out for relief. His pleas are met with a visit from the Lord who does not end Paul's pain, but instead encourages him to re-vision his pain as an opportunity to know God more fully. Paul adopts this radically different perspective: "Therefore most gladly I will rather boast in my infirmities, that the power of Christ may rest upon me. Therefore I take pleasure in infirmities, in reproaches, in needs, in persecutions, in distresses, for Christ's sake. For when I am weak, then I am strong" (2 Corinthians 12:9-10 NIV).

It is not hard to find modern-day equivalents of Paul's benevolent spiritual reframing. For example, a Hindu woman with a congenital neuromuscular disorder described the way she came to view her condition as a spiritual test and opportunity for growth:

> I was told by the swamis early in my study of Vedanta that disability was present in my life so that I could grow in new ways and progress along the path to God consciousness. . . . This life is riddled with physical frustrations but wealthy with opportunities for growth. (Nosek, 1995, pp. 174–175)

Many people going through very difficult situations reframe their suffering in this kind of benevolent spiritual light. For instance, a number of Iranian patients recovering from exposure to mustard gas in the Iraq–Iran war described their medical conditions as divine tests, God's will, gifts from God designed to strengthen their faith, or leading ultimately to divine blessings (Ebadi, Ahmadi, Ghanei, & Kazemnejad, 2009).

A few studies have underscored the value of benevolent spiritual reframing among people going through spiritual struggles. For example, Saritoprak, Exline, Hall, and Pargament (2017) focused on Muslims and Christians struggling spiritually. Both Muslims and Christians, they note, can view spiritual struggles as an opportunity for growth and transformation. Muslims in particular can interpret spiritual struggles as a test that will lead them closer to God, a way to become more devout, and an opportunity to seek out divine forgiveness. The researchers assessed this "transformational trials" outlook and spiritual growth in samples of Christian college students and adult Muslims. In both groups, higher scores on the transformational trials scale were associated with reports of more spiritual growth. These benevolent spiritual appraisals were also tied to less depression and anxiety, and more forgiveness, gratitude, and patience among Muslims. For Christians, transformational trials were related to less depression and anger, and more life satisfaction.

Spiritual Support

Another source of affirmation central to theistically based religions is the promise that people can seek, find, and experience support from God in even the most anguishing of periods. The Book of Psalms contains many powerful expressions of this sentiment. Some of the psalms are directed to those who have reached the limits of their endurance: "The Lord is close to those whose courage is broken and saves those whose spirit is crushed" (Psalm 34:18). Others focus on times when destiny hangs in the balance as we hear in one of the most famous and well-loved psalms: "Yea, though I walk through the valley of the shadow of death, I will fear no evil; for Thou art with me; Thy rod and Thy staff, they comfort me" (Psalm 23:4).

Interest in spiritual support is not a thing of the past. Quite the opposite, a few studies suggest. Wachholtz and Sambamoorthi (2011) reported a sharp spike in the percentage of people who reported that they sought out support from prayer to cope with their own health-related problems from 1993 (13.7%) to 2002 (43.0%) to 2007 (49.0%). Even more recently, when the stark reality of the COVID-19 epidemic began to dawn on people in March 2020, the number of Google searches for the term "prayer" dramatically increased across 95 countries (Bentzen, 2020). It would appear that a significant number of people continue to feel drawn to God in difficult times. This conclusion also applies to times of spiritual struggle, as illustrated by the story of Frank James III. James (2010) recounted the aftermath of a tragedy involving his younger brother, who died after being trapped in a snow cave in Mt. Hood. James did not lack theological breadth and depth; he himself was a pastor. Yet, he was unable to make sense of his brother's death—instead, he was left with unanswered questions. Why, in particular, didn't God come to the rescue when his brother was trapped in the frozen cave? Why did God remain hidden in the tragedy? Why did God continue to remain hidden in his grief that followed? And yet, despite the depth and power of his spiritual struggles, James continued to find himself attracted to God:

> To be sure God is more mysterious and enigmatic than I thought, but still I can't shake loose from Him. There seems to be a kind of gravitational pull to God. . . . I have felt the divine gravity pulling me back toward God, even while I am dumb-struck by his hiddenness. (p. 59)

A number of studies have shown that the search for spiritual support in stressful times is associated with mental health benefits. One study focused on whether people who seek out spiritual support are better protected from the negative effects of spiritual struggles. Among those experiencing high levels of spiritual struggle, people who sought "God's love and care" and "looked to God for strength, support, and guidance" were less likely to report depression and unhappiness (Abu-Raiya, Pargament, & Krause, 2016).

Of course, there is more to spiritual support than seeking it out; as important is the perception that the sacred has responded. Pruyser (1968) described this response as a visitation by a force symbolizing a divine presence that counteracts the visitation by calamity. A supportive response may be perceived as coming directly from God. One woman who had been hospitalized for depression spoke of this experience:

> At one time I reached utter despair and went and prayed to God for mercy instinctively and without faith in reply. That night I stood with other patients in the grounds waiting to be let in to our ward. It was a very cold night with many stars. Suddenly someone stood beside me in a dusty brown robe and a voice said "Mad or sane you are one of My sheep" (Hardy, 1979, p. 91)

Spiritual support can come from other sacred sources as well, such as the spirits of departed loved ones, guardian angels, the soul, nature, or rituals. Listen to the experience of one man grieving the loss of his partner:

> When he first died I felt a very strong presence of him for the first few weeks . . . I remember one time lying on the floor. Just my head down on my arms and I turned my head and all of a sudden he was there. . . . It was a very comforting presence. (Richards et al., 1999)

Whether it is seen as coming from God, the spirits of the deceased, or other sacred sources, the experience of spiritual support has been linked with greater levels of well-being (Benore & Park, 2004). People going through spiritual struggles are also likely to experience benefits from feeling a sense of God's presence and responsiveness.

In sum, both the seeking of spiritual support and the perception that they have received a sacred response contribute to a sense of life affirmation. A study by Exline, Hall, et al. (2016) highlights this point. Working with a sample of Christian undergraduates who reported a spiritual struggle, they measured both positive religious coping efforts initiated on the part of the students and perceptions of helpful actions by God in response to the struggle, such as "God spoke to me" or "healed me" (p. 505). Both the seeking of support and God's perceived response emerged as significant predictors of spiritual growth and posttraumatic growth through the spiritual struggle. Their conclusions underscore the importance of the relationship between God and human for spiritual struggles. On the one hand, Christians can take constructive action themselves through positive religious coping, but it may be equally valuable for them to believe that God is also initiating actions to help them. Working with a larger sample of U.S. adults, Wilt, Stauner, Harriott, Exline, and Pargament (2019) reported similar results.

Within spirituality then we can find deep sources of life affirmation. Of course, some forms of spirituality are more life limiting than life affirming (cf. Doehring, 2015)—we take up this issue in greater detail in later chapters. The central point here is that the positivity embedded within many spiritual expressions may be a powerful stimulus to growth among people experiencing spiritual struggles. Through spirituality, the pain and distress that accompany struggles can be transformed into something of a wholly different character. Chittister (2003) captures this potential for transformation in elegant terms:

> The spirituality of struggle is . . . a spirituality that takes change and turns it into conversion, takes isolation and makes it independence, takes darkness and forms it into faith, takes the one step beyond fear to courage, takes powerlessness and reclaims it as surrender, takes vulnerability and draws out of it the freedom that comes with self-acceptance, faces the exhaustion and comes to value endurance for its own sake, touches the scars and knows them to be transformational. (p. 96)

Now, we shift to a third ingredient of wholeness.

COHESIVENESS

Cohesiveness refers to the degree to which the individual's life journey—its pathways and destinations—is well organized. In a cohesive life, the various bits and pieces of human experience—values, impulses, actions, beliefs, dreams, knowledge, emotions, relationships—are coordinated into a coherent, meaningful pattern, meaningful because they propel the person to a life of enriching purpose and a sense of satisfaction and worth along the way. To paraphrase writer Carlos Castaneda (1971), the cohesive life has "heart." In contrast, incohesiveness is marked by a lack of organization, design, and coherence. This is just the problem Maria was experiencing by virtue of her fragmented personality. With her personas unable or unwilling to communicate, let alone negotiate with one another, Maria was in constant flux, driven here and there by whichever persona was in control at the moment. She came to therapy because she was simply unable to create some sort of order or "oneness" (cf. Edinger-Schons, 2020) out of the disparate pieces of her life.

Cohesiveness is not an original idea. Several psychologists have written about its importance in understanding and helping people whose lives appear to be falling apart. The concept of cohesiveness can also be found within many religious writings. The soul itself has been described as the essential glue that holds the individual together, lending each person a unique identity and humanness. Of course, in practice, religious and spiritual expressions can, at times, foster incohesiveness as well as cohesiveness.

Cohesiveness represents the third ingredient that, along with its two interrelated counterparts—breadth and depth, and affirmation—contribute to wholeness. Below we take a closer look at what goes into a well-organized life.

An Authentic Guiding Vision

Cohesiveness rests in part on a compelling, overarching vision, one that grows out of the individual's orienting system and significant purpose in life. An authentic guiding vision puts life as a whole into perspective and provides a framework that directs the search for significance. We can think of it as a road map of where to go in one's life and how to get there. In one sense, guiding visions are personally created. This is a critical task of adolescence when, as psychologist Erik Erikson (1968) observed, we face the challenge of defining our identities, our place in relation to others and the world, and the life we envision. However, the job of constructing a guiding vision is not limited to adolescence. At any time, we can experience transitions and traumas that call for a reconstruction of our life map.

Guiding visions are created not only out of personal experience and preference but also out of larger forces: social, situational, and spiritual. We are born into our guiding visions by virtue of roles and identities that define in part what it means to be male or female, rich or poor, white or of color, a Muslim or a Christian. Families, institutions, and the larger culture also encourage us, in ways subtle and not so subtle, to adopt certain overarching visions and avoid others. For example, many people who came of age in the 1960s were deeply affected by President John F. Kennedy's call to "Ask not what your country can do for you, ask what you can do for your country" and Reverend Martin Luther King Jr.'s "I Have a Dream" speech. Insular groups, such as the military or religious sects, provide their members with an even more explicit blueprint to follow for significant portions of their lives.

The shaping of guiding visions is a special concern of religion and spirituality. Religious traditions teach their adherents to pursue particular ultimate destinations in life by following particular paths constructed out of various configurations of beliefs, practices, commandments, ethics, and virtues. Consider, for example, the guiding vision so clearly presented to Buddhists in the following daily affirmation:

> Entrusting in the Primal Vow of Buddha,
> Calling out the Buddha-name,
> I shall pass through the journey of life with strength and joy.
> Revering the Light of Buddha,
> Reflecting upon my imperfect self,
> I shall proceed to live a life of gratitude.
> Following the Teachings of Buddha,
> Listening to the Right Path,
> I shall share the True Dharma with all.
> Rejoicing in the compassion of Buddha,
> Respecting and aiding all sentient beings,
> I shall work towards the welfare of society and the world.
> —SENPAI SENSEI (October 12, 2017)

In addition, certain religious rituals are explicitly designed to help individuals discover their own guiding vision. For example, in some Native American communities, adolescents on the precipice of adulthood engage in a "vision quest," a rite of passage in which they spend several days fasting at a sacred site, crying out to the spirits for the vision or dream that will define their purpose in life. Many scriptural verses are also tailored to meet the needs of individuals seeking direction in their lives, as we hear in the following psalm: "Teach me your ways, O Lord; make them known to me" (Psalm 25:4). In less formal ways—moments of contemplative prayer, quiet reflection and meditation, or silent retreats—many people try to discern what God wants for them in their lives. In addition, religious traditions provide their members with spiritual directors, guides, and models for the way a life should be envisioned. These models can be especially valuable to people going through spiritual struggles. In his book on the lives of Roman Catholic saints, James Martin (2006) notes how he found inspiration in their remarkable stories not because the saints avoided the tensions and conflicts of ordinary people but because they showed him how it was possible to remain true to a set of higher values when facing the most profound struggles.

Guiding visions can lend unity and cohesiveness to the varied day-to-day tasks and challenges of living. Not all guiding visions are life enriching or benevolent, though. Parents, organizations, and the larger culture as a whole can impose life visions on people with little sensitivity to their own sensitivities and needs. To discover and hold on to one's own dreams in a less than supportive context is daunting, and many end up living inauthentically—concealing their deepest dreams and desires, engaging in relationships and jobs that violate themselves, or simply losing touch with who they truly are (Palmer, 2004). Major life events can also damage or destroy life visions and plans, triggering a host of psychological problems as well as spiritual struggles. Whether people grow or decline through this time depends in part on whether they can discover, rediscover, or transform authentic, life-enhancing visions for themselves, ones that incorporate their losses and struggles.

A study by King, Scollon, Ramsey, and Williams (2000) illustrates this point. Working with a group of mothers and fathers of children with Down syndrome, the researchers asked the parents to write narratives about their experience of discovering that their child had this condition. They analyzed these stories quantitatively and followed up with the parents 2 years later when they also assessed changes in self-rated growth and ego development. One of the key factors in predicting growth was the parents' willingness to admit their struggles. These admissions could be quite painful, as we hear in the words of one parent when she discovered her baby's syndrome: "I felt as though the earth had opened up and swallowed me. My world seemed to grow (almost tangibly) darker. In that short instant, my normal 'perfect' life disappeared. I thought I would never be happy again. I would never laugh, never have fun" (p. 532). Difficult as it was to acknowledge their pain and disorientation, those parents who were able to integrate their experience of struggle into their narratives and rediscover a vision of themselves and their lives also grew more through their experience. As one parent said, "The pain was so deep. . . . But I did regroup. I did grow. And I did learn to accept the situation. That opened the door for me to bond and love my child. But it took time" (p. 521).

In another relevant study of American adults and undergraduates who were experiencing spiritual struggles, Wilt et al. (2016) found that those who reported that they were able to find a sense of meaning in their struggle experienced more spiritual growth. Moreover, the sense of meaning in struggle was associated with greater life satisfaction and self-esteem, and lower depression and anxiety even after controlling for personality variables and general religiousness.

Weaving Wisdom

Cohesiveness also rests on a particular kind of wisdom: the wisdom of knowing how to weave together the various threads of life into a whole fabric, one that reflects the individual's overarching design and vision. Weaving wisdom, as we call it here, is a higher-order form of mastery, what Baltes and Staudinger (2000) described as a heuristic that "organizes and orchestrates knowledge toward human excellence in mind and virtue" (p. 122). The ability to create wholeness out of the bits and pieces of life is marked by several features.

Knowing When to Do What

The capacity to discern the solutions best suited to particular problems and particular goals within particular contexts is one key. "One-size-fits-all" solutions are not part of the wisdom of weaving. Some situations call for action, while others call for acceptance, tactful retreat, or graceful surrender. Some events require minor adjustments, while others cry out for a major life transformation. Some problems can be handled independently, while others require the support of others. Knowing when to do what has powerful, even life-and-death, implications (Haines et al., 2016). Consider the middle-age man who ignores his persistent chest pains, the mother who enables her heroin-addicted son by giving him money, or the chronic drinker who insists he can "beat this thing" on his own. Problems such as these are commonly presented to psychotherapists whose job is to help people develop their weaving wisdom so they are better equipped to assess problems accurately and tailor solutions to these challenges, including spiritual struggles. Religious and spiritual communities share the job of fostering greater discernment, as illustrated by the popular Serenity Prayer authored by theologian Reinhold Niebuhr: "God, grant me the serenity to accept the things I cannot change, Courage to change the things I can, And wisdom to know the difference" (Shapiro, 2014).

Balancing

A second key feature of weaving wisdom involves the skill of balancing. This is always a work in progress. Permanent equilibrium is impossible because the shifting winds of life throw even the most sure-footed off balance from time to time. Finding balance among the many human motives and attributes can also be complicated when they are treated as adversaries: self-centeredness versus other-centeredness, conservation versus transformation, active versus passive approaches, reason versus intuition, immediate versus delayed gratification, work versus family emphasis, and id- versus superego-oriented responses.

The challenge in finding what Menninger (1963) described as "the vital balance" is not to pick the best of these ostensibly competing elements, for each has an important role to play in human functioning. To select one attribute to the exclusion of others is unbalancing and can manifest itself it in many personal and social problems. Consider these examples: the willingness to sacrifice marriage and family to satisfy cravings for alcohol, drugs, or gambling; denial or minimization of clergy sexual abuse by churches, synagogues, and mosques to protect the larger religious institution; or avoidance of new and challenging situations to prevent anxiety and fear.

Imbalance was certainly part of the problem Maria faced. Because none of her personas could access the redeeming qualities of the others, she was frequently out of kilter. Balance, James (1902) wrote, is the necessary corrective to human excess: "Strong affections need a strong will; strong active powers need a strong intellect; strong intellect needs strong sympathies to keep life steady" (p. 333). Consistent with these theoretical and clinical writings, empirical studies have linked the ability to balance and integrate various life demands to greater well-being and lower levels of anxiety, stress, and depression (e.g., Haar, Russo, Suñe, & Ollier-Malaterre, 2014; Ryan, LaGuardia, & Rawsthorne, 2005).

Balance has also received a great deal of attention within religious traditions. For instance, according to Taoism, all things are said to contain complementary qualities (e.g., light–dark, male–female, strength–gentleness). Rather than oppose each other, these qualities can come together to form a unified and balancing whole as illustrated by the well-known yin–yang figure. Achieving this balance is an essential part of the martial arts, Chinese medicine, and even the artful arrangement of objects (i.e., feng shui). Similarly, virtually every major religion warns against the dangers of extremism and encourages a moderating balance, as illustrated by the middle path in Buddhism and the oft-cited words of Rabbi Hillel: "If I am not for myself, who will be for me? But if I am only for myself, who am I? If not now, when?" (Ethics of the Fathers, 1:14). Psychologist of religion James Jones (2002) has written cogently about the dangers of splitting in the religious realm—that is, an overidealization of religious leaders and institutions purchased at the price of self-debasement. Doing so, he argues, can set the stage for religious fanaticism. What is needed instead is a balancing of religious idealization with realistic appraisals of any religious leader, community, or perspective, as well as one's own strengths and capabilities.

Skill in balancing also applies to the individual's relationship with God. Empirical studies have shown that when people face life crises, working together collaboratively with God may be preferable to less balanced approaches, such as deferring the solutions entirely to God or trying to resolve the problem solely on one's own (Pargament et al., 1988). Two studies have focused in particular on individuals facing spiritual struggles and found that a more balanced collaborative spiritual coping approach was associated with higher levels of struggle resolution and spiritual growth (Wilt, Stauner, et al., 2019) among military veterans, and more posttraumatic and spiritual growth among college students (Hart et al., 2020).

Reconciling Incongruity and Paradox

The process of weaving is especially challenging in a modern world so full of clashing colors, puzzles, and paradoxes. Ours is an age of quantum science in which we wonder how light can be both a particle and a wave, how the act of measuring one quality changes another, and how uncertainty has become a scientific principle. Indeed, our understanding of truth itself has been challenged. "The opposite of a correct statement is a false statement. But the opposite of a profound truth may well be another profound truth," said Danish physicist and winner of the Nobel Prize Niels Bohr (Seldes, 1985, p. 46).

Incongruity and paradox are a part of the lives of individuals as well. As "onion-like" beings, we are made up of layers of contradictory thoughts, feelings, connections, and desires—contradictions we may be only partially aware of. Simultaneously we may love and hate, seek isolation and close connection, pursue pleasures inconsistent with our deepest values, and the list goes on. Contradiction and inconsistency are no less a part of the spiritual realm. Odd as it is, we may feel punished by a God we don't believe in, value love and forgiveness while mulishly holding on to grudges against family members, or see suffering and evil in a world that we insist was created by an all-loving, all-powerful being.

The idea that we are contradictory, paradoxical beings living in a contradictory, paradoxical world is not usually a part of the way we see ourselves. Yet, weaving wisdom calls for the ability not to eliminate but rather to recognize and reconcile incongruities and multiple truths. This capacity is given special emphasis within some religious and spiritual perspectives. The works of Fowler (1981) and Frankel (2005) provide nice examples. Fowler's penultimate stage of faith maturity is "conjunctive faith." This stage is marked by the recognition that the truths we hold are partial and incomplete. In this stage, people shift from "either/or" to "both/and" thinking that is "alive to paradox and the truth in apparent contradictions" (p. 198). Frankel illustrates this perspective through the story of two Jews who seek out a rabbi traveling with his wife to help them resolve a conflict. When the first is finished making his case, the rabbi says, "You are right." When the second has made his argument, the rabbi says, "You are right." Perplexed by her husband's responses, his wife exclaims, "How can they both be right?" The rabbi responds, "You are also right!" (Frankel, 2005, p. 210).

Ultimately, Fowler (1981) maintains, it is the sense of an underlying transcendence that brings unity and wholeness to this human kaleidoscope of contradictory thoughts and feelings. This is the hallmark of reaching the highest stage of religious maturity, "universalizing faith," a level at which people experience a sense of cohesiveness and wholeness within themselves and with others. Frankel (2005) makes a similar point, noting that although we are both body and soul, finite and tied to the infinite, separate and interconnected, we exist "within an ineffable unity in which all our particularities dissolve" (p. 212).

In one of the few empirical studies in this area, Rockenbach and colleagues (2012) worked with college students who were experiencing spiritual struggles and qualitatively analyzed their narratives, journals, and photography. The authors found that their stories of spiritual struggle were "steeped" in contradiction and paradox. Growth, they reported, involved ongoing efforts to reconcile several key contrasts: between ideal and actual selves, between revealed and concealed selves, between self and others, and between one's worldview and lived realities. Rockenbach's students did not find perfect harmony. Instead, they experienced what Kurtz and Ketcham (1992) called a "spirituality of imperfection," a journey in which "the jarring notes, spatial dissonances, and cultural cacophonies [eventually] blend together into a sort of symphony, a chorus of separate, distinct, and sometimes off-key voices harmonizing into a whole . . . not perfect harmony, but harmony nonetheless" (p. 14).

Being Open to Change

Underlying the wisdom of weaving and cohesiveness more generally is an openness to change. Without that, we cannot know when to do what, balance potentially divisive forces, or reconcile incongruity and paradox. In weaving together a life tapestry, we need to find the will, even courage, to reenvision the design, make use of different threads, and at times pull out the old stitches and replace them with new ones. A significant body of psychological theory and research suggests that this kind of flexibility is essential to health and well-being. This should not be surprising. To this point, Kashdan and Rottenberg (2010) conclude their review of the literature from social, personality, clinical, and neuropsychology by noting, "A healthy person is someone who can manage themselves in the uncertain, unpredictable world around them, where novelty and change are the norm rather than the exception" (pp. 875–876). Conversely, inflexibility underlies many kinds of psychological problems, as well as the resistance to meaningful change that is part and parcel of psychotherapy. In the case of Maria, efforts to foster greater wholeness in therapy were often met with stiff resistance, overt and covert, from other facets of her personality, leaving her frozen in her fragmentation.

Although the terms *religion* and *spirituality* may be more likely to bring to mind notions of steadfast commitment than flexibility, openness to change is not alien to religious and spiritual life. Estelle Frankel (2017) has written extensively about this topic in her book *The Wisdom of Not Knowing: Discovering a Life of Wonder by Embracing Uncertainty*. She speaks in particular to the ways openness to change can foster growth through spiritual struggles. The biblical literature, she writes, is replete with tales of spiritual pilgrims willing to venture into unknown territories, as illustrated by the first patriarch and matriarch of monotheism, Abraham and Sarah, who followed God's command to move from their home and family to a strange land. Being open to this kind of change requires several strengths: the ability to let go and mourn the loss of what is familiar, the courage to face anxieties and uncertainties and take a step into the unknown, and the faith that the journey will lead to growth and transformation. This is the courage and faith of the skydiver who free falls into space and trusts that the parachute will open.

Openness to change may be especially important if people are to grow through their spiritual struggles because these times of turmoil signal the need for reorientation and perhaps reevaluation of what is significant. A few research studies speak to this point by examining the ties between a quest orientation and growth following trauma or spiritual struggles. Recall that the quest orientation involves a flexible approach to religious issues, one that values the process of questioning and change (Batson et al., 1993). In one study of college students who had experienced a traumatic event, those who scored higher on the openness to change subscale of the quest measure reported higher levels of posttraumatic growth (Calhoun, Cann, Tedeschi, & McMillan, 2000). In another study among college students who were experiencing spiritual struggles, higher scores on the quest scale were associated with greater posttraumatic growth and spiritual growth (Hart et al., 2020). Paradoxically, higher levels of quest were also tied to reports of greater spiritual decline. Perhaps the process of questing in response to spiritual struggles leads to gains in some areas and declines in others.

Many religious and spiritual figures have also spoken about the dangers of the flip side of openness to change: rigidity. For example, in response to conservative bishops within the Vatican who had failed to embrace his call to welcome homosexuals in the Christian community, Pope Francis (Friedman, 2014, p. 27) warned against "hostile inflexibility—that is, wanting to close oneself within the written word, and not allowing oneself to be surprised by God." Similarly, Frankel (2017) cautions against the rigidity embedded in overcertainty because it "robs us of the space we need to keep on growing" (p. 89). Inflexibility in the face of spiritual struggles may be especially risky. "It is not the struggle itself that kills us," Chittister (2003) writes, "It is allowing ourselves to stay locked in mortal combat with it" (p. 72). Consistent with this point, a number of studies have shown that people who appear to "get stuck" in their spiritual struggles suffer more adverse consequences (e.g., Exline et al., 2011; Pargament et al., 2004; Sherman et al., 2009). For example, in a 2-year study of medically ill older adult patients, those who reported chronic spiritual struggles were more likely than others to experience significant declines in quality of life and significant increases in depression and physical dependence (Pargament et al., 2004).

It is important to note here that openness to change does not imply a lack of deep life commitments. In fact, deep, enduring values and beliefs may create an underlying sense of security that fosters an openness to experimentation and subsequent well-being and growth. In line with this argument, one study found that college students who scored high on both a measure of quest and intrinsic religious commitment manifested the best adjustment to college (McIntosh, Inglehart, & Pacini, 1990).

Ultimately, the courage to persist may accompany the courage to change, and together set the stage for growth in times of turmoil and struggle. Bowland, Biswas, Kyriakakis, and Edmond (2011) highlight this point in their qualitative study of older women who had experienced sexual, physical, or emotional abuse as children and/or adults. Despite their spiritual struggles, the women generally described tremendous persistence in their pursuit of the sacred. One woman said, "It is important to have faith in having faith. It is about keeping on keeping on" (p. 328). At the same time, they demonstrated flexibility and openness in the pathways they took in their spiritual journey. One woman raised in the Catholic church shifted to a non-Christian religious community and to yoga as her regular spiritual practice. Another began to connect to God by sitting beneath a "magnificent caring tree" (p. 328). It was the openness of these survivors to new pathways in the context of their enduring search for the sacred that led to growth and transformation through their spiritual struggles.

CONCLUSIONS

Spiritual struggles often represent a fork in the road. Whether they lead down the path to growth, to decline, or to both depends on the degree to which the person is able to approach the struggles from a place of wholeness. In this chapter, we discussed several qualities of wholeness and brokenness with particular reference to spirituality and spiritual struggles. As described here, wholeness is marked by breadth and depth, life affirmation, and cohesiveness. Brokenness is defined by narrowness and shallowness, harshness, rigidity, and disorganization. At its best, spirituality can lead to greater wholeness. However, it can also be a source of greater brokenness. It is important to stress that much of the thought and research we presented in this chapter is just getting off the ground. Few studies have measured wholeness "as a whole" and more research is needed on the ingredients of wholeness and brokenness. Nevertheless, we believe this line of study has important implications for the way we help people through their times of spiritual struggle. And make no mistake, fostering wholeness and growth in the face of spiritual struggles is a challenging task.

In this day and age in which people are increasingly looking outside religious institutions to create their own individualized smorgasbord of religious and spiritual beliefs, practices, and experiences, many are left with an approach to faith that lacks wholeness, one that leaves them feeling spiritually malnourished and vulnerable to further brokenness when they face stress and struggles. Those who remain within a particular tradition can also be challenged to reconcile seemingly conflicting messages. How, for instance, can fearsome stories of divinely sanctioned violence and damnation be squared with teachings of an unconditionally loving God? These problems are compounded when people accept a hand-me-down religion without personal thought and reflection, resulting in a flimsy faith unable to respond to life's toughest challenges.

In a very practical sense, issues of spiritual struggles, wholeness, and growth often converge in the therapy room. Spiritual struggles can be interwoven into any of the problems that people bring to therapy: anxiety, depression, PTSD, addictions, major mental illness, impulsivity, marital and family conflicts, and personality disorders. And underlying most of these clinical issues is the feeling that something is broken, something is missing, and that life's pieces don't fit together. These were precisely the feelings that led Maria into treatment.

Therapists are enlisted in the process of helping people like Maria identify what is broken, recover what is missing, and put the bits and pieces of life together so that they can find significance. The elements of wholeness and brokenness provide valuable conceptual and practical handholds for therapists grappling with ways to help clients grow through their times of stress and struggle. In subsequent chapters, we see how therapists can foster the ingredients of wholeness in their clinical work. We begin with some basic guidelines for work with clients who come to therapy in the midst of spiritual struggles.

PART II

CLINICAL CHALLENGES
OF SPIRITUAL STRUGGLES

CHAPTER 7

How to Address Spiritual Struggles in Clinical Practice

Recently, at a workshop on spiritually integrated psychotherapy, a participant commented that when it comes to spirituality and spiritual struggles in particular, the mental health field is suffering from a "professional dissociation disorder." He made a good point, unfortunately. As we have stressed, mental health professionals cannot afford to dissociate themselves from spiritual struggles in clinical practice. Let's review the reasons why. First, a significant body of research has shown that spiritual struggles are commonplace among people, including those who seek out psychological treatment. Second, spiritual struggles are robustly linked to signs of emotional distress and serious psychological, social, and physical problems, and they represent risk factors for poorer outcomes. Third, spiritual struggles are pivotal times in the lives of clients that can lead to growth, decline, or both. By addressing spiritual struggles in therapy, practitioners have the opportunity to deepen the therapeutic conversation and shape their clients' trajectory toward greater wholeness and growth. Finally, many clients would like the chance to discuss spiritual matters, including spiritual struggles, in their mental health care. Doing so may enhance the effectiveness of their treatment.

Yet, in spite of these good reasons to integrate spiritual struggles into clinical work, many practitioners may not know how to do so. In this section of the book, we focus practically on how to address spiritual struggles in treatment. This chapter provides some guidelines for clinical work with spiritual struggles of all kinds. In the chapters that follow, we concentrate on specific types of spiritual struggles and how practitioners can understand and assist people who are dealing with these particular tensions and conflicts.

AN ORIENTATION TO SPIRITUAL STRUGGLES
IN PSYCHOTHERAPY

Ted was raised by his grandmother following a car accident that killed his father and left his mother severely incapacitated. At an early age, Ted began to fill his time by caring for living things. He started his own "animal clinic" where he did his best to treat dogs with limps and birds with broken wings. Ted liked going to church and listening to the stories, especially the story of Jesus as a healer. He became close to his pastor and together the two often tinkered around with various gadgets: a lawn mower, a washing machine, an old Victrola record player. Ted also volunteered to spend time with children whose parents were staying in a homeless shelter. One day, Ted remarked to his pastor, "Boy, I wish helping people was as easy as repairing broken machines." The pastor put down his tools and said, "You know, Ted, our job is to do what we can in the world, but Jesus is the one who does the heavy lifting when it comes to healing. If you do your part, he'll do his." Ted was comforted by these words. He stayed involved in the church and moved through adolescence trying to be a good Christian, doing what he could to heal the damage in the world.

Ted saw the terrorist attacks of 9/11 as another opportunity to heal. He decided to join the Army, in spite of the advice of his grandmother, a widow of the Vietnam War. Not surprisingly, Ted became a medic. In Iraq, Ted felt he had entered a totally different world—the place, the people, the climate, the language, the religion—all alien. And as the war began to go poorly, Ted encountered things he had never faced before: people willing to destroy themselves and the innocent men, women, and children around them; the looks of pure hatred directed his way by those he only wanted to help; the chaos of day-to-day life in Iraq, indeed the uncertainty of whether he himself would live out the day. Ted's work routinely put him in danger since it was his job to treat soldiers under attack.

One day, while on a routine patrol with his unit, Ted was sitting in the second of two light vehicles. Suddenly, a violent explosion rocked his truck, and the vehicle in front of him disintegrated before his eyes. Ted raced to the truck, but there were no survivors; no one was even recognizable. The thought came to him: "Even Jesus can't put this back together."

The remainder of his tour in Iraq passed in a blur. He continued his work, but his heart was no longer in it. He isolated himself from others, lost weight, and was unable to sleep. At night he was flooded with images of the destruction he had witnessed and questions he was unable to answer: Where had all of this hatred and evil come from? What difference had all of his talents made? He had done his part, why hadn't God done his? How could a place and a people be so broken? Was the world, in fact, beyond repair? Was he himself beyond repair? How could he go on? What real purpose did he now have in life? Ted returned to the United States with PTSD and deep spiritual struggles. His symptoms worsened, and Ted became increasingly vegetative. At the strong urging of friends, he sought therapy.

What approach should therapists take when clients, like Ted, come to treatment with serious psychological problems that are exacerbated by their spiritual struggles? Psychological and spiritual concerns are so interwoven here, it would seem impossible to try to disentangle these threads and attend only to the psychological symptoms. Even if it were possible, that type of therapeutic "spiritual dissociation" may not be effective. So what is the alternative?

Fortunately, the alternative does not have to be overwhelming. Work with spiritual struggles does not require a totally new form of treatment. Rather, it calls for a spiritually integrated approach in which the clinician is alert and open to addressing spiritual struggles. The therapist can and should make use of tools from existing treatments. Having said that, it is also the case that therapy must be tailored to the distinctive nature of spiritual struggles.

In this regard, it is vital for therapists to remember that spiritual struggles are not a form of pathology in the spiritual realm. They are, instead, a critical but natural part of spiritual development, a crossroads that can lead in the direction of growth, decline, or sometimes both. (If a magical pill were developed that promised a "cure" for spiritual struggles, we would hope it does not receive Food and Drug Administration [FDA] approval!) To simply eliminate the struggle would also eliminate an opportunity for positive transformation and growth. The job of the practitioner is not to treat spiritual struggles as if they were another diagnostic category of mental illness but to help people achieve a positive reorientation through their struggles. This reorientation often involves first restoring the client's sense of equilibrium and then considering deeper changes in his or her life pathways and destinations. The general goal of this clinical work is to help spiritual strugglers address the problems that brought them to therapy and move to greater wholeness and growth. With this perspective in mind, we begin by examining some of the issues involved in assessing spiritual struggles.

HOW TO ASSESS SPIRITUAL STRUGGLES

On the face of it, assessing for spiritual struggles in psychotherapy should be a pretty straightforward task. Simply ask the client whether he or she has been experiencing tensions, strains, or conflicts about spiritual issues and listen to the response. Right? Not really. Assessing for spiritual struggles is not necessarily straightforward, for several reasons. First, spiritual experiences, including spiritual struggles, may be difficult to describe. Deep spiritual conflicts within the individual, with the supernatural, or with others, can be especially hard to put into words. Second, people may not be fully aware of their spiritual struggles. Like other painful emotions and conflicts, spiritual struggles can be suppressed or repressed. Direct questions about spiritual struggles, then, may not always lead to an informative response. Third, as Exline and colleagues (Exline & Grubbs, 2011; Exline, Kaplan, & Grubbs, 2012) have found, spiritual struggles can elicit personal feelings of shame and guilt, and fears of criticism and disapproval by others or God. As a result, clients may be reluctant to admit their spiritual struggles to their therapists. Finally, although many clients would welcome a chance to discuss their spiritual struggles, others may have questions about whether spiritual struggles are an appropriate topic of conversation in psychotherapy. Are therapists qualified to talk about these issues? Will therapists be open-minded or will they have a particular "axe to grind"? Given the lack of training of many mental health professionals in the area of religion and spirituality (Saunders et al., 2014), and the fact that mental health professionals are considerably more secular than those they serve (Shafranske & Cummings, 2013), the clients' questions are reasonable enough. For these reasons, the process of assessing spiritual struggles calls for sensitivity and care. Drawing from Pargament's (2007) more general model of spiritual assessment, let's consider five steps in the assessment of spiritual struggles.

Step 1: Setting the Stage for Assessing Spiritual Struggles

It takes remarkable courage for clients to walk into a therapy office and share the intimate details of their problems with a stranger, even if that stranger is a mental health professional. To encourage the client in this process, the therapist must create a welcoming space for conversation. Warmth, genuineness, empathy, and openness on the part of the therapist are all necessary to foster this welcoming space and to build the strong working alliance that sets the stage for progress (Horvath, Del Re, Flückiger, & Symonds, 2011).

Special sensitivity is needed to welcome dialogue about topics as deeply personal as spirituality and spiritual struggles in particular. We suggest that at least four factors are important in this regard. The first involves the therapist's genuine curiosity about the spiritual life of the client. Nothing is likely to shut off talk more quickly than signs of disinterest from the therapist—be it a yawn, a glance at the clock, or a quick change of subject to more familiar ground—when the subject of spirituality comes up. Conversation can also be closed off when the therapist communicates that he or she already understands the client's spiritual struggles, which could imply a failure to appreciate the distinctiveness of each client's spiritual experience (Doehring, 2015). And dialogue can be shut down when practitioners respond to a client's struggles with quick fixes. These may take the form of false reassurances that the struggles will soon pass, facile religious sayings, such as "God doesn't give us more than we can handle," or premature efforts to lift the client's spirits, as illustrated by the title of Kenneth Haugk's (2004) book *Don't Sing Songs to a Heavy Heart: How to Relate to Those Who Are Suffering.* Quick fixes, however well-intended, are inadequate responses to spiritual struggles, for they may communicate the therapist's own discomfort, delegitimize the client's pain, and short-circuit efforts to help the client explore the deeper meaning and potential life-transforming value of his or her spiritual struggles. When clients raise spiritual struggles, a therapeutic response of "That's really interesting, I'd like to hear more," is far more likely to open the door to further conversation. Patience on the part of therapist and client will be needed to explore spiritual struggles in treatment.

Humility on the part of the therapist is a second foundation to building a welcoming space for spiritual dialogue and assessment. A humble approach steers clear of assumptions that a client's spiritual story can be fully understood by knowing his or her denomination or level of engagement in spiritual practices. Humility, instead, rests on the recognition that the therapist does *not know* about the client's spirituality, that each client has a distinctive spiritual story to tell, and that the therapist needs to learn more, to be taught, in essence, by the client.

Spiritual self-awareness is a third factor that sets the stage for the assessment of spirituality and spiritual struggles. Few people are emotionally neutral about spirituality—it is a subject of tremendous power for many therapists, as well as clients. Consider, for example, your own initial emotional reactions to the following possible therapeutic scenarios: the rape victim who feels she was being punished by God for an abortion she had in high school, the Muslim couple at odds because the husband wants his wife to wear a hijab (head covering), the college freshman who left her parents' church and has become involved in an on-campus pagan group. Emotional reactions, positive or negative, to scenarios such as these are an inevitable part of treatment. Therapy, after all, is not a value-free enterprise (Bergin, 1991). But spiritual self-awareness on the part of the therapist represents an important corrective to religious and spiritual biases of all kinds that can interfere with the process and outcomes of treatment.

Finally, a welcoming space for spiritual conversation grows out of the therapist's respect for the client as a human being, including his or her spirituality and struggles. Therapist Russell Jones (2019) puts it well: "Make sure your struggler feels met as a person, not as a problem to be solved" (p. 113). Respect does not imply agreement. Murray-Swank and Murray-Swank (2012) note that, although they may find it difficult to hear traumatized clients say things such as "This is God's will for me," they remind themselves of the many clients who find strength, meaning, and purpose from this system of meaning (p. 240). Respect for the client simply acknowledges the place of spiritual values, beliefs, practices, and struggles in the individual's world. Respect also rests on the belief that, as in other areas of life, the client is the final arbiter of his or her spiritual choices. Attempts to convert or counterconvert clients toward or away from any religious perspective are simply inconsistent with the most basic values and ethics of psychotherapy. The American Psychological Association and other mental health professions codify respect for religion and spirituality as part of their ethical standards (e.g., American Psychological Association, 2017). This is not to say that practitioners should not address religious or spiritual concerns when they become sources of harm to clients or others in their lives. The challenge here is to do so in a way that remains sensitive to the client's core spiritual beliefs, practices, and values. In this regard, it is noteworthy that greater sensitivity to clients' spirituality is more predictive of change in therapy than the degree of spiritual similarity between clients and therapists (Wade, Worthington, & Vogel, 2007).

Step 2: Initial Spiritual Assessment

The initial spiritual assessment is just that, initial. It consists of a few basic questions that offer a preliminary glimpse into the role of religion and spirituality in the life of the client and the presence of spiritual struggles (see Table 7.1). Rather than "red-flagged" or set apart as somehow overly sensitive or unusual, these questions are interwoven into the host of information the clinician gathers about the life of the individual: mental health, physical health, personal and family history, orienting system, significant values and purpose, resources and burdens, social context, and the elements of wholeness and brokenness. The assessment of spiritual struggles is also embedded in a broader clinical evaluation of spiritual life, including those spiritual resources and elements of wholeness that may facilitate the process of change.

For example, in learning about the client's identity, the therapist can ask whether the person sees him- or herself as a religious or spiritual person. In discussing the individual's social ties, the therapist can ask whether the client is part of a larger religious or spiritual community. In talking about the ways the client handles problems, it is reasonable to ask how his or her religion or spirituality

---

TABLE 7.1. Initial Spiritual Assessment Questions

- *Salience of spirituality*

   Do you see yourself as a religious or spiritual person? If so, in what way?

- *Salience of religious affiliation*

   Are you affiliated with a religious or spiritual denomination or community? If so, which one?

- *Salience of spirituality to the problem*

   Has your problem affected your religious or spiritual life? If so, in what way?

- *Salience of spirituality to the solution*

   Has your religion or spirituality been involved in the way you have coped with your problems? If so, in what way?

- *Presence of spiritual struggles*

   Have you been experiencing tensions, conflicts, questions, or struggles about religion or spirituality? If so, in what way?

Note. Adapted from Pargament (2007).

has been involved in coping. And when considering how the person has been impacted by his or her problems, it is easy to raise a question that may point to the spiritual impact of the problem: Has your problem affected you religiously or spiritually? Any of these questions may generate responses that suggest the client is experiencing spiritual struggles, in which case it is important to raise the most direct question: Have you been experiencing tensions, conflicts, or struggles about religion or spirituality?

Many clients respond to some of these initial spiritual questions with expressions of spiritual disinterest or uninvolvement. Even so, they may still be experiencing spiritual struggles. In this vein, one study showed that spiritual struggles were as common among religiously nonaffiliated patients with psychiatric diagnoses as they were among religiously affiliated patients (Rosmarin et al., 2014). Thus, follow-up questions to those who are secular or religiously disaffiliated are quite appropriate. Rosmarin (2018) provides a compelling illustration in his work with a 26-year-old single female who had been repeatedly sexually assaulted by her father when she was a child:

> As a teenager, the patient disaffiliated completely from her family's religion and remained completely secular when she presented for treatment. [She denied] that S-R (spirituality and religion) was personally important. However, when asked about the clinical relevance of S-R to her symptoms, she welled up with tears and disclosed that she felt very angry at God and her religious community for letting her experience untold suffering. . . . She further reported that encountering S-R stimuli (e.g., seeing members of her faith, passing by places of worship) would invariably elicit a host of negative emotions for her, and had even been a trigger for self-injury in the past. (pp. 106–107)

Apart from the context of individual psychotherapy, it can be useful to screen for spiritual struggles to identify people who might be good candidates for other struggle-related programs and activities, such as psychoeducation, group counseling, and hospital chaplaincy visits. Several brief screening methods have been developed.

- The Brief RCOPE (see Chapter 1 for items) has been used to screen for spiritual struggles, but as noted earlier, these items focus largely on divine spiritual struggles.

- To screen for a wider range of spiritual struggles, Exline and colleagues developed summary descriptions of each of the six types of spiritual struggles identified in the 26-item Religious and Spiritual Struggles (RSS) scale (see Table 7.2). Shorter forms of the RSS are now under development, including a 14-item version (Exline, Pargament, Wilt, Grubbs, & Yali, 2021; see Table 1.2 for the items) as well as six-item and one-item brief screeners (Exline, Pargament, & Wilt, 2020).

- Murphy et al. (2016) classified older adults with depression as spiritual strugglers if they indicated that they receive less than they need from religion/spirituality and make less use of religion/spirituality to cope than they once did. Using this method, 18% of a sample of patients with blood and marrow transplants were identified as potential spiritual strugglers (King, Fitchett, & Berry, 2013). The importance of this kind of screening was underscored by the finding that spiritual struggles were not identified by any regular psychosocial assessments of these patients.

- In a comparison of ways of screening for spiritual struggles among adult survivors of cancer, King, Fitchett, Murphy, Pargament, Harrison, et al. (2017) found that the most sensitive screening method consisted of a combination of positive responses to a question about self-described struggle ("Do you currently have what you would describe as religious or spiritual struggles?") and a question about a lack of meaning and joy in life ("Do you struggle with the loss of meaning and joy in your life?"; p. 479).

Whatever conclusions that are drawn from the initial spiritual assessment should be held tentatively. Even if spiritual and religious issues do not come to the surface in the initial assessment, don't assume they will not arise later. In their debriefings of 200 Marines returning from duty in Iran, military chaplains reported the ironic finding that those who most strongly voiced no need for debriefing had the most to say about the deeper conflicts raised by their war-related experiences (Drescher, Smith, & Foy, 2007). Conversely, if these spiritual issues do come up in the initial assessment, don't assume that they will be important parts of therapy. The perspective on spirituality gained from the initial assessment can shift and change over the course of therapy.

TABLE 7.2. Screener for Spiritual Struggles

Divine struggles (e.g., anger or disappointment with God; feeling punished or abandoned by God)

Struggles involving the devil or evil spirits (e.g., feeling attacked by the devil; worried that problems you were facing were caused by the devil or evil spirits)

Moral struggles (e.g., wrestled with attempts to follow your moral principles; felt guilty for not living up to your moral standards)

Doubt-related struggles (e.g., feeling confused about your religious/spiritual beliefs; feeling troubled by doubts or questions about religion/spirituality)

Struggles of ultimate meaning (e.g., feeling as though your life had no deeper meaning; questioning whether life really matters)

Interpersonal spiritual struggles (e.g., conflicts with other people about religious/spiritual matters; feeling hurt, mistreated, or offended by religious/spiritual people; anger at organized religion)

Note. Adapted from the 26-item scale in Exline, Pargament, Grubbs, and Yali (2014).

Step 3: Implicit Spiritual Assessment

The initial assessment may reveal that the client is indeed struggling with religious or spiritual issues and, if so, the therapist can move directly to Step 4, which involves a more extensive and explicit conversation about these concerns. However, as we noted, a lack of response to the initial spiritual assessment questions does not preclude the possibility of spiritual struggles. Clients may not see their struggles as particularly spiritual in nature, so direct questioning using religious and spiritual language may not generate meaningful responses. For example, moral or ultimate meaning struggles could be understood and experienced without reference to spirituality. Clients may also keep their spiritual tensions and conflicts to themselves for many reasons, as we have noted.

In any case, therapists should remain alert to the possibility of spiritual struggles in their assessment. An implicit spiritual assessment represents another way of examining this possibility by raising a few questions that hint at deeper spiritual tensions and conflicts. In Table 7.3, several of these questions are presented. Note that none of these questions makes explicit mention of religion or God. Instead, by use of "psychospiritual" terms, such as *greatest despair and suffering, deepest questions,* and *shaken faith,* the questions suggest that there may be a more profound dimension to the client's problems. Practitioners should listen carefully for similar "psychospiritual" language in their client's responses. Heartfelt pleas, such as "Why is this happening to me?" "I feel contaminated," "My world is falling apart," "Life is so unfair," "I'm feeling punished," "When will my suffering end?" and "I feel so violated" strongly signal a deeper, potentially transcendent dimension to the client's pain. In therapeutic conversations about topics fraught with such deep emotion and power, the focus can transition, at times quickly, into more explicit spiritual dialogue and assessment.

Let's return to the case of Ted, the Iraqi veteran presented earlier in this chapter, for an example. Recall that Ted was clearly experiencing a spiritual struggle as a result of his trauma.

TABLE 7.3. Implicit Spiritual Assessment of Spiritual Struggles

- What are the deepest questions your situation has raised for you?
- What causes you the greatest despair and suffering?
- How has this experience changed you at your deepest levels?
- What have you discovered about yourself that you find most disturbing?
- How has this situation shaken your faith?
- What has this experience taught you that you wish you had never known?
- What are your deepest regrets?
- What would you like to be able to let go of in your life?

Note. From Pargament (2007).

In the initial spiritual assessment, Ted offered only brief responses to the religious and spiritual questions. He was mainly concerned about his symptoms of PTSD: flashbacks, insomnia, trouble concentrating, and anxiety. Not until later in therapy did the topic of spiritual struggles come up. It arose in the context of a very emotional session in which Ted spoke of his feelings that his world had been shattered physically, socially, and emotionally. Hearing the psychospiritual tone in Ted's words, the therapist responded not only with empathy and compassion, but also with an implicitly spiritual question: "What is the source of your greatest despair and suffering?" At that point, Ted recounted what his pastor had said to him many years ago: "If you do your part, Jesus will do his." Tearfully, Ted went on to describe his profound disappointment in himself, his pastor, his church, and God: "What my pastor taught me was just not true." Ted began to realize that he had been deeply shaken spiritually. At this point, the therapy moved forward to a more explicit spiritual assessment.

Step 4: Explicit Spiritual Assessment

When the initial or implicit spiritual assessment indicates that the client may be experiencing spiritual struggles, the therapist moves to a more extensive and explicit assessment of spiritual struggles and the place of spirituality in the client's life more generally. This assessment will likely extend beyond the first session and, in fact, may become a part of the conversation in several sessions over the course of therapy. It is important to remember, however, that this kind of spiritual questioning is *not* appropriate when the client has expressed disinterest in this area or a preference to avoid the topic.

To encourage conversation about spiritual struggles and spirituality, we recommend the use of exploratory spiritual questions. These questions are intentionally open-ended because they are designed to help the client tell his or her spiritual story. Toward this end, there is no need to raise all of these queries. In fact, too many questions can shut clients down rather than open them up. Neither should therapists use the same set of questions with every client. To take one obvious example, asking about God would generally not be appropriate for clients who are nontheists. These questions are simply starting points to lead the client into a spiritual conversation and should be tailored to the individual. Similarly, the therapist should listen carefully to the words clients use to convey their spiritual experiences and try to become more conversant in their languages, perhaps speaking in some instances of values and worldviews rather than religion or spirituality, higher power rather than God, existential or ultimate concerns rather than spiritual struggles, or cherish rather than hold sacred.

Exploratory Questions about Spiritual Struggles

One set of exploratory questions focuses on spiritual struggles (see Table 7.4). The therapist can begin by delving into the kind of spiritual struggles the client has been experiencing. The therapist may learn that the client is encountering a particular kind of struggle (e.g., divine, demonic, doubt related, ultimate meaning, moral, interpersonal) or some combination of these spiritual struggles. And the therapist may discover that the struggle has been long-lasting or relatively recent, a singular event or one of a series of struggles the client has faced in life.

The therapist should also explore the ways in which the client has been disoriented by his or her struggles. Disorientation, as we noted earlier, is a natural consequence of spiritual struggles. But to help the client regain some degree of equanimity and stability, it is important to pinpoint the ways in which the client has been shaken by spiritual struggles. The therapist should examine those aspects of the individual's orienting system that may have been disrupted. Perhaps the struggles have affected the client's core beliefs, daily practices and routines, close relationships, and/or emotional stability. Or perhaps the spiritual struggles have shaken the client's sense of significance and configuration of purposes for living. Even in the early stages of therapy, however, the therapist should be alert to signs of positive changes and growth that the client may begin to experience through spiritual struggles.

TABLE 7.4. Explicit Spiritual Assessment: Exploratory Questions about Spiritual Struggles

- *Exploring the kind of spiritual struggles*

  Could you tell me more about your spiritual struggles? What or who do you feel you have been struggling with? How long have you been struggling? Could you tell me about other spiritual struggles you may have had in the past?

- *Exploring struggle-related disorientation*

  How have you been shaken? What kinds of questions has your spiritual struggle raised for you? How have your spiritual struggles affected the person you were and the life you led prior to your struggles?

- *Exploring the relationship between spiritual struggles and the presenting problem*

  What do you feel led to your spiritual struggles? How have the problems that brought you to therapy contributed to your spiritual struggles? How have your spiritual struggles affected the problems that brought you to therapy? How have you changed for better or worse as a result of your spiritual struggles?

- *Exploring resources for coping with spiritual struggles*

  How have you tried to make sense of your spiritual struggles? Where do you turn to for help and support in coping with your spiritual struggles? What ways of coping have been most helpful? What ways of coping have been least helpful?

- *Exploring barriers to a resolution of spiritual struggles*

  Do you try to think about your spiritual struggles or try to avoid thinking about them? What kinds of feelings do your spiritual struggles raise for you (e.g., guilt, shame)? If you have shared your struggles with others, how have they responded? How do you feel other people would react if they knew about your spiritual struggles? Have your shared your struggles with God? How do you feel God would respond if you did?

In a related vein, the therapist must look into the relationship between the client's spiritual struggles and the problems that brought him or her to therapy. In most cases, people do not seek out therapeutic help for spiritual struggles alone. Rather, the spiritual struggles are interwoven into the issues that have led to psychotherapy. As yet, research on the links between specific spiritual struggles and specific psychological problems is just developing. At this point, it is safest to assume that any presenting problem, symptom, or diagnosable disorder could be potentially associated with any kind of spiritual struggle.

When examining spiritual struggles it is also important to determine whether they are an end result of psychological problems (secondary struggles), a cause of psychological problems (primary struggles), or both a cause and an effect of psychological problems (complex struggles). The answer to these key questions can shape the course of treatment. When spiritual struggles are an expression of a more basic psychological disorder, the struggles could mask the primary psychological problem. Moreover, successful treatment of the psychological problem alone could potentially alleviate the pain of spiritual struggles. For example, psychotropic medications may be sufficient to soothe the spiritual struggles of a patient who hears God's voice commanding him or her to hurt him- or herself. In cases of primary spiritual struggles, however, focusing exclusively on the psychological problem to the neglect of the client's spiritual struggles would be ineffective because the struggles are perpetuating and even exacerbating the emotional difficulties. Progress in therapy would depend on the practitioner's willingness to deal directly with the client's spiritual struggles. Of course, many spiritual struggles are likely to be complex, calling for attention to both spiritual and psychological dimensions of the case.

Therapy is rarely the first place people turn to when they face problems, including spiritual struggles (e.g., Exline, Prince-Paul, Root, & Peereboom, 2013). Often, they have attempted a variety of ways of coping on their own, with limited degrees of success. By examining how clients have already tried to cope with their struggles, the therapist can avoid methods that haven't proved to be helpful. Questions about where the client turns to for support, comfort, meaning, hope, and transformation to cope with his or her struggles can be quite fruitful. Given the transcendent character of spiritual struggles, it is especially important to explore spiritual ways of coping that the client may have tried or overlooked.

Finally, like other psychological concerns, spiritual struggles can be resistant to change. Some clients may be reluctant to talk about their spiritual conflicts because they trigger feelings of guilt and shame. Others may fear rejection by others, including religious figures, if they admit their spiritual struggles. Still others may worry about how God will react to their negative spiritual feelings. And some may prefer to avoid their spiritual struggles altogether rather than face them directly. In the explicit spiritual assessment, the therapist should explore potential barriers such as these that could interfere with efforts to address spiritual struggles.

Exploring the Spiritual Life of the Client

Because spiritual struggles are only one of the processes that contribute to the spiritual life of the client, it is important to examine spiritual struggles within the context of the client's spirituality as a whole. Toward this end, the therapist should raise questions that encourage the client to tell his or her larger spiritual story. Once again, there is no need to burden the client with a long list of questions. A relatively small number of questions are often enough to elicit the client's spiritual narrative.

We have presented some illustrative queries in Table 7.5. They include questions that explore the client's spiritual history; questions that shed light on the way the client understands and relates to God, or whatever he or she holds sacred; questions that help the client reflect on his or her most sacred purposes in life; questions that delve into aspects of the client's spiritual orientation; and questions that address the ways in which the client's spirituality has proven to be a source of growth or decline.

Let's return to the illustrative case of Ted.

Once his therapist recognized that Ted was grappling with spiritual concerns, the two began to talk about spirituality more explicitly and extensively. The conversations were quite revealing. The therapist learned that Ted was experiencing several types of spiritual struggles: feelings of being let down by Jesus, doubts about whether his fundamental religious beliefs were in fact true, considerable uncertainty about the ultimate meaning and purpose of his life, and questions about whether good was really stronger than evil in the world. These were deeply disturbing tensions and conflicts, and they were producing a great deal of disorientation both in terms of Ted's most important goals and purposes in life and the pathways he was taking to realize his dreams. Ted's struggles appeared to be complex in nature; they were both a result of his traumatic exposure and PTSD, and a source of greater psychological symptomatology. The therapist also sensed that Ted's struggles might be even more deeply tied to the absence of his father and incapacitation of his mother as he was growing up. Perhaps Ted's traumatic experience in Iraq had reawakened the feelings of helplessness and hopelessness he had experienced as a young child. Any efforts to help Ted address his struggles, the therapist realized, would be complicated by Ted's mixed set of feelings of embarrassment and shame—embarrassment that he could have been so naïve as to believe that Jesus would protect him from serious harm, and shame that he was letting down his minister and religious community. Ted's grandmother had died, and he had cut himself off from important sources of support for his problems and struggles. Nevertheless, Ted did have a base of coping resources he could potentially access and build on, including his friendships,

TABLE 7.5. Explicit Spiritual Assessment: Exploratory Questions about the Spiritual Life of the Client

- *Exploring the client's spiritual history*

  Could you describe the religious or spiritual tradition you grew up in? How did your family express its spirituality? How did you discover or learn about God or the sacred?

  How did you understand God or the sacred as a child? What types of spiritual beliefs or practices did you engage in as a child? How have your spiritual beliefs and practices changed over time?

- *Exploring the client's vision of God and sacred purposes in life*

  How do you envision God now? What do you hold sacred in your life now? How would you describe your relationship with God or the sacred? What do you seek from your spirituality and faith? What do you feel God wants from you? Do you feel you have a higher purpose in life and, if so, what might that be?

- *Exploring the client's spiritual orientation and pathways to the sacred*

  What has helped you nurture your spirituality or faith? What has been damaging to your spirituality or faith? Who supports you spiritually and how so? What do you do and where do you go to practice your spirituality or feel the presence of the sacred?

  What aspects of your spirituality are particularly uplifting or meaningful?

- *Exploring the effectiveness of the client's spirituality*

  How has your spirituality changed your life for the better? How has your spirituality changed your life for the worse? In what ways would you say you have grown or not grown spiritually?

Note. Adapted from Pargament (2007), Griffith and Griffith (2002), and Hodge (2001).

church involvement, healthy lifestyle, and desire to make a meaningful contribution to the world.

Step 5: Putting It All Together—Assessing Spiritual Struggles in the Larger Context of Wholeness and Growth

The final step of the assessment process is a challenging one, calling for what we have described as weaving wisdom on the part of the therapist. In this step, the therapist must place the client's presenting problem and spiritual struggles within the larger context of the client's life, in particular within areas of wholeness and brokenness in the client's life. In the previous chapter, we reviewed three critical ingredients of wholeness and brokenness: (1) breadth and depth—the client's ability to see and approach life in its fullness; (2) life affirmation—the degree to which the client's life is infused with positivity toward the self, others, the world, and the sacred; and (3) cohesiveness—the extent to which the bits and pieces that make up a life are coordinated into a coherent, well-organized pattern. Evaluations of these ingredients of wholeness and brokenness can be understood as part of the "subtext" of the assessment process. While exploring the client's problems, struggles, and life more generally, the therapist is simultaneously evaluating ways in which the client is more and less whole. These evaluations play an essential role in the development of a treatment plan to address the client's problems and struggles, and to foster greater wholeness and growth. Consider how Ted's therapist "put it all together" in the final step of the assessment.

Ted's psychological problems and spiritual struggles, his therapist concluded, were partly rooted in a lack of breadth and depth in Ted's orientation to the world. Particularly important, the therapist believed, was Ted's limited ability to understand and come to terms with suffering. Traumatized as a child by the death of his father and incapacitation of his mother, Ted tried to find some solace and a greater sense of control and mastery in life by becoming a healer. At some level, he may have dreamed of being able to return his mother to health. As he grew, Ted had to confront his own limited powers to heal, but he was buoyed through this time of initial struggle by his pastor, who reassured him that if he did his part, Jesus would do his. While these words were tremendously comforting to Ted, they left him with a false sense of confidence that he would be able to avoid tragic loss in the future. Thus, Ted moved into young adulthood unequipped to anticipate and deal with tragedy and suffering. In Iraq, he encountered a trauma that would have shaken anyone. Ted, however, was particularly vulnerable to its psychological and spiritual effects because it revealed the underlying fragility of his worldview and the experience he lacked in facing and grieving his losses.

Ted's therapist was also struck by the disparity in the kindness and caring Ted showed to others and the compassion he was unable to find for himself. Even though he had always been there for the people around him in difficult times, Ted had separated himself from the support they might have offered him in return. This lack of support extended to members of his church who were unaware of Ted's traumatic experience and struggles, and to his relationship with God. Ted's prayers had always centered on divine requests for the healing of others, never for himself. As altruistic as he was, Ted was limited by his inability to affirm himself.

Clearly, Ted was experiencing a great deal of disorientation, confusion, and disorganization. He had lost his guiding vision and was flailing in his effort to regain a sense of direction and balance. In his therapist's assessment, the problem resided not in Ted's dream of healing others, certainly a noble goal, but in the overidealization of the dream, one in which he, with the help of Jesus, would be able to heal the world. Key questions for therapy were whether Ted would be able to find a more realistic and sustainable vision. Could he accept, for example, the dream of making a world a better place rather than a perfect place? As importantly, could he accept himself as a wounded healer who required the same compassion and caring for himself—psychological, social, and spiritual—that he offered others?

Progress and growth in treatment, the therapist felt, would rest on Ted's willingness to learn more about himself. Ted was not practiced in self-reflection. He had not considered how his life had been shaped by the early loss of his parents, how his understanding of suffering might be limited, how his guiding purpose in life might be problematic, and how his difficulty finding compassion for himself could leave him vulnerable to times of stress and struggle. In short, Ted was largely unaware of how and why his world had been shaken and how he might change the trajectory of his life. And yet, Ted's therapist was optimistic. A good-hearted, bright, and motivated young man, Ted had several of the raw tools and resources he would need to reach a place of greater self-awareness and greater wholeness in his life.

As can be seen below, the therapist's preliminary treatment plan for Ted integrated each of these elements: the psychological problems that brought Ted to therapy, his spiritual struggles, and his areas of wholeness and brokenness.

Therapeutic Plan for Ted

1. *Reestablish psychological stability.* As a first step in treatment, basic crisis-oriented services are needed to combat Ted's vegetative symptoms, reestablish the regular rhythm of his life (e.g., eating, sleeping, exercising, talking to people), and regain his emotional equilibrium by offering reassurance and hope.

2. *Address symptoms of PTSD.* Exposure therapy is necessary to help Ted face rather than avoid his images and memories of destruction.

3. *Evaluate the need for medication.* Referral to a psychiatrist and consultation is called for to discuss the value of antidepressant medication for Ted's symptoms.

4. *Education about spiritual struggles.* Psychoeducation is needed to address Ted's feelings of embarrassment and shame about his spiritual struggles, to help him reframe his struggles in a more hopeful light, and to foster greater understanding that spiritual struggles, though painful and disruptive, are a normal part of life, and can be a source of growth and positive transformation.

5. *Broaden understanding of pain and suffering.* Reflective-oriented therapy would help Ted develop a deeper understanding of the darker sides of life, including pain, unfairness, trauma, and mystery. This reflective work could be supplemented by readings about suffering. Pastoral counseling could also prove helpful to Ted.

6. *Foster greater self-compassion.* Support-oriented therapy is needed to encourage Ted to cultivate and access sources of compassion in his life, including friends, members of his church, God, and himself. Supportive prayers from Ted's tradition and self-compassion meditative exercises may be especially valuable.

7. *Explore a sustainable guiding vision.* Meaning-centered therapy is necessary to help Ted examine the guiding vision of his life and consider whether it is viable or in need of change. In particular, can he find a significant purpose that encompasses his core commitment to caring for others with the need to experience care for himself?

8. *Encourage greater self-awareness.* Mindfulness approaches would help Ted develop greater awareness of his thoughts and feelings. Insight-oriented therapy could foster a deeper understanding of the forces that have shaped Ted's development, his response to trauma, and his spiritual struggles. This self-awareness could also help Ted make more active and informed choices about both his life goals and pathways to attain them.

Through the spiritual assessment, Ted's therapist had developed an ambitious therapeutic plan. It was (1) multidimensional, targeting thoughts, behaviors, relationships, emotions, struggles, symptoms, and ingredients of wholeness; (2) a plan that cut across time, covering developmental and traumatic events in the past, experiences in the present, and visions for the future; (3) multimodal, drawing on a variety of therapeutic tools and resources that come from diverse treatment orientations; and (4) attentive to both immediate needs for stability and conservation, and longer-term needs for more substantive transformation and growth. Like all therapeutic plans, this one would require adjustments depending on the client's own goals, response to the plan, interest in short-term versus long-term treatment, time constraints for therapy, and new information and insights that accumulate over the course of care. However, preliminary as it is, the plan would provide the therapist with a necessary road map to help guide the direction of psychological care.

HOW TO ADDRESS SPIRITUAL STRUGGLES

We switch gears now to consider what therapists should do when their clients bring spiritual struggles into psychotherapy. Our focus here is on the basic practices that apply to the full range of spiritual struggles. In the chapters to follow, we consider how to respond to more specific types of spiritual struggles. Although we place primary attention on spiritual struggles, it is important to keep in mind that psychotherapy with spiritual struggles does not replace the need for attention to other aspects of the clinical case. In the case of Ted above, the therapist's treatment plan called for crisis intervention, evaluation for psychotropic medications, and exposure therapy for symptoms of PTSD, as well as interventions to help Ted grow through his struggles. Clinical work with spiritual struggles is simply one part, albeit an often neglected yet integral part, of the larger process of psychotherapy.

Become a Trusted Guide

What determines whether people make positive changes in psychotherapy? In many cases, the best predictor of change does not appear to be whether the client receives a particular form of psychotherapy (e.g., psychodynamic, CBT, ACT) but rather the strength of the working relationship between client and therapist

(Horvath et al., 2011). Regardless of whether the therapist is working from a psychodynamic, CBT, or ACT model, he or she is unlikely to be effective if the client does not feel a sense of security and safety in the relationship. To venture into areas of vulnerability and uncertainty, such as spiritual struggles, it takes a great deal of trust in the therapist's ability to provide caring guidance.

"Guidance" here is not meant to suggest that the therapist knows what is best for the client, what purposes he or she should pursue, or how best to realize those ends. Instead, guidance refers to the therapist's skill in helping the client explore, discover, and achieve his or her own significant goals in living. The ultimate goal of this process is for the client to become more self-guiding along the path to greater wholeness and growth. Bergin (1991) speaks well to this point:

> The [client] being influenced becomes stronger, more assertive, and independent; the person learns ways of clarifying and testing value choices; the influencer decreases dependency, nurturance, and external advice; and the person experiments with new behaviors and ideas until he or she becomes more mature and autonomous. (p. 395)

In becoming a trusted guide, the therapist becomes a part of the client's orienting system, offering a sense of new possibilities, direction, and inspiration to the client who is feeling disoriented and downhearted. As part of the client's orienting system, the therapist can model qualities of wholeness, including a broad and deep approach to living, an ability to infuse life with hope and compassion, and the capacity to weave the threads of life together into a more unified tapestry. As therapy unfolds, the therapist has opportunities to demonstrate how to look beneath the surface of oneself and one's world, how to discover and hold on to a guiding vision in difficult times, how to welcome rather than avoid change, how to find balance between competing needs and interests, how to respond to challenging situations with discernment and sensitivity, and how to live with ambiguity and paradox.

In working with spiritual struggles, Jones (2019) offers the useful metaphor of the therapist as a midwife guiding the client through the waxing and waning of contractions:

> Sometimes working with a spiritual struggle requires incredible focus—going deep with a client and staying there as long as it takes. And sometimes it requires taking a break, giving you and your client some time to catch your breath, affirming the good labor that's happening, and preparing yourself to ride the next wave. (p. 6)

Becoming a trusted guide is an important task for all forms of psychotherapy. It is, however, especially important with clients who feel overwhelmed by their struggles.

Be Present to Spiritual Struggles

Few therapists go through their careers without encountering clients who have experienced tremendous loss, trauma, and subsequent struggle. Consider this example.

Janelle, a 64-year-old African American woman and deacon in her African Methodist Episcopal (AME) church, came to therapy severely depressed. Over the past 5 years she had served as caregiver to both of her parents with dementia; suffered the loss of her adult daughter from a degenerative neuromuscular disorder; and undergone her own surgery, radiation, and chemotherapy for breast cancer. To top it all, Janelle's husband of 45 years had recently suffered a stroke that left him paralyzed on one side and unable to speak. Janelle felt immobilized by not only this series of cascading crises but by the questions they raised for her faith. Why?, she continually asked herself. Why had God taken these loving people, good Christians all, from the world? Why had God allowed this suffering? Members of Janelle's church had only made matters worse, suggesting that surely her misfortunes were a sign that she had stepped out of God's good graces. In an effort to provide some spiritual support, Janelle's therapist commented on the parallel between Janelle's cataclysmic losses and the biblical story of Job. This attempt at support backfired, provoking an angry response from Janelle: "No, I'm no Job and I don't expect God to replace my good fortunes like He did Job's. I don't expect Him to give me more children. And I don't expect Him to let me live another 140 years. I'd be happy if God just left me alone."

Janelle's therapist was certainly working out of a desire to provide some emotional and spiritual relief. And yet, her attempt at spiritual support was premature. What Janelle needed most of all was the simple presence of someone who could sit quietly with Janelle, listening to her painful story, bearing witness to her suffering without comment. This is the lesson Karff (2015) shares from his years of grief counseling with families: "In the freshness of such tragedy, families aren't in need of our theology as much as they need our caring presence, our listening ear, and our responsive heart" (p. 184).

Responding with presence to spiritual struggles often entails silence on the part of the therapist, but this is no easy task. For one thing, it is hard to sit quietly by while others are anguished. For another, listening to the client's story may vicariously trigger the therapist's own unresolved spiritual struggles and wounds. To avoid these difficult issues, the therapist can be sorely tempted to offer a few words of reassurance. It is important, however, to rein in this desire. Hard though it may be to provide, the therapist's silent presence in the face of spiritual struggles conveys a recognition that some aspects of life are beyond human comprehension and that the client's inner turmoil cannot be assuaged by simple though well-intended words of comfort (Frankel, 2017). Sitting quietly with a client does not mean that the therapist is distant or disengaged. As

Doehring (2015) has written, the silence of presence communicates compassion, and the sense that the therapist is suffering along with the client. The presence of the therapist can also be experienced as a conduit to a divine presence. Being present to the client's spiritual struggles is profoundly relational: it expresses the therapist's willingness to accompany the client as he or she experiences life's deepest mysteries and sources of suffering (Karff, 2015). Being a willing companion may also eventually facilitate a shift in emphasis in the therapist's role from silent presence to conversational partner with the client.

Name and Normalize Spiritual Struggles

Often, people going through stressful times feel as if they are "going crazy." This point holds true for spiritual struggles as well because they can be so distressing and disorienting. Not only that, owing to their focus on core religious beliefs, practices, and commitments, spiritual struggles may also be interpreted by clients as signs of a weak faith. It is important, then, to give a name to spiritual struggles so clients have a way of grasping what can feel truly bewildering. Practitioners can also provide clients with basic education about spiritual struggles as normative life experiences. In this vein, it is helpful to point out that spiritual struggles are not unusual, as we noted in Chapter 1. They can be found among illustrious religious figures, past and present, in foundational religious writings, and in the reports of diverse people in the general population today.

At an appropriate point in the process of therapy, therapists might also consider disclosing spiritual struggles they may have experienced themselves. By choosing to disclose their own struggles, therapists could help validate or normalize the client's experience, thereby enhancing the client's sense of support in treatment (e.g., Exline & Grubbs, 2011). However, it is important to stress that decisions to self-disclose are a matter of professional judgment and personal preference; if done, they should be thoughtfully timed and contextualized, with the aim of any therapist self-disclosure not to shift the focus to the practitioner's struggles but rather to help normalize the client's struggles.

Spiritual struggles can also be normalized by placing them in their larger developmental context. We have stressed that growth is not possible without times of turmoil and struggle. Therapists can draw on many metaphors to reframe spiritual struggles in this bigger picture. Spiritual struggles can be likened to a time of darkness that is necessary for growth, just as the darkness of the womb is necessary for growth and birth (Kidd, 2016). Spiritual struggles can serve as a reminder that life is cyclical with endings leading to new beginnings, just as the planted seed must break apart before grain can emerge from it (Frankel, 2005). And spiritual struggles can be reframed as a part of the larger cup of life that has to be emptied out at times to pour something new in; the cup cannot always be full (Rupp, 1997). As a group, these metaphors provide a way to make initial sense of what may otherwise seem totally nonsensical. Reframing spiritual struggles in any of these benevolent and ultimately hopeful fashions can get tricky, though. If offered prematurely or in an insensitive way, clients may perceive the therapist as attempting to minimize or discount their pain. That is not the purpose of reframing. The research and clinical literature make clear that pain and problems are often intertwined with spiritual struggles. In reframing spiritual struggles, the therapist conveys that, even though distress, disorientation, and turmoil are often part and parcel of spiritual struggles, these experiences also carry with them a larger potential for renewal, positive transformation, and growth. Reframing suggestions then can be offered in an open, tentative manner by noting that some people find it helpful to think about spiritual struggles in alternative ways and that perhaps the client might as well.

There are some important exceptions to the rule of normalizing spiritual struggles. In the case of secondary spiritual struggles, religious and spiritual tension and conflict are the result of more basic psychopathology. The most central focus in these instances must be on treating the underlying psychological disorder. Griffith (2010) describes how he explains the need for psychiatric treatment of illnesses that are creating religious conflicts for patients:

> It is my best judgment that the strain from this illness upon your body is making it difficult for your brain to think clearly. I would like you to take a medication that will make it easier for you to organize your thoughts, to concentrate, and to think clearly. (p. 222)

Griffith also tries to draw on healthier aspects of the patient's religious life to mitigate the powerful negative emotions that can accompany mental illness.

Facilitate Acceptance and Reflection

Naming and normalizing spiritual struggles may help people accept and reorient themselves to the reality that they are in fact wrestling with important spiritual issues. In the previous chapter, we described research showing how important it is to acknowledge and accept rather than suppress and avoid spiritual struggles (Dworsky et al., 2016). Therapists can foster acceptance by encouraging clients to notice and observe the thoughts and feelings that accompany spiritual struggles as they would other disturbing experiences. The key message here is that it is okay to struggle, to feel unsettled and experience the myriad feelings and thoughts that are part of struggle. Kornfield (1993) has written a mindfulness exercise of special relevance to acceptance in the face of spiritual struggles. After having the individual sit quietly and breathe naturally, Kornfield instructs:

> Cast your attention over all the battles that still exist in your life. . . . If you have been fighting inner wars with your feelings . . . sense the struggle you have been

waging. Notice the struggles in your thoughts as well. Be aware of how you have carried on the inner battles. Notice the inner armies, the inner dictators, the inner fortifications. . . .

Gently, with openness, allow each of these experiences to be present. Simply notice each of them in turn with interest and kind attention. In each area of struggle, let your body, heart, and soul be soft. Open to whatever you experience without fighting. Let it be present just as it is. Let go of the battle. Breathe quietly and let yourself be at rest. Invite all parts of yourself to join you at the peace table in your heart. (p. 30)

The acceptance of spiritual struggles opens up vital opportunities for self-reflection and analysis. As Murray-Swank and Murray-Swank (2012) point out, it is not enough to accept and express spiritual struggles; clients also need help in making meaning of the struggles. To that end, therapists can help clients examine how their spiritual struggles developed. Recall that struggles grow out of many factors: life crises, the client's spiritual and more general orienting system, and the client's significant purposes. Clients can also be encouraged to explore how they have been impacted by their spiritual struggles: psychologically, socially, physically, and spiritually. Because spiritual struggles are manifestations of core rifts and conflicts in the individual's world, explorations of these struggles can be a source of "sacred revelation" (cf. Frankel, 2017, p. 240).

Even so, this kind of reflection can be challenging; clients may have little experience with self-reflection, particularly in the spiritual part of their lives. Doehring (2015) has noted that many people hold a set of beliefs, values, and attitudes toward religion and spirituality that are largely implicit and preconscious. Guidance and encouragement may be necessary if clients are to develop greater conscious awareness of their spiritual perspective and move from their "embedded theology" to what Doehring (2015) calls a more "intentional theology."

Difficult though it may be to achieve, the process of reflecting upon spiritual struggles can offer deep insights into areas of brokenness in need of repair and areas of wholeness in need of development. With critical self-awareness, clients can use their spiritual struggles to make more conscious and intentional choices about the destinations they seek and the paths they hope to take in their lives.

Help Access Resources

Clients rarely come to therapy empty-handed. They carry along with them many personal and social resources. In the midst of their turmoil, however, they often lose touch with what has worked for them in the past, and forget even the most basic, such as eating and sleeping regularly, talking to friends and family, and going to work. One of the simplest but most important gifts therapists can give clients is to remind them of the resources they already have available to them, and encourage them to tap more fully into these sources of support and strength. This point applies to spiritual struggles, too. We explore these resources in greater detail in chapters to come. Below we highlight two sets of resources: social and spiritual.

Because spiritual struggles can be alienating, one important task of therapy with struggling clients is to help them reestablish connections (Murray-Swank & Murray-Swank, 2012). Clients can be encouraged to seek out support from others who have also struggled spiritually. For example, some religious congregations have begun to create "a communal space for complaint" by offering "Doubt Nights," a time when members can come together to share their questions and doubts about matters of faith, without fear of judgment or criticism (Beck, 2007, p. 77). Support of this kind can be reassuring to clients who feel alone in their struggles. Here are the words of one college student who participated in Winding Road, a group therapeutic psychoeducational program for spiritual strugglers (Dworsky et al., 2013):

> Being able to talk about my spiritual struggles is not something I get to do . . . to just talk about my spiritual struggle without being judged and just being able to get it all off my chest without someone going "well, this is what you need to do" or "oh, I don't agree with that" . . . I felt better. It made me stronger . . . realizing I was not alone. (p. 329)

Group support for spiritual struggles, however, may be hard to find. If it is not available, clients can also look for one or two people in their own network who could provide a listening ear and, as importantly, share their own experiences with spiritual struggles.

Jung (1954/1985) once said that "religions are psychotherapeutic systems in the truest sense of the word, and on the grandest scale" (p. 172). It may seem paradoxical, though, that a client's religion or spirituality could be a valuable resource for tensions and conflicts embedded in religion and spirituality. As we have stressed, however, spiritual struggles can touch particular areas of spiritual life, leaving others unaffected. This helps to explain how religion and spirituality can at times be both a problem and a solution. Research by Abu-Raiya, Pargament, and Krause (2016) illustrates this point. They identified several religious factors (e.g., spiritual coping, seeing life as sacred, religious hope, and commitment) that helped to cushion the effects of spiritual struggles on unhappiness and depression (Abu-Raiya, Pargament, & Krause, 2016). Also, relevant here is a study by Schnitker et al. (2021) who found that two virtues—gratitude and patience in the face of hardships in life—tempered the relationship between struggles of ultimate meaning and the risk of suicide in a sample of Christian psychiatric inpatients. Perhaps similar effects would occur with other forms of spiritual struggles.

McGee, Zhao, Myers, and Eaton (2018) illustrate the point that religion and spirituality can be both a problem and a solution in their description of Mrs. A, a 58-year-old African American woman diagnosed with early-stage Alzheimer's disease. In addition to her loss of cognitive functioning, Mrs. A was experiencing spiritual struggles, particularly a sense of "spiritual desolation" when she felt mistreated by members of her meditation group and then had to move into an assisted living center. With the encouragement of her therapist, Mrs. A found support from several spiritual resources: a small group that read Scriptures and inspirational books; involvement in a Unitarian church; and spiritual practices, such as walking a labyrinth to remind her that she remained on a meaningful path in her own life. This is simply one example. Practitioners have begun to integrate other religious and spiritual resources—prayer, meditation, spiritual coping, theodicy, and forgiveness—into intervention programs to address spiritual struggles and trauma. These efforts have shown promising results in clinical evaluation studies.

One set of interventions focuses specifically on ways to address spiritual struggles and wounds. These include programs for military veterans who are traumatized (Harris et al., 2011; Starnino et al., 2019), patients with HIV/AIDS (Tarakeshwar, Pearce, & Sikkema, 2005), adult survivors of sexual abuse (Murray-Swank & Pargament, 2005), college students (Dworsky et al., 2013), and people with psychiatric problems (Reist Gibbel, Regueiro, & Pargament, 2019). Another set of programs incorporates a spiritual struggles component within a broader set of spiritual and nonspiritual interventions. Programs of this kind have been developed for people with cancer (Cole & Pargament, 1999), older adult survivors of trauma (Bowland, Edmond, & Fallot, 2012), individuals with major depressive disorder and medical illness (Pearce & Koenig, 2016), and child survivors of modern-day slavery in Haiti (Wang et al., 2016).

It is important to consider the possibility that other psychological interventions, not designed with spiritual struggles in mind, may in fact impact this process. In this regard, Loewenthal (2019) described how the topic of spiritual struggles arose spontaneously in eye movement desensitization and reprocessing (EMDR) therapy with orthodox Jewish women who had experienced trauma. EMDR reportedly helped participants resolve not only their psychological distress but their spiritual difficulties as well. We examine some of the programs that address specific spiritual struggles in more detail in subsequent chapters.

CONCLUSIONS

Because spiritual struggles are often fundamentally disorienting, one aspect of therapy with strugglers focuses on helping them regain a sense of equilibrium. Important as it is, though, regaining equilibrium is only part of the clinical task in working with spiritual struggles, and perhaps the easier part at that. By their very nature, spiritual struggles are also revealing of the client's deepest longings, most fundamental beliefs, and greatest questions. Therapy with spiritual struggles, then, often goes beneath the surface, deepening the process of psychotherapy as a whole. This work can be challenging and difficult, but it also opens up possibilities for fundamental changes, changes that can lead to greater wholeness and growth.

In this chapter, we provided some guidelines for how to address spiritual struggles in clinical work. Our review here was brief and basic. We explored the steps involved in assessing spiritual struggles within the larger context of clinical assessment, and we considered some of the general methods practitioners can apply to their work with clients who struggle spiritually.

Until this point in the book, our focus has been on spiritual struggles as a group. Yet, as we noted in the first chapter, spiritual struggles are plural as well as singular. We have identified six distinctive, albeit interrelated, types of spiritual struggle (Exline, Pargament, Grubbs, & Yali, 2014). As we will see, each struggle represents tensions, conflicts, and strains about a different core set of religious and spiritual issues. In the chapters that follow, we delve more deeply into the ways practitioners can address each of these types of spiritual struggles. We review cutting-edge research and practice in these areas. Chapters 8–13 are organized similarly according to (1) what we are learning about each type of struggle through emerging study, and (2) how practitioners can apply this knowledge to each form of struggle.

CHAPTER 8

Divine Struggles

Where is God? This is one of the most disquieting symptoms . . . go to Him when your need is desperate, when all other help is vain, and what do you find? A door slammed in your face, and a sound of bolting on the inside. After that silence. You might as well turn away. . . . Not that I am (I think) in real danger of ceasing to believe in God. The real danger is of coming to believe such dreadful things about Him.
—Lewis (1961, pp. 9–10)

At the core of spirituality is the human yearning for a relationship with something larger or deeper than our limited selves, something sacred. Most people, especially those who come from monotheistic traditions, think about the sacred in personal and relational terms. People seek a relationship with what they perceive as divine. Like other ties, however, the individual's relationship with the divine can be marked by conflict, tension, and strain, as we hear in the words above from C. S. Lewis (1961) following the death of his wife. Lewis's example also highlights that even the most devout individual—Lewis was a lay theologian and Christian apologist—can have "winter experiences" with God in which they experience a full range of negative emotions (Beck, 2007). The emotions that accompany struggles with the divine can add to the pain and distress of the psychological problems people bring to therapy, but they may also be a source of positive transformation and growth. Of all the various types of spiritual struggles, divine struggles have received the most attention from researchers and practitioners. However, it is important to note from the outset that, with rare exceptions (e.g., Exline, Kamble, & Stauner, 2017), the vast majority of this attention has focused on the struggles of monotheists as opposed to polytheists or those who envision the sacred in nonpersonal forms, such as karma or natural forces. We begin our focus on specific spiritual struggles by considering divine struggles—what we have learned about them from systematic study and, building on this knowledge, how to approach them in psychotherapy.

WHAT WE KNOW ABOUT DIVINE STRUGGLES

Divine struggles revolve around questions, conflicts, and tensions about the individual's understanding of and relationship with the divine. It might be tempting to dismiss these kinds of strains as exceptions to the rule of the close connection many people feel toward God, and, in fact, positive feelings toward the divine are far more common than negative ones (Exline et al., 2011). Nevertheless, though they may be among the least common of all spiritual struggles (Abu-Raiya, Pargament, Krause, et al., 2015; Exline, Pargament, Grubbs, & Yali, 2014), struggles with God are not at all unusual. Stories of divine struggle can be found in sacred texts and in modern-day narrative accounts. In our empirical work with several subsamples that total over 18,000 people, we asked how often in the past few weeks they had experienced struggles related to God, such as anger, disappointment, and feeling punished or abandoned by God. We found that 32.6% reported some degree of divine struggle over the past few weeks (Exline, Pargament, & Grubbs, 2014). Groups dealing with major life stressors may be even more likely to encounter divine struggles (Winkelman et al., 2011). In short, the individual's relationship with the divine is not infrequently marked by times of tension, strain, and conflict.

Let's take a closer look. Research on divine struggles is still in its early stages of development, but we have learned some important things.

Divine Struggles Revolve around a Variety of Negative Emotions and Are Not Unusual

Just as people can experience a range of emotions in their interpersonal relationships, they can have a variety of feelings toward the divine, including negative emotions. It is useful to delineate three interrelated subtypes of divine struggles that center on different negative emotions: anger toward God, concerns about divine punishment or disapproval by God, and alienation from God.

Anger toward God

One form of divine struggle, anger toward God, has been reported by people for thousands of years. The anger may take milder forms of feelings of frustration, disappointment, or impatience, or stronger forms, such as rage and hatred. The Hebrew Bible is filled with the voices of religious figures expressing their discontent with God, from Moses's complaints about God's mistreatment of the Israelites enslaved by the pharaoh in Egypt to perhaps the ultimate example of

Job, who boldly calls God to account for his suffering: "Does it seem good to you to oppress, to despise the work of your hands and favor the schemes of the wicked?" (Job 10:3).

Contemporary examples are not hard to find, either. One mother whose daughter had survived many medical procedures as an infant, only to be murdered as an adult, expressed her anger toward God:

> The hatred that I had, that God let me down. . . . Here was this baby, one pound, three ounces. He [God] didn't even take her every time she went under anesthesia. That He could have taken her any time He wanted, but yet He let her be murdered, stabbed to death the way she was. (Johnson & Armour, 2016, p. 282)

Animosity toward God has also been portrayed in modern literature. One of the most striking literary expressions of anger toward the divine can be found in Elie Wiesel's (1979) play *The Trial of God*, in which God stands accused and ultimately convicted of the brutal Chmielnicki pogroms in which 100,000 Jews were murdered. Wiesel reportedly based the play on an actual small trial of God he witnessed in the concentration camp of Auschwitz where God was also accused and found guilty of crimes against humanity by a small group of inmates.

Surveys also underscore the commonality of anger toward God. Much of the research on anger toward God has been pioneered by Julie Exline and her research group. Working with a nationally representative sample of Americans obtained through the 1988 General Social Survey, they found that 62% indicated that they sometimes feel angry toward God (Exline et al., 2011). Among groups facing major life stressors, substantial numbers of people report at least some anger toward God, including 40% of those who lost a loved one (Exline et al., 2011) and 60% of Israeli women with breast cancer (Baider & Sarell, 1983).

Concerns about Divine Punishment

While the divine struggles of some people are marked predominantly by anger toward God, the struggles of others are defined more by feelings that God is angry with, displeased with, or is punishing them. To place this type of struggle in context it is important to note that stories of compassion, kindness, and mercy abound in scriptural writings across religious traditions. Within monotheistic religions, these accounts center around a divine being often depicted as a loving and just parent. Like a parent, the divine is actively involved in rewarding people for their good behavior but may also punish people for their transgressions. In the Hebrew Bible, divine punishments are well known, from the banishment of Adam and Eve from the Garden of Eden after eating fruit from the Tree of Knowledge (Genesis 3:11-24) to the great floods that destroyed much of humanity because of their wickedness (Genesis 6:1-7). The New Testament also contains vivid descriptions of the punishment awaiting those who engage in immoral acts: "But the cowardly, the unbelieving, the vile, the murderers, the sexually immoral . . . they will be consigned to the fiery lake of burning sulfur" (Revelation 21:8). Similarly, sacred Islamic texts offer powerful descriptions of divinely based disasters visited on communities that take the wrong path, such as the people of Ad: "And the Ad, they were destroyed by a furious wind, exceedingly violent" (al-Haaqqa, 6-8).

Steeped in this sense of God's potential for retribution, many people today struggle with feelings that their misfortunes are punishments by God. These struggles are often accompanied by guilt, shame, confusion, and uncertainty about the potential for further divine retribution. For example, a 21-year-old woman wondered whether a disabling stroke she had experienced came as the result of an offense against God: "She felt that she no longer knew God. God had never let serious harm come to her. Now she didn't know what to think. Had she done something to displease God?" (Magyar-Russell et al., 2013, p. 132). Attributions to a punishing God can also be applied to the misfortunes of others, as we hear in the words of one woman to another who had been diagnosed with cancer: "Surely, there's something in your life which is displeasing to God. . . . You must have stepped out of His will somewhere. These things don't just happen" (Yancey, 1977, p. 13).

Reports of feeling punished by God are not uncommon but they vary considerably from culture to culture. Winkelman et al. (2011) found that 22% of patients with advanced cancer in the United States agreed to some degree that their cancer was a punishment from God for their sins and lack of devotion. However, a different picture emerges outside of the United States. Among people with sickle cell disease in the West Indies, a strikingly higher number (74%) strongly endorsed a similar item (Morgan et al., 2014). Likewise, 57% of Salvadoran earthquake survivors attributed the disaster to "God's punishment of Man's evil behavior, violence, or lack of prayers and respect"; this was the most common of all explanations (Vazquez, Cervellón, Pérez-Sales, Vidales, & Gaborit, 2005, p. 318). Culture appears to count when it comes to the divine struggle of feeling punished by God.

Feeling Isolated from God

A third subtype of divine struggles centers on feelings of being isolated from or even abandoned by God. Adherents of the world's major monotheistic traditions learn from the sacred texts that God is available and present in their lives. Yet, the same texts contain expressions of isolation and alienation from the divine. The psalmist asks, "How long, O Lord? Will you forget me forever? How long will You hide Your face from me?" (Psalm 13:1). On the cross at the end of his life, Jesus cries out his own powerful feelings of divine abandonment: "My God, my God, why has though forsaken me?" (Matthew 27:46).

These expressions of alienation are not a thing of the past. Consider, for example, part of the prayer of lamentation written in memory of the six million Jews killed in the Holocaust: "Why didst thou forsake us, O our God? Why didst thou stand afar at the time of our distress? Why didst though keep silent when the tyrants spilled our blood like water?" (Fundaminsky, 2000, p. 349). In recent years, we have discovered that Mother Teresa experienced an intense and prolonged sense of alienation from God throughout her years of selfless devotion to the women, men, and children living in the slums of Calcutta. At one point, she wrote,

> The place of God in my soul is blank. There is no God in me. When the pain of longing is so great—I just long and long for God—and then it is that I feel—He does not want me—He is not there—The torture and pain I can't explain. (Teresa & Kolodiejchuk, 2007, p. 210)

A relatively small but still noteworthy number of people in the United States describe feeling isolated from God to some extent. Among college students, 27% reported that over the past few months they had felt as though God had abandoned them (Exline, Pargament, & Hall, 2014b). Twenty-nine percent of U.S. adults with advanced cancer indicated wondering to some degree whether God had abandoned them (Winkelman et al., 2011). As with the findings related to struggling with a punishing God, a larger percentage of people in other cultures report struggles of isolation from God. In their study of people with sickle cell disease from the West Indies, 74% reportedly wondered whether God had abandoned them (Morgan et al., 2014).

Additional Points to Consider

Three additional points are important to consider when we think about these different kinds of divine struggles. First, the figures we presented on the commonality of various types of divine struggles may be underestimates. As stressed in earlier chapters, people may be unaware of or reluctant to admit to their negative emotions toward God because they believe these feelings are morally unacceptable or a potential source of social stigma (Exline & Grubbs, 2011; Exline et al., 2012). In addition, conflicts with the divine may lie beneath the surface of conscious awareness.

Second, the three subtypes of divine struggles that we just considered are not independent of one another. In fact, they are often interconnected, as research has shown. For example, in a largely Hindu university sample, anger toward God was correlated significantly with views of God as cruel, distant, and punishing (Exline, Kamble, et al., 2017).

Finally, we have to think very carefully about the relationship between experiences of divine struggles and nonbelief. On the one hand, divine struggles do not typically signify a lack of belief in God. Many of the examples of divine struggles we presented above came from exemplary religious figures: Jesus, Job, King David, C. S. Lewis, and Mother Teresa. Their conflicts, protests, and challenges to God rest on an underlying hunger for a relationship with the divine. On the other hand, we cannot assume that nonbelief in God necessarily frees people from divine struggles. In fact, Exline et al. (2014b) found that 25% of nonbelieving college students voiced some anger around the idea of God, and 16% reported concerns about God's disapproval. How do we explain these puzzling findings? Nonbelievers may hold negative feelings around a current, hypothetical image of God (e.g., Bradley et al., 2015), or they may recall past experiences of anger toward God when they believed in God (Bradley et al., 2017). Some might also feel anger around the idea of a God they reject consciously but continue to struggle with unconsciously. C. S. Lewis, in his 1955 autobiographical book *Surprised by Joy,* said this about an earlier phase of his life: "I had maintained that God did not exist. I was also very angry at God for not existing" (p. 111). In psychotherapy, then, it is important to remain open to the possibility of divine struggles among people who span the full spectrum of religiousness—from the most to the least devout.

Divine Struggles Are Accompanied by Distress, Disorientation, and Serious Consequences

Struggles with the divine can pose a challenge to individuals' sources of greatest value and purpose, and to their core beliefs, practices, experiences, and connections that guide and orient them toward significant ends. Each type of divine struggle targets particular areas of significance and life orientation. In the experience of anger toward God, the individual grapples with questions about whether God and life more generally are fair. Feelings of being punished or disapproved by God can elicit guilt, shame, and questions about self-worth. The struggle of feeling distant from or abandoned by God raises basic concerns about whether the individual is a part of the world or apart from it and whether God actually exists (Exline, Grubbs, & Homolka, 2015). Beneath the surface of these struggles with the divine we can often find unfulfilled longings for protection, connection, fairness, self-esteem, control, and a repaired relation with the divine itself. No surprise then that, like spiritual struggles more generally, divine struggles are accompanied by distress and disorientation, as well as potentially more serious consequences.

The research is clear here: divine struggles as a group are associated with higher levels of psychological distress and/or lower well-being across a variety of groups facing a variety of problems. Just a few examples of these include patients with breast cancer (Gall, Kristjansson, Charbonneau, & Florack, 2009); survivors of the 1993 Midwest floods (Smith, Pargament, Brant, & Oliver, 2000);

Christians bereaved by homicide, suicide, or fatal accidents (Neimeyer & Burke, 2017); people facing acute financial stressors (Gutierrez, Park, & Wright, 2017); adolescents who have been sexually abused (Jouriles et al., 2020); and Hindus in the United States coping with major life stressors (Tarakeshwar et al., 2003). Conflicts with the divine, these studies show, can be disconcerting and disorienting.

Some studies also suggest that divine struggles may be especially problematic for people who are more religious (Pargament, Tarakeshwar, Ellison, & Wulff, 2001) and have a closer religious bond in their marriages (Jung, 2020). Because these individuals may center their lives more around God, struggles with the divine may be particularly disruptive.

Divine struggles can have significant consequences that go beyond distress and disorientation. A case study by psychiatrist Larkin Kao and her colleagues illustrates this point (Kao, Shah, Pargament, Griffith, & Peteet, 2019). The patient, Mr. W, was seen in the hospital following a self-inflicted gunshot wound. Mr. W had had a history of major depression and heavy drinking. He said that he had been feeling terribly guilty about how his alcohol use and marital infidelity had damaged his marriage and his relationship with his children. Not only that, he struggled deeply with whether his transgressions meant that he could no longer be loved by God. So he decided to put the question to a test by "gambling with God" (p. 66). Loading a revolver with a random set of blanks and bullets, he put the gun to his head and told himself that if he fired a blank, it would mean that God loved him. Unfortunately, the gun went off. Mr. W sustained multiple injuries but survived. In this case, struggles with feelings of divine alienation and insecurity had life-threatening consequences.

Research studies have shown that, in some cases, intense struggles with God can be linked with serious mental health symptoms. These include suicidality among U.S. veterans (Raines et al., 2017) and men recovering from substance use disorders (Currier et al., 2020); symptoms of PTSD among African survivors of torture (Leaman & Gee, 2012) and Americans following the 9/11 terrorist attacks (Meisenhelder & Marcum, 2004); and behaviors associated with disordered eating, such as purging, excessive exercise, and fasting (Exline, Homolka, & Harriott, 2016).

The findings from these cross-sectional studies have been supplemented by a few longitudinal studies that suggest that divine struggles may play a primary role in the development of problems. One study showed that struggles with God were tied to a higher risk of subsequent hospitalizations and depression among patients with chronic heart failure (Park et al., 2011). Another 12-month longitudinal study of adults with cystic fibrosis revealed that feelings of alienation and isolation from God were associated with increases in depression (Sherman et al., 2021). Finally, among older patients who were medically ill, the risk of dying over the next 2 years was greater for those who endorsed two divine struggles items: "wondered whether God has abandoned me" and "questioned God's love for me" (Pargament, Koenig, et al., 2001).

Are There Any Benefits of Divine Struggles?

The general pattern of findings here links divine struggles to distress, disorientation, and potentially serious negative consequences. But is this the full story? Are there any benefits of divine struggles? Recall that, from the perspective of our spiritual model, divine struggles, like other spiritual struggles, can be a source of benefits, including growth and transformation.

As a case in point, feelings about a punishing God could conceivably constrain destructive behaviors. Griffith (2010) offers the illustration of a suicidal middle-age woman who had suffered a head injury in a car accident. Although she felt that God was responsible for her injury and unconcerned with her present suffering, her fears about God kept her from hurting herself: "She could not imagine God feeling compassion for her, but feared God's judgment if she were to commit suicide" (p. 102). Shariff and Norenzayan (2011) provide another illustration of the constraining value of a punishing view of God in two laboratory studies of college students. They found that students who saw God in more punitive terms (e.g., harsh, vengeful) were less likely to cheat on what they felt to be an anonymous computer task. Along similar lines, some research shows that countries with a higher proportion of people who believe in hell manifest significantly lower crime rates (Shariff & Rhemtulla, 2012).

These findings need to be considered in light of several other studies that link feelings of divine punishment with clearly negative outcomes, such as faster disease progression over 4 years among patients with HIV (Ironson et al., 2011) and less independent physical functioning among older individuals who are medically ill over 2 years (Pargament et al., 2004). Groopman (2004) provides the poignant clinical example of a 29-year-old Jewish woman who had been diagnosed with breast cancer. She believed that the cancer was a punishment from God for an affair she had had, and refused to seek chemotherapy or help of any kind. She died in silence.

We are left then with the question of what determines whether feelings and beliefs related to a punishing God may be beneficial (at least in some ways) or harmful. One key may lie in the degree to which God is seen as punishing in a loving corrective fashion, akin to an authoritative but kindly parent, or punishing in a harsh, mean-spirited, capricious way. The experience of struggles with a punishing God may well center more around the latter than the former type of appraisal.

What about the potential for more wholesale growth through divine struggles? The "dark night of the soul"—those periods of deep despair and desolation in relation to the divine—were perceived by many exemplary religious figures (e.g., Saint Augustine, Saint Teresa of Ávila, Mother Teresa) as chances to develop in the virtues, purify one's soul, deepen in self-understanding, and form a stronger union with God (Durà-Vilà & Dein, 2009). Unfortunately, systematic study is lacking as yet on this important topic. The weight of the evidence we do have makes clear that divine struggles are tied to disorientation, distress, and serious negative consequences. This underscores how important it is for therapists to be able to understand and assist people wrestling with divine conflicts. Learning more about the roots of divine struggles is another key part of that understanding.

Roots of Divine Struggles

According to our model of spirituality (see Chapter 2), spiritual struggles generally grow out of three interrelated factors: life events and transitions, the significant purposes the individual seeks in life, and the individual's orienting system. Below we consider how these three factors set the stage for divine struggles in particular.

Negative Life Events and Transitions

Empirical studies have shown that divine struggles are more likely to follow encounters with more severe, disruptive life events (e.g., Exline, Homolka, & Grubbs, 2013; Exline et al., 2011; Lyons et al., 2011). Some of the strongest evidence of this effect comes from survivors of physical and sexual abuse (Fallot & Heckman, 2005; Gall, 2006; Korbman, Pirutinsky, Feindler, & Rosmarin, 2021), who are apt to suffer a myriad of negative feelings toward God following their traumas. This is how one survivor of incest vents her rage toward God:

> How could you in all your greatness have abandoned me, a little girl, to the merciless hands of my father? . . . I have been faithful, and for what, to be raped and abused by my own father? I hate and despise you . . . your name is like salt on my tongue. I vomit it from my being. I wish death upon you. You are no more. You are dead. (Flaherty, 1992, p. 101)

People can point the finger of blame toward God in many situations. Like the survivor of incest, many may blame God for their suffering even when humans are clearly responsible, such as instances of assault, wartime atrocities, pregnancy following a rape, and divorce (Exline, 2020). God can also be blamed for the individual's moral weaknesses by having created him or her in this way (Grubbs & Exline, 2014). Other negative events that cannot be pinned on human misconduct—natural disasters, freakish accidents, and untimely deaths—can be even more easily blamed on God or attributed to a punishing or abandoning God. In addition, as Exline et al. (2011; Exline, Homolka, et al., 2013) have noted from studies and conversations with strugglers, less momentous stressful situations (e.g., rain on a special occasion, an injury that prevents participation in an athletic event) can trigger divine struggles.

Why do people experience conflicts and negative emotions related to God across such a wide range of situations? Based on a variety of empirical studies, Exline (2020) maintains that the key theme underlying divine struggles (and anger toward God in particular) is the perception that God is somehow complicit in undeserved suffering. God is generally counted on to offer protection from mistreatment and unfairness, and when innocent people suffer or evil acts go unpunished, people get mad at God. To put it in a nutshell, anger occurs when God is seen as failing to live up to peoples' expectations. In a related way, feelings of punishment by God may be grounded in the perceptions that the individual has failed to live up to the expectations God holds for him or her. Thus, major life events may elicit divine struggles, at least in part, because they threaten, challenge, or damage the individual's underlying set of foundational beliefs, practices, social connections, or values. To understand the roots of divine struggles, then, we must also consider the individual's orienting system and significant purposes in living.

Orienting System and Significance

Several characteristics of the orienting system and significant life purposes leave people vulnerable to divine struggles, especially in the context of life events and transitions. Although many factors are important here (see Chapter 3 for a lengthier discussion of the roots of spiritual struggles as a group), emerging theory and research point to three characteristics of the orienting system that may be especially relevant to the development of divine struggles. First, perhaps not surprisingly, individuals who have difficulties regulating their emotions generally are also more likely to experience emotional conflicts with God. In several empirical studies, divine struggles have been associated with indicators of emotional dysregulation, such as neuroticism (Werdel, Dy-Liacco, Ciarrocchi, Wicks, & Breslford, 2014), emotional exhaustion and depression (Büssing, Baumann, Jacobs, & Frick, 2017), and trait anger (Exline, Yali, & Lobel, 1999). Self-views are often linked to emotion regulation (see, e.g., Grubbs & Exline, 2014), and divine struggles have been tied to certain self-views, including low levels of self-esteem, self-compassion, and humility (Grubbs & Exline, 2014; Grubbs et al., 2016, 2017).

Second, divine struggles are partially rooted in limited representations of God. One example involves the lack of a cohesive picture of God. Psychodynamic theorists have underscored the multilayered, multidimensional nature of God representations (Hall & Fujikawa, 2013; Rizzuto, 1979). Like an onion, new layers of beliefs and emotions about the divine are created over older layers over the lifespan. While some people are aware of their divine representations and able to form a cohesive whole, others are not. Earlier embedded beliefs (cf. Doehring, 2015) may be repressed or fall outside of conscious awareness. This creates the potential for what LaMothe (2009) described as an internal "clash of Gods" in which people struggle with confusing and contradictory beliefs, emotions, and desires about the divine, such as the sense of divine betrayal experienced by an atheist who has not believed in God for many years, or the inability of a devout Christian to feel divine comfort from a God who has been intellectually understood as a constant loving presence.

Another limited representation involves "small gods," in the words of J. B. Phillips (1997). As discussed in Chapter 3, small gods become problematic because they do not prepare people to deal with the full range of life experiences. As a result, beliefs in small gods are more easily shaken when difficult problems come up. For example, beliefs in the "God of absolute perfection"—who insists on error-free performance—can be a precursor to struggles of feeling punished by God when the individual makes a mistake. Beliefs in a "distant star God"—who is no longer intimately involved in peoples' lives—can trigger struggles of isolation from the divine. And beliefs in God as a "heavenly bosom"—who can always be counted on for protection, love, and support—may result in anger toward the divine following experiences of profound violation or loss, when suffering continues unabated, and prayers go unanswered. The potential downside of seeing God as a heavenly bosom in times of trouble is illustrated by a finding in the Currier et al. (2020) study of recovering substance users: among those with more loving concepts of God, divine struggles were more strongly related to suicidality.

Beliefs in these small gods offer at best a limited, less-than-compelling response to the very thorny challenge of reconciling suffering and evil in the world with beliefs in God, particularly beliefs in a loving, just, and all-powerful divine being. This is the challenge of theodicy. Well over 2,000 years ago, the Greek philosopher Epicurus articulated the key questions of theodicy:

> Either God wants to get rid of evil, but he can't, or God can, but he doesn't want to; or God neither wants to nor can, or he both wants to and can. If God wants to, but can't, then he's not all-powerful. If he can, but doesn't want to, he's not all-loving. If he neither can nor wants to, he's neither all-powerful nor all-loving. And if he wants to and can—then why doesn't he remove the evils? (summarized in Zuckerman, 2012, p. 38)

Narrow concepts of God and limited responses to these difficult questions of theodicy have been linked to divine struggles in a few empirical studies. For instance, in research with college students and adults, beliefs that God is cruel and distant were associated with higher levels of current and lifetime struggles with the divine (Exline, Grubbs, et al., 2015). In another study, Wilt et al. (2016) examined the relationship between theodicies and struggles with the divine in samples of college students and adults. As predicted, participants who saw God's role in suffering as weak, malevolent, punitive, or uninvolved were more likely to experience struggles with the divine.

Third, struggles in an individual's relationship with God appear to be nested partly in the individual's more general style of attachment to key figures and God. In his seminal book *Attachment, Evolution, and the Psychology of Religion,* Lee Kirkpatrick (2005) articulated important linkages between the quality of the individual's attachment relationships with parents and the character of the individual's relationship with God. Drawing on John Bowlby's attachment theory, Kirkpatrick described how secure attachments with parents and God can provide the individual with (1) a safe haven of protection when he or she is feeling distress, and (2) a secure base that fosters the confidence to engage in explorations of the world and develop new skills. Insecure attachments, on the other hand, predispose the individual toward anxiety and avoidance in relation to other people and the world.

Research has shown that these different attachment styles have important implications for the development of divine struggles. With respect to parental attachment and struggles with God, homeless men who reported poorer relationships with fathers and mothers, historically and currently, also described more perceived problems in their relationship with God (Smith & Exline, 2002). Another study of adults and college students revealed that viewing one's mother or father as cruel was associated with greater anger toward God and feelings of God's disapproval toward the self (Exline, Homolka, et al., 2013). Other studies on the links between divine attachment styles and divine struggles have yielded similar findings. For example, working with people in the hospital waiting for loved ones undergoing surgery, Belavich and Pargament (2002) reported that a secure attachment to God was associated with less divine struggle; conversely, avoidant and ambivalent attachments to God were tied to more divine struggles.

Finally, our model of spiritual struggles suggests that divine struggles are more likely following situations in which the individual's significant purposes have been challenged, violated, or lost. Little research has been done yet on this topic. In one exception, Appel, Park, Wortmann, and van Schie (2020) found that divine struggles were more likely when the individual had experienced events that interfered with his or her ability to pursue meaningful goals.

In sum, divine struggles grow out of a complex array of situational, personal, and social forces that we have only touched on here. Of course, as we described in our model of spirituality, the spiritual journey does not end with spiritual struggles, divine and otherwise. When they develop, struggles with God are not crystallized into a fixed and final form. Instead, they create possibilities for reorientation, greater wholeness, and growth. This includes the potential for shifts throughout the lifespan in the ways the individual understands and relates to the divine. Building on what we are learning from theory and research, we turn now to ways the practitioner can address divine struggles in therapy.

HOW TO ADDRESS DIVINE STRUGGLES IN PRACTICE

In the remainder of this chapter, we discuss how therapists can approach divine struggles in clinical work, focusing on several of the ingredients of wholeness that can help the client move from distress, disorientation, and brokenness to growth.

Talk about God

We cannot help clients who are struggling with the divine, unless we can talk with them about God. Yet the idea of talking about God in psychotherapy may fill some practitioners with dread. One fear may be that of overstepping the proper boundaries of psychotherapy by venturing into the realm of theology. (The "supernatural lens" concept from Chapter 1 is relevant here.) An additional concern may be the possibility of facing one's own painful or unresolved issues about God. And yet another fear may arise about entering into unfamiliar spiritual territory, especially for therapists who do not believe in God. We cannot, however, afford to give in to these fears. Divine struggles are an appropriate, indeed, a potentially vital, topic for psychotherapy—as we have seen, the client's struggles with God can hold important implications for his or her health and well-being, and should not be ignored. It is true that therapists may need to face their own difficult spiritual issues or unresolved struggles when they work with clients who are wrestling with God, but this offers an opportunity for therapists to grow professionally and perhaps personally as well. Granted, many therapists, including atheists, may find it uncomfortable to discuss spiritual or religious topics in therapy. However, practitioners should remember that they can still talk about spiritual struggles using what we have called the psychotherapy lens (see Chapter 1). In doing so, they can discuss spiritual issues with clients in a psychological framework, without feeling the need to disclose their own beliefs, challenge the beliefs of clients, or try to answer ultimate questions about the existence or nature of a deity. Drawing on their general clinical skills, practitioners can approach a conversation about divine matters with the same openness, interest, patience, and sensitivity as they would apply to any other important, emotionally loaded subject in therapy, be it parents, divorce, sexual orientation, or illness.

Of course, the client also has to be willing to enter into a conversation about God and divine struggles. Our own clinical experience, supported by survey research, suggests that many clients welcome the chance to talk about spiritual issues, including their beliefs about God. Some clients, though, may be surprised when they hear about the possibility of including God in the therapeutic dialogue. For them, a brief rationale can be helpful. Here is one example:

> "I am getting the sense that your problems may be related in part to some struggles you may be experiencing in your relationship with God. You're

not alone—we are psychological, social, physical, and spiritual beings—and many people encounter struggles with God or others aspects of spirituality at points in their lives. I think it would be helpful to enlarge our conversation to include your thoughts and feelings about God. What do you think?"

If the client is willing, then God can enter the therapeutic conversation. One key to facilitating meaningful talk about God is asking good questions. Many of the exploratory questions that were presented as part of the explicit spiritual assessment in Chapter 7 can be easily adapted to focus specifically on divine struggles. These include questions such as "Can you tell me more about your struggles with the divine? What are they like? How have your struggles with God affected you? What do you feel led to your struggles with God? Where do you turn to for help and support in coping with your divine struggles?" The conversation generated by these questions should foster greater general awareness of the client's divine struggles and more concrete insights into how to help the client deal with these conflicts.

God talk is often hard talk for clients, and they will need encouragement, time, and patience from the therapist to go down this road. As we noted in the previous chapter, the therapist must create a safe and welcoming space for all of the client's tensions, conflicts, and emotions—including spiritual struggles. This point is especially relevant to struggles with God, which can be a source of shame, embarrassment, and fear of criticism from others, including the therapist (Jouriles et al., 2020).

Here is a sensitive approach that hospital chaplain Katherine Piderman (2015) takes toward Angela, a 17-year-old client who suffered paralysis through a car accident that raised profound questions and concerns about God. Why, Angela asks, did God do this to her? Surely, she feels, she must have done something wrong. And why was God leaving her prayers unanswered? Piderman encourages Angela to explore these questions, but patiently and methodically:

> Suffering is so hard to understand. We always have more questions than answers in the midst of it. Usually any answers we have aren't enough to take away the pain, but still somehow it seems important to voice the questions and the feelings we have about them. I'm so glad that you're doing that with me. Would you like to take a question or two and work with them and see if we can find some light, some hope as we do? (p. 77)

Therapists can also encourage conversation by normalizing divine struggles. After all, as we have seen, painful questions about God are not uncommon in the general population. Furthermore, exemplary religious figures experienced and openly expressed their own divine struggles (e.g., Jeremiah, Job, Jesus). In addition to making these points, therapists can suggest readings about divine struggles or, for those involved in a religious institution, encourage conversations with clergy who could normalize struggles. For example, in his writing, pastor George Zornow (2014) encourages clients to lament. God, he says, is big enough to hear the full range of human feelings, negative as well as positive. What makes Zornow's own work with congregation members especially noteworthy is that he models this process by sharing some of his own divine struggles and lamentations.

Being able to talk about God is a prerequisite to effective work with divine struggles. Earlier, we reviewed research showing the value of facing and accepting rather than avoiding spiritual struggles. This point holds true for divine struggles. In a study of patients with breast cancer in the United Kingdom, Thuné-Boyle, Stygall, Keshtgar, Davidson, and Newman (2013) found that divine struggles increased anxiety and depression to a greater extent among people who coped by more denial and less acceptance, respectively. On the other hand, people appear to benefit by more direct expressions of struggle with God. In this vein, Exline, Krause, and Broer (2016) studied a group of patients seeking treatment for chronic headaches and found that those who voiced more protests toward God (e.g., arguments, complaints, questions) showed a significant reduction in distress and an increased sense of meaning before and after treatment. Interestingly, anger toward God was predictive of sustained distress over time. These findings underscore the importance of distinguishing between the *experience* of anger toward God and the *expression* of anger toward God. Talking about God and divine struggles may also contribute to a repaired relationship with God. As Karff (2015) has written, people can "move from God the enemy to God the companion and friend by going through that confrontational mode. God can handle our negative thoughts" (p. 184).

Explore Benevolent Spiritual Reappraisals

Because divine struggles can be distressing and disorienting, therapists may need to stabilize and reorient the client early in treatment. Toward that end, therapists can help clients examine the disturbing questions about God's character and intentions that are often bound up in divine struggles. Is God to blame for misfortune? Is the individual experiencing divine retribution, fairly or unfairly? Has God chosen to turn away from the person? Of course, the therapist cannot know the mind of God—whether God is, in fact, to blame; whether the individual is, in fact, suffering the divine consequences of misbehavior; whether God has, in actuality, abandoned the person. Therapists can, however, explore these dark questions (as they would any sensitive issue) and, in the process, encourage clients to consider a broad range of possible explanations for their stressors, struggles, and suffering. In this regard, benevolent spiritual reappraisals deserve consideration as one hopeful response to the distress divine strugglers may face. Benevolent spiritual reappraisals are typically conservational in nature; they soften the experience of divine struggles by placing them within a larger benevolent framework of meaning and, in the process, they allow the individual to sustain life-affirming, core beliefs embedded in his or her orienting system and significant purposes in life. Benevolent spiritual reappraisals can take different forms.

First, divine struggles and the events and distress associated with them can be reappraised as rooted in divine mystery rather than divine maliciousness. Some things go beyond human understanding from this perspective. The story of Corrie ten Boom (1971) provides a case in point. She and her father were placed in a concentration camp during World War II by the Nazis for their role in harboring Jews. After the death of her father in the camp, the guard derisively asked, "What kind of God would let that old man [her father] die here in Scheveningen?" Ten Boom responded with words her father had shared with her: "Some knowledge is too heavy . . . you cannot bear it . . . your Father will carry it until you are able" (p. 163). By attributing her loss to the will of a God she could not fully know or understand, ten Boom was able to hold on to her deep faith in a caring being. Note that she did not reach any definitive insight into how a loving God could have allowed her father to die. Instead, she came to an understanding that there were larger, unknowable but ultimately benevolent forces at work in life.

Second, divine struggles and the emotions and situations surrounding them can be appraised in more benign spiritual ways that permit clients to preserve their beliefs in a well-intentioned God. For example, struggle and suffering can be reframed as divine challenges rather than divine punishments. This is the approach Frankl (1959) took in his clinical work with an older woman dealing with depression and anxiety in her dying days:

> PATIENT: You see Doctor, I regarded my suffering as a punishment. I believe in God.
>
> FRANKL: But cannot suffering sometimes also be a challenge? Is it not conceivable that God wanted to see how [you] will bear it? And perhaps He had to admit, "Yes she did so very bravely." (p. 144)

Third, rather than continue to wrestle fruitlessly with efforts to find satisfying answers to the questions of God's role in suffering and struggle, questions of "why" can be sidestepped entirely by shifting the focus to questions of "how" the individual should move forward in life. Simply listening to clients as they express their divine struggles may facilitate this shift in focus. In her clinical work with a mother who was angry at God for the loss of her daughter, Frankel (2005) sat quietly and listened as the mother expressed her rage. With time, Frankel noted that the unresolved questions of "why" that had so preoccupied the mother gradually evolved into no less profound but perhaps more constructive questions about who she will become if she's not a mother, and what part God should play in her life. Therapists can also encourage clients to postpone the difficult questions of "why" until they have had a chance to regain their emotional equilibrium.

In short, benevolent spiritual reappraisals appear to have potential value for divine strugglers. The clinical stories and anecdotes presented here are also supplemented by some research. Exline (2002a), for example, conducted a study of undergraduates who reported negative feelings toward God following a distressing event. Many felt that they had been helped in their divine struggles by various types of benevolent spiritual reappraisals, including positive reappraisals of God's intentions, seeing the event as God's will, and seeing something good come out of the event.

In spite of these positive findings, we caution therapists to approach benevolent spiritual appraisals carefully. Efforts to appraise spiritual struggles and their accompanying distress and disorientation in a more positive light could be offputting if clients feel their therapists are minimizing the reality of their pain and suffering. Appraisals of these kinds might also inadvertently contribute to denial, avoidance, and repression of spiritual struggles, responses that are more likely to make matters worse than better. Benevolent spiritual reappraisals are designed to help clients regain their footing and emotional equilibrium following struggles with the divine. They are not designed to mask, eliminate, or foreclose these conflicts with God because, though research is scant, these struggles may be a source of insights that can lead to growth in the most fundamental beliefs, practices, and values of clients, including their understanding of and relationship with the divine. As with other sensitive topics in therapy then, benevolent spiritual reappraisals must be approached with care and sensitivity to the particular goals, needs, and values of the client.

Facilitate Spiritual Connectedness

Divine struggles are generally marked by feelings of a frayed or broken relationship with God. Therapists can help clients interested in repairing that connection through a variety of practices. Many people find prayer to be helpful to them in dealing with their struggles. Ironically, their relationship with God can offer a solution to the problems in their relationship with God. Flaherty (1992) illustrates one prayer written by a survivor of sexual abuse that helped her reconnect with God in the midst of her struggles:

> Oh God, hear me! Come down from your mighty throne and fill the emptiness of my soul. This is Sandy. I know you remember my name; you hear me when I call. Meet me in the wasteland of my tears, wrap me up in your mighty arms, and rock me to sleep. Be my father, my mother, my savior, whisper to me echoes of healing, words of comfort in my despair. Touch me, call me by name, say that you have knowledge of my pain. (p. 51)

Because prayer involves communication with a partner who is not there in a physical sense, it may be difficult for many clients. Therapists, however, can help concretize this process by drawing on a few other clinical methods. Visualization can facilitate a sense of connection to the sacred. Flaherty (1992) encourages abused Christian women to picture themselves weeping outside the empty tomb of Jesus, as Mary Magdalene did in the story of the resurrection, and respond to Jesus's question: "Woman, why are you weeping?" (p. 56). "Recount for Jesus the multitude of reasons for your tears," Flaherty instructs. "Speak to him honestly about the loss of innocence, loss of family, loss of self, share with him the heart-wrenching question, 'Why?'" (p. 56). Visualizations can be adapted to the many ways people understand and imagine the sacred.

The empty-chair technique is another concrete way to build a sense of intimacy with God in times of divine struggle (Murray-Swank & Murray-Swank, 2012). Developed from Gestalt psychology, this technique can be adapted to the spiritual context by having clients express their feelings to God or another sacred figure sitting in the formerly empty chair, and then taking the sacred seat and imagining God's response. Murray-Swank and Murray-Swank present a powerful example of this method in their work with a 24-year-old woman who had been sexually abused over several years as a child by her stepfather. With the encouragement of the therapist, she voices her confusion and anger toward God in the chair:

> Have I done something wrong to deserve this? Why didn't you protect me? I was a little girl. I hate you, yet I love you. You can heal me, why don't you? Where is the justice? All I feel is alone and in despair. There is no end to the pain. (p. 234)

The act of venting her rage to God was transformational for this client. For the first time, she experienced a sense of spiritual support and God's presence. Her therapist went on to help her process these feelings. Murray-Swank and Murray-Swank (2012) note that this wasn't the end of therapy but rather a new start. The client was able to find greater peace through deeper understandings of herself, her abuse, her stepfather, and her relation with God.

Other clients struggling with God may reconnect with the divine through less direct methods. From drawing and music to sitting silently in an empty church and simply being outdoors, people have found many conduits to God. For example, Price, Kinghorn, Patrick, and Cardell (2012) recount the experience of a physician who, following a stroke, struggled with questions about God and the meaning of life. He was able to reengage with God as the result of a sacred encounter with nature:

> I was driving up the street toward our house [during] springtime. A forsythia was in blossom . . . and . . . I was thinking theologically about . . . the nature of God. Did God inflict this stroke on me? Is that the kind of God there is? And then I said to myself, but still there is beauty. And the fact that there's beauty says I think God is loving and wants to give us pleasure. And that was helpful. (p. 114)

Meditation is another way spiritual strugglers can reconnect to the sacred or the divine. Oman et al. (2007) evaluated the effects of two 8-week interventions for college students that centered around passage meditation and mindfulness meditation. It is noteworthy that even though these meditations were not explicitly theistic, both groups of meditators reported significant declines in their levels of divine struggle over the course of the program and at 8-week follow-up.

Still others may be more affected by the written word, be it from scriptures, classic religious writings, or popular literature. As Kushner (1989) notes, readings may be helpful not so much for intellectual reasons as for the experience of the divine they stimulate:

> People do not start to see the world different because someone has written a book giving them good reasons for doing so. They do it because they feel they have been touched by the presence of God incarnated sometimes in words, sometimes in stories, sometimes in memories triggered by a written passage. (p. 45)

Table 8.1 presents illustrative classic and popular readings on divine struggles. Practitioners can discuss and process these readings with clients.

Finally, social connections can foster the sense of spiritual connection. In an Internet survey on God's role in suffering, Exline and Grubbs (2011) zeroed in on a subsample of people who reported anger toward God and then disclosed their feelings to others. Those who felt that they had received a supportive response from others were more likely to draw closer to God, feel their faith was strengthened, and report fewer doubts about God's existence. Therapists then might encourage clients struggling with the divine to seek out social support, with an important caveat: Not everyone necessarily responds positively to the divine struggles of other people. Angela, the adolescent we presented earlier who had suffered a permanent spinal cord injury, provides an example:

> I think the worst thing is that people are telling me that this is all part of God's plan. I don't get it. I don't deserve it. Why did God do this to me? . . . And why does God think I can take it? . . . I'm praying for a miracle and lots of other people are, too. But my mom says that I just don't have enough faith or I'd be healed already. (Piderman, 2015, pp. 77, 81)

These less than favorable responses are not without consequence. In the Exline and Grubbs (2011) study noted above, about half of the sample reported that they received responses that were at least partly unsupportive, in which people felt judged or shamed for being angry at God. These unfavorable responses were tied to greater substance use; more chronic anger along with more attempts to suppress it; and more exit behaviors toward God, such as rebellion and withdrawal from God and questioning God's existence. Other researchers have also found that a lack of social and religious support in response to divine struggles was associated with poorer outcomes (Harris, Erbes, Winskowski, Engdahl, & Nguyen, 2014; Webb, Charbonneau, McCann, & Gayle, 2011). It follows that

TABLE 8.1. Classic and Popular Readings on Divine Struggles

Bloomfield, H., & Goldberg, P. (2003). *Making peace with God: A practice guide.* New York: Tarcher/Putnam. (Interfaith)

Chittister, J. D. (2003). *Scarred by struggle, transformed by hope.* Grand Rapids, MI: Eerdmans. (Christian/Roman Catholic)

The cloud of unknowing and other works. (2001). Translated by A. C. Spearing. New York: Penguin Classics. (Christian mysticism)

De la Cruz, J. (1916). *The dark night of the soul.* London: Thomas Books. (Christian)

Flaherty, S. M. (1992). *Woman, why do you weep? Spirituality for survivors of childhood sexual abuse.* New York: Paulist Press. (Interfaith)

Jaffe, H., Rudin, J., & Rudin, M. (1986). *Why me? Why anyone?* New York: St. Martin's Press. (Jewish)

Kushner, H. S. (1981). *When bad things happen to good people.* New York: Random House. (Jewish)

Novotni, M., & Petersen, R. (2001). *Angry with God.* Carol Stream, IL: Tyndale House. (Christian)

Yancey, P. (1977). *Where is God when it hurts?* Grand Rapids, MI: Zondervan. (Christian)

when seeking support for struggles with God, clients should be careful to look for those who are more likely to respond in a caring way.

Because people can take so many different pathways to connect to God, therapists cannot assume that any particular pathway will be of value to all or most clients who are experiencing divine struggles. Rather, therapists should help each client explore and identify the ways that may facilitate his or her connection with the sacred.

Consider New Ways to Understand the Divine

For many clients, struggles with God disrupt what was once a secure and meaningful connection. In these cases, therapists can help clients reconnect to God and thereby conserve their relationship through methods we just described. For other clients, however, divine struggles reveal old understandings of God to be no longer viable. Among some trauma victims, for instance, prior representations of the divine, regardless of their nature, become so deeply associated with the memories of the crisis, that God, as once understood, cannot be approached without reexperiencing the trauma. God, in essence, becomes a trauma (cf. Mogenson, 1989). Divine struggles can also reveal fundamental limitations in the ways God was once envisioned. This is just the kind of struggle Rabbi Harold Kushner (1981) described in his classic book *When Bad Things Happen to Good People.* Kushner was unable to reconcile the tragic death of his young son with his prior beliefs in God as an omnipotent, all-loving Being who ensures that bad things will not happen to good people. To sustain that belief, Kushner wrote, he would have had to reframe the loss of his son as (1) a justified punishment for his or his son's transgressions, or (2) some type of blessing in disguise. Kushner was unable to see the death of his son from either perspective. He could find nothing his young son or he himself had done to warrant a divinely imposed death sentence, and he could find absolutely no benefit in the loss of his son. Instead, Kushner arrived at a dramatically different understanding of God as a loving, but limited Being. He concluded:

> I believe in God. But I do not believe the same things about Him that I did years ago, when I was growing up or when I was a theological student. I recognize his limitations. He is limited in what He can do by laws of nature and human moral freedom. I no longer hold God responsible for illnesses, accident, and natural disasters, because I realize that I gain little and I lose so much when I blame God for those things. I can worship a God who hates suffering but cannot eliminate it, more easily than I can worship a God who chooses to make children suffer and die, for whatever exalted reasons. . . . Because the tragedy is not God's will, we need not feel hurt or betrayed by God when tragedy strikes. We can turn to Him for help in overcoming it, precisely because we can tell ourselves that God is as outraged by it as we are. (p. 134)

To put it in the terms of our spiritual framework, Kushner (1981) created a transformation in his spiritual orienting system and, more specifically, his way of thinking about God. This could also be described as a fundamental change in Kushner's global meaning system (cf. Park, 2005).

Kushner (1981) illustrates only one of many possible ways people can transform their understandings of God. Regardless of its form, therapists have a role to play in this transformational process, not as theologians or members of the clergy committed to a particular set of beliefs, but as supportive guides who help interested clients explore alternative visions of God that promote the resolution of divine struggles and greater wholeness and growth.

Frankel (2005) provides an apt illustration in her clinical work with Rebecca, a middle-age woman grappling with a severe autoimmune disease. Her physical symptoms and pain were compounded by periods of depression and anxiety in which she engaged in unrelenting self-criticism and self-blame. God too, she felt, was punishing her for her worthlessness through her illness. What became clear over the course of therapy was that Rebecca's image of God was a reflection of her view of her parents who had severely abused her emotionally growing up, and justified their abuse by telling her that she was a bad child. In an effort to differentiate her view of God from that of her parents, Frankel asked Rebecca to engage in a loving-kindness meditation, envisioning herself through the eyes of a caring, compassionate God rather than the eyes of her cruel parents. This led to a "radical shift" in her view of herself: "Instead of seeing herself as damaged goods, she began to experience herself as a beloved spark of the divine" (p. 191).

In her book on the spirituality of survivors of childhood sexual abuse, Flaherty (1992) provides other compelling examples of radical transformations in representations of God. She notes how the images of God developed in childhood are simply inadequate to the challenges faced by women who have been sexually abused. Visions of an all-powerful, male, controlling Being that are so widespread in mainstream religious traditions can become painful reminders of the suffering survivors experienced at the hands of powerful, controlling men. Flaherty encourages women to explore more immanent, feminine pictures of God: "When we experience the immanent God," she writes,

> we begin to view God's relation to our abuse in a new way. God did not stand by and do nothing as we experienced sexual abuse; rather God was one with us in this tragedy. As we were abused so also was God—broken and wounded. As we heal, God heals with us; as we become enraged as a result of our violation, so does God experience anger. (p. 109)

In some cases of human-inflicted trauma, any personal image of God may be a source of further pain rather than solace. Murray-Swank (2003) found it helpful to offer survivors of sexual abuse a life-giving, but nonpersonal image of God:

> Picture God as a waterfall within you . . . pouring down cool, refreshing water . . . the waters of love, healing, restoration throughout your body . . . a cool, refreshing, waterfall washing down over your head, your face, your shoulders, your neck, out through your arms, down your legs, out through your toes, refreshing, bringing life, quenching thirst . . . renewing, refreshing, restoring. (p. 232)

Transformations of the ways people understand God do not have to be radical; they can build on the client's existing perspective but move toward a more comprehensive representation of the divine. As we noted earlier, through their religious socialization or through their selective abstraction from their religious traditions, many people develop "small" images of God. Virtually every religious tradition, however, offers larger representations of God that could help clients move from narrow to broader images. For example, punitive views of God can be complemented by more compassionate divine images. Comforting, undemanding visions of God can be supplemented by those in which God is seen as challenging people to improve themselves and the lives of others. Kass (2017) presents the illustration of Hasna, a 17-year-old Algerian American Muslim, who was struggling with feelings of anger and disappointment in God following the death of her father, the decision to have sex with her boyfriend, and the development of psychosomatic reactions. Why hadn't Allah protected her from these ordeals, she wonders? Was he punishing her for her misdeeds? Eventually, Hasna recognizes that she is seeing God in narrow, masculine terms. As she explores Islam further, she comes to a transformational insight that Allah is not one thing. She writes:

> I have discovered a sweet surprise. There are 99 other names that are listed for Allah within the Quran. Here are some: The giver of life, The taker of life, Protecting

Friend, Creator of the Harmful, The Preventive of Harm, The Maker of Order, All Compassionate, The Patient One, the Avenger, The Forgiving, The Just—and the list goes on. Perhaps the message is clear. There is no need to look elsewhere for a creator, when it is present in everything. (p. 297)

The process of transforming the way God is understood can be painful. Even if they are no longer adequate to the individual's changing life experiences, beliefs about the divine are often deeply established and have the comfort of the familiar. Letting go of old images can leave a vacuum and sense of spiritual emptiness for a period of time. Efforts to help clients through this transformational time then may be met with frustration and resistance. Therapists should remember that it is not their job to convince the client of the need for change. For some clients, God-related beliefs may represent core values that are inviolate and off the table for discussion in therapy, and therapists must respect these fundamental beliefs, values, and choices. Other clients, though, will be interested in talking about the ways their image of God has developed and changed over time, even if this discussion is, at times, difficult. And just as they might engage clients in a conversation about their parents, romantic attachments, or their understanding of themselves, therapists can help clients explore and perhaps reconsider their relationship with God.

In fact, the therapist's caring presence, openness, and receptivity to the client's experience of divine struggles and unfolding relationship with God may, in itself, be a source of transformation. Psychologist Lauren Maltby provided a powerful clinical example in her work with Maggie, a 26-year-old Christian woman, with a history of trauma at the hands of both of her parents (Maltby & Hall, 2012). In the course of treatment, Maggie was raped and experienced a divine struggle with strong feelings of anger toward and fear of abandonment from God. These feelings were enacted in therapy. At a critical point, Maggie became angry with Maltby and threatened to leave the session and cancel her next appointment. Sensing that Maggie feared she would be abandoned in therapy and was pushing away, Maltby responded with caring and acceptance, saying, "I will care about you just as much if you come once a week, once a month, or every day. I will care about you" (p. 307). When Maggie did storm out of the office, Maltby looked for her in the bathroom of the clinic and then quickly returned a phone call from Maggie that night. These were pivotal experiences for Maggie. In the next session, she said:

I felt like me and you was, for a second, this replication of what God does for me, how here you are and I am not the greatest and you're here with me in this. And then I turn, and I leave. I literally left. I left. But then you looked for me! Not only did you look for me, then I called you and you're like "it doesn't matter" I'll still be here no matter what. . . . I felt like for the first time I have a tangible example of what that looks like . . . I'm not comparing you to God, but that relationship dynamic was just like it. (p. 308)

Through the therapist's uncritical acceptance and caring, Maggie experienced a deeply felt, transformed connection with God that addressed her anger and sense of divine abandonment.

Integrating Divine Struggles into a Cohesive Whole

For some people, divine struggles reflect a life out of kilter. The bits and pieces of experience, including the individual's relationship with God, don't come together into an organized cohesive whole. Positive feelings are not integrated with negative feelings. Past cannot be woven into the present. Actions are inconsistent with significant goals and values. Personal experience is disconnected from interactions with other people. Treatment in these instances cannot focus solely on the symptoms of distress, but must also address the need for greater cohesiveness, especially the place of the divine in the whole of life. Consider the case of Roger.

"You know when I broke both my legs, I wasn't completely surprised," Roger said. "I feel like I have been teetering my whole life."

I [K. I. P.] had been seeing Roger, a 45-year-old pastor from the Presbyterian church, for several months as he was recovering from surgery on both legs following a bicycle accident. He had been dealing with depression, anxiety, and periodic bouts of heavy drinking for much of his adult life, and his symptoms had intensified following his accident. But he had sought me out for therapy because he was also experiencing struggles with God and in his role as a clergyman.

"What do you mean by teetering?" I asked Roger.

"Well, as a child, I never knew when my parents would be around," Roger responded.

"My father was on the road a lot and it was hit or miss when he'd be home. And my mother had her moods, when she pretty much shut herself off in her bedroom with just her bottles of wine. We had some wonderful times as a family, but I always felt like I was on the edge, waiting for the rug to be pulled out and then left alone—I hated that feeling."

"How did you handle those feelings?" I asked Roger.

"I'm not sure I did," he responded. "I was an anxious kid, but my parents didn't really want to hear it. They were each others' biggest cheerleaders. My father would tell me how lucky I was to have a mother who loved me so much. And my mother would tell me how lucky I was to have a father who was such a good provider. When my anxiety got worse as an adolescent and I started to have times of real panic, I began to drink. I ended up going to church indirectly when I attended a 12-step program in a congregation and started talking with the pastor. I found myself drawn to the idea of a God who was always there with you and for you. You know, like a substitute parent."

"Did that discovery of God make a difference in your life?" I asked.

"Yes and no," Roger said. "There were times when I felt a sense of connectedness that I'd never had in my family. That's the reason I went into the ministry—to hold on to that feeling and share it with other people."

"I hear a 'but' coming," I said.

"Yeah," Roger replied. "The 'but' is I couldn't hold on to that feeling. And when I lost that sacred feeling, I felt abandoned, totally isolated, and hopeless. I would get—no, I still get—furious at God, for playing such a mean cat-and-mouse game with me."

"Do you still have times when you feel a sense of God's presence?" I asked.

"Yes, and those are the best times of my life," he said, "but they don't happen very often."

I asked Roger whether he had talked to other people about his struggle.

"No," he responded, "and I feel like a damned fraud preaching about God's love when all I've got inside me is nothing."

Roger exemplified someone at war within himself spiritually. In a recapitulation of his relationship with his parents, Roger had been unable to find a way to reconcile his experiences of divine love and connection with those of divine abandonment and emptiness. His attempts to build his spiritual resources, "pray away" his negative feelings, and focus on the positive had proven unsuccessful; they seemed only to amplify his anger, anxiety, and emptiness in relation to God (and his parents). Rather than try to help Roger minimize his negative feelings, I focused on helping him integrate them into a larger more cohesive orientation to life.

In one key session, I came back to the image of Roger "teetering" in his life: "It sounds like there are times when you are teetering on one leg, feeling angry and abandoned, and then you teeter on the other leg when you feel there is a God who loves you and cares about you. Is that right?" I asked.

"That's about it" Roger said and then went on: "It's hard keeping your balance when you're always standing on one leg."

"Yes, that must be really tough. . . . What do you think it would be like to stand on both legs?" I asked.

"I'm not sure I know what you mean," Roger responded.

"Well, I guess I'm asking what it might be like to experience both sets of feelings that you have toward God: anger and abandonment, and love and care."

Roger paused for a while and then said, "I'd have to think about that. I've spent so much time in my life trying to eliminate all the pain and hurt I've felt. But that's only backfired on me—I get totally caught up in the dark stuff, except for those times when I sense that God has come to me."

"Kind of like feast or famine," I commented.

Roger began the next session by noting that he was struck by my last "feast or famine" comment. "It brought to mind the story of Joseph in Egypt who interpreted the pharaoh's dream to mean Egypt would face 7 years of feast followed by 7 years of famine. And I realized that, like the pharaoh, in times of feast, I could still prepare for times of famine ahead. And in times of famine, I could still hope for better times ahead."

This was the beginning of an important shift for Roger, from all-or-nothing thinking about God and parents to both-and thinking. In the sessions that followed, we explored how Roger might be able to "keep two feet on the ground," by recognizing and accepting both his positive and negative feelings toward God and his parents.

Switching to another metaphor, I said, "We're all onions made up of layers of thoughts, feelings, behaviors, and motives, many of them involving God. I don't think we can excise any layer, but it's easier to live with ourselves when we're more aware of them."

Roger was receptive and even joked, "I know this onion has given me of a lot of tears."

Roger became more comfortable talking about the incongruities, polarities, and paradoxes in his life—how he could feel so distant and yet so close to his parents, how God could be present and absent to him, how he could experience great clarity at times and confusion at others. He started reading books by authors who also spoke of the important place of paradox and imperfection in creating lives of greater wholeness—for example, *The Promise of Paradox* by Parker Palmer (2008) and *The Spirituality of Imperfection* by Ernst Kurtz and Katherine Ketcham (1992).

Over the 2 years of therapy, Roger experienced a gradual reduction in his symptoms of depression, anxiety, and his cravings for alcohol. He continued to have periods of feeling abandoned by God, but they no longer troubled him as much and he began to take more satisfaction from his ministry. Toward the latter part of therapy, I raised the possibility of sharing some of his own divine struggles with members of his church. After giving it some thought, Roger opened up about some of his struggles to members of the Men's Study Group at church. Their response was positive and led to a deeper level of conversation and sharing about the spiritual struggles others in the group were experiencing. In the last session, Roger said he was thinking about giving a talk to the entire church on spiritual struggles, including his own.

There is no single ingredient in the recipe for fostering cohesiveness among people struggling with the divine. It involves helping clients by (1) developing greater awareness and acceptance of multiple representations of God; (2) going beyond inflexible black-and-white thinking; (3) finding greater balance among competing thoughts, feelings, behaviors, values, and guiding visions; (4) beginning to share personal struggles with others; (5) living with paradox, incongruence, and imperfection; and (6) encouraging the wisdom to weave the different threads of life together into a meaningful overarching orientation to life. This process can take time. But, as the case of Roger suggests, greater cohesiveness represents one vital contributor to greater wholeness for those struggling with the divine.

CONCLUSIONS

Do therapists really have any business talking with clients about God? This is a question some readers might be asking. Certainly, it is not the place of therapists to tell clients whether to believe in or what to believe about God. That has not been the approach we have encouraged in this chapter. Instead, working from a psychotherapeutic lens, we focused on how to help clients deal with their tensions, strains, and conflicts about the divine—however the divine may be understood, experienced, or related to. Why? Because divine struggles can be interwoven into the problems people bring to treatment and are associated with distress, disorientation, and decline, as well as the possibility of growth. Thus, as would be true of any conflict, struggles with the divine are a potentially relevant topic for therapy.

Addressing divine struggles in treatment is likely to be new and challenging territory for therapists—theists as well as nontheists. Including God in the therapeutic conversation may seem strange to many therapists who do not believe in God. But psychotherapy often involves work with both seen and unseen presences, particularly when they are sources of conflict and strain. Unseen presences can take the form of departed loved ones, childhood memories, former partners or spouses, or people clients refuse to speak to. God is another unseen presence that, at times, requires therapeutic attention when clients struggle. Therapists who believe in a higher power face their own challenges, such as the need to guard against the presumption that clients experience and relate to God in the same way they themselves do. We have emphasized that people envision the divine in myriad ways. As with other topics, the task in therapy is to learn about the client's distinctive way of understanding God and the client's distinctive struggles with the divine. With that understanding, therapists will be better able to help clients use their struggles as a launching pad to greater wholeness and growth.

We are about to shift our focus to other spiritual struggles. However, we are not leaving divine struggles far behind, for as we will see, divine struggles are frequently implicated in other spiritual struggles, and other spiritual struggles, in turn, can set the stage for divine struggles. We turn our attention now to another important type of struggle: struggles of ultimate meaning.

CHAPTER 9

Struggles of Ultimate Meaning

> When F_____ told me about his dream [that he would soon be
> liberated from the concentration camp], he was still full of hope
> and convinced that the voice of his dream would be right. But as
> the promised day drew nearer, the war news . . . made it appear
> very unlikely that we could be free on the promised date. On
> March twenty-ninth, F_____ suddenly became ill and ran a high
> temperature. On March thirtieth, the day his prophecy had told him
> that the war and suffering would be over for him, he became delirious
> and lost consciousness. On March thirty-first, he was dead. To all
> outward appearance, he had died of typhus.
>
> —FRANKL (1959, p. 96)

The ultimate cause of death in this case was not typhus but rather loss of faith in the future, loss of a reason to go on living, according to psychiatrist Viktor Frankl. From his careful observations of fellow concentration camp prisoners, Frankl (1959) concluded that "having a why to live for" could make the difference between life and death. Frankl tried to foster this sense of purpose and significance among fellow inmates. "Whenever there was an opportunity for it," he wrote, "one had to give them a why—an aim—for their lives, in order to strengthen them to bear the terrible how of their existence. Woe to him who saw no more sense in his life, no aim, no purpose, and therefore no point in carrying on. He was soon lost" (pp. 97–98). Over the next decades, Frankl went on to develop a theory and method of treatment, logotherapy, that grew out of the assumption that the will toward meaning is as important a human motive as the will toward pleasure.

Frankl's (1959) observations and theories have since been supported by a large body of theory and research. In our own model (see Chapter 2), for example, we have stressed that even though people are driven by biological, social, and unconscious forces, that is not the full story; people are proactive as well as reactive beings, striving to attain purpose and significance in their lives. Many empirical studies have shown that having significant goals in life and a sense that one's life matters are important predictors of mental health, physical health, and longevity (e.g., Alimujiang et al., 2019; King, Heintzelman, & Ward, 2016; Krause & Hayward, 2012c). On the other hand, a lack of strong purpose and feeling that one's life is meaningless can be fundamentally disorienting and destabilizing, as we read in the story of F above. Meaninglessness "places a trembling animal at the mercy of the entire cosmos," Ernest Becker (1973, p. 26) wrote in his book *The Denial of Death*. Not surprisingly, then, studies indicate that meaninglessness increases vulnerability to a wide array of problems (e.g., Berg, 2011; Galek, Flannelly, Ellison, Silton, & Jankowski, 2015; Park & Baumeister, 2017).

It oversimplifies things, however, to treat significant purpose as a fixed and final state, something we either have or don't have. In contrast, in this book we have emphasized that the search for significance is an ongoing dynamic process with people trying to find and hold on to meaning. And in this process, people occasionally experience tensions, strains, and conflicts—in short, they struggle. Struggle with meaning occupies a place of its own, one that lies between a rock-solid, life-directing sense of purpose on the one hand, and a sense of meaninglessness that leaves the individual feeling hopelessly bereft of purpose on the other. Wilt, Stauner, et al. (2017) found support for this point in a factor-analytic study: the measure of struggles with ultimate meaning loaded on a separate factor from a measure of presence–absence of meaning. Regardless of the degree to which people have or lack a sense of significance in their lives, they may struggle to more fully realize, broaden, deepen, discover, recover, or rediscover their purpose for living. We believe that struggles of meaning represent an unrecognized but important dimension of the search for purpose and significance.

UNDERSTANDING STRUGGLES OF ULTIMATE MEANING

In this chapter, we make what has been largely implicit in the field more explicit by focusing our attention on struggles of meaning and purpose. Consistent with the theme of this book, we pay particular attention to struggles of *ultimate* meaning. The first section of this chapter examines what theory and research have to teach us about ultimate meaning struggles. Building on this knowledge, the second portion of the chapter considers how practitioners can help people struggling with questions of ultimate meaning.

The Meaning of Ultimate Meaning Struggles

Ironically enough, the term *meaning* has many meanings (e.g., George & Park, 2016; Martela & Steger, 2016; Wong, 2017). It has been used to describe the cognitive process of making sense or meaning out of life, the motivational process of searching for meaning and purpose, and the affective process of experiencing a sense of meaningfulness. This multiplicity of definitions can lead to some confusion, as several authors have noted (e.g., Martela & Steger, 2016). The individual who says, "My life has no meaning," could be referring to problems in making any sense of life, in finding a purpose to life, or in feeling that life really matters. To reduce this potential ambiguity, we do not use the term *meaning* in this chapter to refer to the cognitive process of meaning-making (this topic is taken up in other chapters, particularly struggles with doubt). Instead, we focus on the motivational and affective qualities of meaning: the search for significant purpose and the experience of a sense of significance.

But why focus on *ultimate* meaning? Recall in Chapter 2 we noted that significant goals and purposes come in many shapes and sizes. Not all of these purposes are created equal, however, as William James (1902) observed. Among the range of possible life goals—from least to most worthwhile—spiritual goals and strivings are often near or at the top of the list. By spiritual strivings, we are referring to motivations to transcend oneself, relate to what is perceived to be sacred, or form and maintain a connection with a higher power (Emmons & Schnitker, 2013; Mahoney et al., 2005). Spiritual strivings emerged as the most valued of possible life goals in a study by Emmons (1999). Similarly, in a survey of Americans who were asked to indicate their most important source of meaning in their lives, religious faith ranked second, exceeded only by spending time with family (Pew Research Center, 2018). Even this ranking may be an underestimate when we remember that seemingly secular strivings—such as family, work, and spending time outdoors—can take on spiritual value when they are imbued with sacred qualities (Pargament & Mahoney, 2005).

Transcendent goals have often been compared favorably to more mundane or self-centered purposes. Wong (2017), for instance, writes, "In a paradoxical way, self-transcendence points out that we have to redirect our focus from self-interest to others, in order to live the good life. It is in awakening and cultivating our spiritual values of will to meaning and self-transcendence that we find a sense of fulfillment and significance" (p. 87). Similarly, Seligman (2014) said that "a purposeful life is a life that joins with something larger than we are, and the larger that something is, the more meaning our lives have" (p. 70).

Several research studies have also underscored the exceptional power of sacred purposes, aspirations, and strivings, as we saw in Chapter 2. As sources of self-definition and social identity for many people, spiritual strivings can help organize and integrate lower-level goals into a more coherent whole (Emmons et al., 1998). The pursuit of spiritual goals and strivings has also been associated with a variety of mental health benefits (see Mahoney et al., 2013, for a review). For example, in a longitudinal study of young adults, Chen, Kim, Koh, Frazier, and VanderWeele (2019) found that having a sense of mission or calling in life was predictive of many positive changes in mental health and less depression over time. Working with a national sample, Krause, Pargament, Ironson, and Hill (2017) compared the roles of having a religious, God-given purpose and meaning in life to that of having a purpose measured more generally. They found that religious purpose buffered the effects of financial strain on the drug use of participants, while general purpose in life did not.

In short, sacred purposes occupy a place of special importance and power. It follows that struggles in the domain of ultimate meaning are likely to have special importance and power as well. It also follows that where we find significant psychological problems of the kinds people bring to therapy, we may also find struggles of ultimate meaning. We focus then in this chapter on tensions, strains, and conflicts around one's ultimate purpose in life. These struggles can involve challenges of letting go of a sacred purpose that is no longer attainable, recovering an ultimate source of meaning, realizing a higher purpose in life, or discovering a new and greater destination of significance.

The Prevalence of Ultimate Meaning Struggles

In her powerful account of the aftermath of the atomic bomb dropped on Nagasaki to end the second World War, Southard (2015) details how several survivors tried to come to terms with their losses of family, friends, physical and mental health, occupations, material possessions, and institutions. The survivors also shared in the experience of lost hopes and dreams. And, as a group, they agonized over whether "human effort and personal values were ultimately meaningless" (p. 183). One woman, for example, hid herself for 8 years, questioning day after day what, if anything, could replace all that she had lost and what, if anything, she could devote herself to.

How well do these stories apply to people in less dramatic circumstances? Frankl (2000) suggested that they may be more common than imagined. Tension and strain, he insisted, are built into the search for ultimate meaning because, although the will toward meaning is universal, human beings have only a limited capacity to comprehend their larger transcendent purpose. Frustration then is part of the existential condition. Perhaps that is why portrayals of people wrestling with questions of ultimate purpose and meaning are so common in great literature, from the works of Shakespeare and Dostoevsky to Thornton Wilder and Virginia Woolf.

What does the research tell us? Initial systematic studies suggest that ultimate meaning struggles, like other spiritual struggles, are not unusual. In our large study of adults in the United States (Exline, Pargament, & Grubbs, 2014), 52% indicated that they had experienced some degree of ultimate meaning struggles, such as questioning whether life really matters, over the past few weeks. It is important to add that struggles of ultimate meaning do not appear to be strongly related to demographic factors, such as age, gender, and ethnicity

(Exline, Pargament, Grubbs, & Yali, 2014). Instead, they seem relevant to people from diverse backgrounds.

The Consequences of Ultimate Meaning Struggles

Like other spiritual struggles, struggles of ultimate meaning may potentially result in distress, disorientation, and decline, and/or growth and positive transformation. Let's take a look at these possible trajectories.

Ultimate Meaning Struggles and Decline

Existential frustrations and crises of meaning, Frankl (1959) wrote, can create a vacuum of purposelessness, one that leaves the individual vulnerable to what he called "noogenic neuroses," marked by despair, suicidality, depression, anxiety, and addictiveness. Dysfunctional as they are, these symptoms, he said, represent attempts to fill that existential vacuum.

Several studies have linked struggles in finding a purpose for living to significant psychological problems. Dees, Vernooij-Dassen, Dekkers, Vissers, and van Weel (2012) interviewed a group of Dutch patients who had asked for euthanasia to identify what contributed to their perceptions of "unbearable suffering." The most frequently mentioned theme involved struggles around purpose and hope leading to despair. One patient said, "I can't do anything anymore. I used to like music, participated in social clubs, all so very companionable, I had to say farewell to all of it. It feels so awful just waiting to become bedridden and then waiting to die" (p. 732). Other studies have tied struggles with ultimate meaning to indicators of poorer mental health, including greater anxiety, depression, anger, loneliness, and lower levels of life satisfaction and resilience (Exline, Pargament, Grubbs, & Yali, 2014; Wilt, Stauner, et al., 2017). As noted earlier, one study reported that struggles of ultimate meaning were associated with greater risk of suicide; these effects were buffered by higher levels of gratitude and patience in the context of life's hardships (Schnitker et al., 2021). Among atheists, too, a study found that struggles of ultimate meaning were associated with greater depression, anxiety, and lower life satisfaction (Sedlar et al., 2018).

In comparison to the other forms of spiritual struggles, struggles with ultimate meaning appear to be particularly strong predictors of declines in mental health (Currier, Foster, Witvliet, et al., 2019; Currier, McDermott, McCormick, Churchwell, & Milkeris, 2018; McCormick et al., 2017). For example, among the six types of spiritual struggles, ultimate meaning struggles were most consistently related to depression and anxiety among parents whose infant had been in a neonatal intensive care unit (Brelsford & Doheny, 2020). Similarly, ultimate meaning struggles emerged as an especially strong predictor of suicidal behavior (Currier, McDermott, McCormick, et al., 2018) and of increases in manic-depressive symptoms and declines in positive mental health (Currier, Foster,

Witvliet, et al., 2019). These latter studies were longitudinal in design, and the findings were consistent with a primary spiritual struggles model in which ultimate meaning struggles led to declines in mental health.

All in all, these findings highlight the risks that struggles of ultimate meaning hold for an individual's psychological health and well-being. Is that the full picture? Could struggles of ultimate meaning have a brighter side?

Ultimate Meaning Struggles and Growth

From Frankl's (2000) point of view, struggles of ultimate meaning provide an opportunity for growth. The capacity of humans to raise questions of meaning is one of the ways that people differ from animals, he said. And through experiences of existential frustration and vacuum, he believed, people could potentially transform their lives. Grappling with questions of meaning and meaninglessness then represents "an achievement rather than a neurosis," according to Frankl (p. 134).

A number of narrative accounts suggest that ultimate meaning struggles can indeed lead to growth and positive transformation. Frankel (2017) recounted one striking example: the story of Laura Stachel, a successful obstetrics and gynecology physician, who developed a degenerative spinal condition that forced her to give up the practice she loved. Having lost what had given her life meaning and direction, Stachel went through a period of struggle to find new purpose. Eventually, she decided to return to school to get a degree in public health and traveled to Nigeria to study why maternal mortality rates were so high. There, she learned that women experienced complications at childbirth often due to a lack of reliable electricity that often forced them to deliver in conditions of near darkness. Returning to the United States, she and her husband developed a portable electric device, a "solar suitcase," to illuminate the delivery areas in homes and hospitals. This turned into the founding of an international organization, "We Care Solar," that has provided solar suitcases all over the world. Painful as Stachel's time of struggle was, it led eventually to a new mission in life for her, one that became a source of greater joy and fulfillment than she could have imagined.

Others have had similar stories to tell. Chow and Nelson-Becker (2010) conducted a qualitative study with 11 female stroke survivors from Hong Kong. As a group, the survivors experienced a full range of spiritual struggles, including deeply felt questions about whether their lives continued to hold any purpose. Several of the survivors reported that, through Chinese spiritual practices that emphasized balance and harmony, they achieved a transformation of significance from more material concerns, including their own bodies, to caring and nurturing their loved ones.

Unfortunately, quantitative studies have not been conducted as yet that might shed further light on what might be the brighter side of ultimate meaning struggles. Nevertheless, if we take narrative accounts such as these seriously, then struggles of ultimate significance may lead eventually to a life of transformed purpose. Once again, however, these findings have to be considered with other research in mind that links ultimate meaning struggles to distress and decline. We would say that growth that takes place following struggles of ultimate meaning may not be a sure thing, and if it does occur, it may not be achieved without real pain. For practitioners, this raises the key question of how best to help clients struggling with ultimate meaning find greater wholeness and growth rather than brokenness and decline. We turn to that question shortly. First, however, we examine how ultimate meaning struggles develop.

The Roots of Ultimate Meaning Struggles

Joseph, a 62-year-old Jewish man, came to therapy for depression following the loss of his job. Largely housebound, he had cut himself off from family and friends, and was irritable and moody. Much of his time at home was spent playing online poker. It became clear in therapy that Joseph's depression was wrapped up in a struggle of ultimate meaning. He had worked his way up from a salesman to vice president of sales in an airplane parts manufacturing company. But in an effort to cut costs, the company had trimmed its staff. "I can't believe they let me go," he said.

> "I gave them everything I had. And for what? I spent my life helping them sell parts to airlines that overcharge people for flights that treat people like they're sardines in a can. What a waste! And now what? No one wants to hire a 62-year-old guy. I'm still reasonably healthy—how am I going to fill the next 20 years of my life? I don't have a clue. Why am I even alive?"

As the therapist got to know Joseph better, he learned that Joseph's struggle had deeper roots. Joseph had been a musically gifted child: "My first memories were of songs and sounds. And growing up I spent every minute I could listening to music and playing piano. Those were the best years of my life." Joseph's grandfather, a professional violinist in his own right, had recognized and encouraged his grandson's talents. "God gave you a gift," his grandfather would remind him, "and you must share it with others." Joseph took that message to heart. His parents, however, felt differently. A working-class couple that struggled to make ends meet, they felt that, while music was a fine hobby, it wouldn't put bread on the table. They strongly encouraged Joseph to be more practical. However, after Joseph won a national competition at the age of 12, they accepted his dreams of a career in music.

When he was 16, Joseph developed a benign tumor on his hand that needed to be removed surgically. Unfortunately, the surgery left Joseph with restricted movement in his hand, damage that could not be corrected by physical therapy. Joseph's dream of a career as a concert pianist was shattered. He severed any connection with music. The idea of playing another instrument, teaching music, or simply listening to music was too painful. Joseph lost interest in his studies and went on to college only because he couldn't think of what else to do with his life. "Nothing else had any appeal. And no one was there to help me figure things out; my grandfather had died, God had turned his back on me, and I was on my own." Joseph majored in business, as his parents had recommended, and took a job in sales as soon as he graduated. When asked how he felt about his work, Joseph shrugged and said, "It put food on the table. It paid for my kid's college. And it kept us out of the poor house."

Ultimate meaning struggles, like other forms of spiritual struggle, grow out of the interplay among three forces: life events and transitions, the significant purposes we seek, and the orienting system. In the earlier chapter on the roots of spiritual struggles (see Chapter 3), we reviewed these forces in some detail, and much of that discussion applies here. In this section, we examine some of the roots that are particularly relevant to struggles of ultimate meaning, drawing on the story of Joseph, as well as research and theory.

Life Events and Transitions

Part of what makes life events stressful lies in their power to damage and disrupt our dreams, and call into question our reasons for living. In this vein, Janoff-Bulman and Frantz (1997) observed that the struggles of trauma survivors shifted over time from questions of "Why did this happen to me?" to the challenge of finding purpose. Similarly, the conflicts Joseph brought to therapy centered less around why he had lost his purpose in life and more around what, if anything, still mattered. The damage he had suffered to his hand as an adolescent destroyed what had become for him a sacred vision: the opportunity to share his God-given gift with others. When Joseph lost his job decades later, he reexperienced his earlier struggles and grief over lost meaning and purpose that had remained unresolved for much of his life.

Studies illustrate how major life transitions and crises can shake our sense of greater purpose (McCormick et al., 2017; Van Tongeren, Hill, Krause, Ironson, & Pargament, 2017). Among older adults, for instance, Kopacz and Connery (2015) note how life transitions—retirement, children leaving, changes in physical health, death of friends and family—can result in questions of ultimate meaning of the kind experienced by Joseph: "Who am I now?"; "What's the purpose of life?"; and "What is my role in the future?" (p. 63). Life events that damage or violate sacred aspirations, as in Joseph's dream of becoming a concert pianist, may be especially likely to trigger struggles of ultimate meaning (Pargament, Magyar, et al., 2005).

Major life events can take more abstract existential forms. According to some existentialists, the encounter with what is perceived as an absurdly meaningless world creates a decisive moment in life when the individual chooses one of two options: give up in the pursuit of meaning and reach a place where it no longer matters that nothing matters or, paradoxically, struggle to find a reason for living in a meaningless universe (Camus, 1946; Sartre, 1948; Yalom, 1980). Consistent with this perspective, Wilt, Stauner, et al. (2017) studied large samples of adults and college students and found that people who continued to search for meaning in spite of a low sense of meaning were more likely to report struggles of ultimate meaning.

In sum, one place struggles of ultimate meaning can be found is in the aftermath of major life trauma or transition when a deep source of significant purpose has been shaken, damaged, or revealed to be inadequate.

Problems of Purpose

William James (1902) once said, "It makes a great deal of difference to a man whether one set of his ideas, or another, be the centre of his energy" (p. 193). Joseph's life, for example, took on a very different character when he was no longer able to pursue his musical dream and instead settled for a job without passion, one that merely "put food on the table." Like Joseph, many people strive toward goals in life that do not offer a sense of deep purpose and fulfillment. For example, in response to an open-ended question on the Pew Survey (2018) about what provides respondents with a sense of meaning, only 7% mentioned helping others and only 11% spoke of learning as giving meaning to their lives. Brooks (2019) wrote, "It's as if people no longer see life as something that should be organized around a specific vocation, a calling that is their own way of doing good in the world."

Many writers have commented on the downside of lives that lack deeper purpose. For example, Frankl (1985) enumerated the psychological costs of "having means to live but no meaning to live for" (p. 1221). Similarly, Tillich (1957) maintained that the life exclusively devoted to pleasure and material gain cannot offer ultimate meaning. As necessary as these goals are, they are preliminary rather than ultimate concerns, and cannot bear the weight of the sacred (Jones, 1991). When they become the centerpiece of life, they may result in the sense that one is living an inauthentic life.

Research on the topic is lacking, but we believe that struggles of ultimate meaning are more likely when people strive toward limited purposes. Exclusively materialistic and hedonistic goals illustrate the problem of purposes that lack depth. In addition, difficulties can arise in balancing important goals that, at times, compete with each other, such as the needs of family and job-related demands. People who pursue a narrow purpose in life, even if it is imbued with sacred value, can also be vulnerable to ultimate meaning struggles when they are no longer able to realize their single dream, as was the case with Joseph's hopes of becoming a concert pianist. Struggles of ultimate meaning then grow in part out of a limited set of purposes in life, including those that lack depth, balance, and breadth.

Limitations of the Orienting System

Ultimate meaning struggles can also be rooted in social, personal, and spiritual limitations in the individual's orienting system. Social forces, large and small, play a part in shaping the dreams people can and cannot pursue. At one extreme, terrorist groups promulgate extremist visions of ultimate meaning that, if accepted by vulnerable individuals hungry for a sense of significance, can lead to personal and social destruction (Webber & Kruglanski, 2018). Opportunities to seek out a greater purpose can also be closed off by economic deprivation and institutionalized forces of racism, sexism, and religious prejudice. For example, the father of one of us (K.I.P.) was unable to pursue his dream of going to medical school, blocked by the informal quota system of medical schools for Jews in the first half of the 20th century. (His thwarted dream had ripple effects over time, with two of three of his children, and three of six of his grandchildren becoming physicians). In less obvious ways, the values and norms of culture at large can affect what people choose to strive for. Numerous social scientists have described a shift away from more communal values to more individualistic values in the United States (Brooks, 2015; Putnam, 2000; Twenge & Campbell, 2009). For example, Brooks (2019) maintains that meaning in life has been "miniaturized" in the United States. "The upper registers of moral life—fighting for freedom, struggling to end poverty," he says, "have been amputated for many. The awfulness of the larger society is a given. The best you can do is find a small haven in a heartless world" (p. 21).

Closer to home, family and friends can also shape purpose in life for better or worse. For instance, Joseph gave up on his hopes for a life that offered ultimate meaning, in part because he had lost his spiritual model: the grandfather who had encouraged him to tend to his divine spark. Without the support of his grandfather, Joseph fell back on the advice of his parents to take the safer route and go into business.

These social forces, large scale and more immediate, can constrict opportunities for people to realize their higher potential, leading them instead to goals that are inconsistent with their deeper values, interests, and character. As a result, they become more vulnerable to questions, tensions, and conflicts about their ultimate meaning in life.

Personal and spiritual factors can also contribute to the development of struggles of ultimate meaning. People who are out of touch with themselves, overly influenced by external forces, or lacking the sense of self-efficacy to make their dreams a reality may be especially prone to these struggles because they are unable to be true to themselves. Wilt et al. (2021) examined the implications of this kind of inauthenticity for ultimate meaning struggles and the presence of meaning in a college student and large adult sample. Although the findings were complex, people who reported greater inauthenticity generally described greater struggles of ultimate meaning and a lower sense of meaning. This makes good sense. After all, how can people find fulfillment if they are alienated from their own desires, living the lives others want for them rather than what they want for themselves, or lack the resources to get what they truly want out of life?

It is important to add that, from many religious or spiritual perspectives, authenticity involves more than being true to oneself, but also true to the special purpose God is said to have for every individual. "Each of us is said to carry a divine spark," 19th-century Hasidic Rabbi Israel of Rizin said (cited in Lynberg, 2001, p. 34). Discovering that ultimate meaning rather than creating it, Frankl (1959) famously asserted, is the critical task of life. However, the process of discerning this divine mission may be easier said than done. Pain and suffering may make it difficult to locate any greater purpose. For example, feeling that God had abandoned him, Joseph was unable to identify another higher meaning for himself.

Other people experience conflicts between what they feel God wants for them and their own needs and desires. Martínez-Taboas (2018) illustrates this point through the case of Nancy, a 21-year-old religious Puerto Rican woman, who came to therapy with disabling seizure-like movements in both legs. Seizure medication, however, was ineffective, leading the therapist to look for any psychological roots to her problem. Three years earlier, the therapist learned, Nancy had felt a vocation to become a nun. Not long after though, she began to feel unsure whether she would be able to control her strong sexual urges as a nun. As a result, Nancy had started to have serious regrets about her decision. However, she feared disapproval of her parents, family, and church if she changed her mind. Nancy's somatoform disorder, her therapist suggested, represented an unconscious expression of her inner struggles to realize a purpose in life that was authentically hers. With support and encouragement, Nancy was able to talk openly and honestly with family and friends about her change of heart, and her seizures dissipated. Nancy did not reject her faith, but instead reenvisioned marriage and motherhood as more fitting expressions of her spirituality. In this sense, she found a way to harmonize her own desires with what she felt to be God's purpose for her.

Generally, those who have a stronger religious and spiritual commitment may feel more confident that they have found their higher purpose, whereas those who are less religious and spiritual may be more likely to struggle in their search for a greater meaning, as Exline, Pargament, Grubbs, and Yali (2014) found. Consider the words of a 19-year-old who had exited from Christianity:

I had a purpose and a direction. Losing that made me really feel like, lost. . . . Like, well, if I'm not so sure that there is this Christian God or if like the Bible is the word of God, then like what am I doing here? What am I supposed to be? And . . . I still don't necessarily have a clear sense of purpose for my life. Which is something that I miss. (Zuckerman, 2012, p. 130)

In this section, we have reviewed how ultimate meaning struggles may be rooted in life events and transitions, problems of purpose, and limitations of the orienting system. Research in this area is only just underway. Preliminary though they may be, these emerging insights into the prevalence, consequences, and roots of ultimate meaning struggles can help guide practitioners' efforts to foster greater wholeness and growth rather than brokenness and decline. We now turn to these practical issues.

ADDRESSING STRUGGLES
OF ULTIMATE MEANING IN PRACTICE

Few people come to psychotherapy presenting struggles of ultimate meaning as their main problem. Even so, these tensions and strains may be very much a part of problems that are commonly presented in counseling, such as depression, anxiety, trauma, addiction, and relational conflicts. Meaning-related struggles may be easy to overlook though because clinical work tends to focus on "what's the matter" rather than "what matters." Considering questions of meaning in therapy, however, broadens the conversation from issues of the past to visions of the future. It becomes as important to "take a future" (cf. Pargament, 2007) as it is to take a history. The range of topics expands from the depths of human experience to its potential heights, as Frankl (2000) noted. By broaching issues of ultimate meaning, then, therapy becomes more fully dimensional and new possibilities for wholeness and growth may emerge. Let's take a closer look.

Exploring Ultimate Meaning Struggles

I worry that my life is hopeless"; "I wonder why I'm here in this world"; "Half the time, I don't know who I really am"; "I'm afraid that when I leave this world, no one will remember me"; "Every day seems like the same old, same old. Why don't I feel more alive?" These are the kinds of complaints practitioners often hear from clients who are feeling depressed, anxious, and demoralized. But in each of these phrases, we can also hear questions, tensions, and doubts about purpose, meaning, significance, hopes, and dreams. By attending to these implicit signs, therapists can open the door to a more explicit conversation about struggles of meaning. Listen to how Joseph and the therapist began to explore these struggles:

THERAPIST: Losing your job really shook you up, Joseph, as it would anyone. But I wondered how rewarding you found your job to be.

JOSEPH: Well, like I said, it "put food on the table." I wasn't crazy about the work. I mean anyone who liked selling airplane parts would really have to have their head examined. But the job kept us out of the poor house and helped get my kids through college.

THERAPIST: It sounds like your family's really important to you.

JOSEPH: They always have been, even though I don't think they know it. I spent so much time at work my kids used to call me "the invisible dad."

THERAPIST: Ouch!

JOSEPH: Well, they were kind of right. I wasn't fully there even when I was there, if you know what I mean.

THERAPIST: I'm not sure I do. What was it was like to be there but not fully there?

JOSEPH: It was like being on the outside looking in. My wife and kids would be laughing, crying, yelling, or joking, and I'd watch, but like from a distance.

THERAPIST: And how were you feeling as you watched from a distance?

JOSEPH: I'm not sure I really noticed. I didn't pay much attention to my feelings.

THERAPIST: You sound kind of subdued right now, maybe even a little sad.

JOSEPH: I do?

THERAPIST: Yeah. How long do you think you've felt on the outside?

JOSEPH: I don't know. Maybe most of my life.

THERAPIST: Can you recall a time when you felt more . . . engaged, more alive?

JOSEPH: I guess when I was a kid playing music. Those were the best times of my life. I . . . I . . .

THERAPIST: Yes?

JOSEPH: [*Head down*] I don't want to talk about it anymore.

THERAPIST: You look really sad now. But we don't have to talk about it if you'd rather not. [*Pauses*] Do you have anything happening that's exciting in your life right now?

JOSEPH: Well, this may sound even sadder. [*Pauses*] The most exciting thing I have going on is my online poker. I spend so much time now in my den gambling. My wife doesn't like it and it seems pretty pathetic to me, too. It fills the time though.

THERAPIST: [*Pauses*] You know, I wonder about your gambling. You don't seem comfortable with it yourself, but maybe it's serving a purpose for you. Maybe it's a way to fill not only your time but the gap that was left when you lost your job, when your kids grew up and left home, and maybe some earlier gaps, too.

JOSEPH: I'm not sure what you mean.

THERAPIST: I could be off base, but it seems like you've been missing something really fulfilling in your life for quite a while. And now, you're worried about how you're going to fill the years you have remaining. You're struggling to find some kind of larger purpose.

JOSEPH: I think that's true, but I'm not sure that's even possible.

THERAPIST: Okay, let me inject a note of hope here. If you're willing to keep talking about these sensitive issues, I think you have a chance now to make these latter years some of the *best* years of your life.

JOSEPH: Well, I'm glad one of us is an optimist. [*Laughs*] I'll see you next week.

———

By exploring struggles around ultimate meaning, clients can begin to learn more about the potentially deeper side of their problems. Joseph, for example, was introduced to the idea that his feelings of depression and anxiety might be tied to the loss of his sense of significance. The problem of gambling was reframed as an attempt to fill that gap. And a name was given to the idea of "struggle." Efforts such as these to help people like Joseph explore their struggles have been tied to greater well-being and growth in research studies (Desai & Pargament, 2015; Wilt, Stauner, et al., 2019).

With a greater understanding of these struggles, the client can start to feel a glimmer of hope that there may be a way out and that things may get better. Not only that, the outline of a road map for change may begin to emerge. With respect to this road map, therapy involving struggles of ultimate meaning often takes one of two directions (and sometimes both): conservation, which involves holding on to or more fully realizing current sources of meaning; and transformation, which involves letting go of sources of meaning that are no longer viable and discovering new sources of meaning in their place (Pargament, 1997).

Conservation: Holding on to Ultimate Meaning

Because the confusion and disorientation that accompanies struggles of ultimate meaning can be so distressing, strugglers often need to find some goal they can hold on to as they work through their questions of purpose. Therapists can help them in this process. Consider once again the case of Joseph.

———

THERAPIST: Something you said last week stuck with me. You talked about how much you love your family and then added that you don't think they know it, that you're the invisible man. I wonder if it has to be that way.

JOSEPH: Well, that ship has already sailed. My kids are grown and out of the home.

THERAPIST: Do you have any grandchildren?

JOSEPH: Yes, two, the youngest just turned 1 and the other is 4.

THERAPIST: Are they close by? How often do you see them?

JOSEPH: Yes, they live in town but I only see them every few months.

THERAPIST: Here's a thought: What if you started to stop by more regularly?

JOSEPH: I guess I could. My daughter is always asking me to come over.

THERAPIST: Maybe you have a chance now to be a more visible loving parent.

Joseph began to drop over occasionally to see his two grandchildren and found that he enjoyed his time with them. When his daughter mentioned that she was thinking about going back to work and would need a part-time babysitter, Joseph volunteered. His daughter was surprised, but happy to take her father up on his offer. A while later, when I asked Joseph whether he still felt like the invisible man, he responded, "Running after kids, feeding them, and being peed on when you change a diaper would make anyone visible." As he invested more of his time and energy in something that truly mattered to him, Joseph's mood began to lighten and he began to spend less time gambling.

Relevant to Joseph's case, Russo-Netzer (2019) conducted a research study that showed how prioritizing meaningful activities in daily life can enhance well-being. Working with two samples of Israeli adults, she found that those who devoted more of their time to activities that reflected their goals and purposes in life experienced a number of benefits, including more life satisfaction, happiness, positive emotions, gratitude, and a sense of meaning in life. "Focusing on and prioritizing engagement in activities that are inherently value-congruent," she concluded, "offer a promising route to experiencing well-being" (p. 1887).

Of course, holding on to one's reasons for living may be easier said than done. As we have noted, life can create obstacles that make it quite difficult to realize personal dreams. Nelson Mandela's remarkable life story provides a case in point. In his autobiography *Long Walk to Freedom*, Mandela (1994) described his lifelong struggle against apartheid to achieve freedom and democracy for South Africans. Along the way, he spent 28 years in a tiny prison cell where he faced separation from family, the cruelty of guards, and hard physical labor. His ability to hold fast to his larger spiritual vision in the face of personal suffering, conflict with white oppressors, and clashes with other black freedom fighters who advocated for racial violence accounts, in part, for his heroic status today as the father of democratic South Africa.

In the context of therapy, many clients need support, encouragement, and hope if they are to persist in the pursuit of their own meaningful goals. This support may come directly from the therapist, who at times can help by simply cheering the client on, or from other sources, including spiritual resources. Years ago, one of K.I.P.'s clients with bipolar disorder described the support and direction she experienced from God when she felt directionless and lost:

> "If I did not believe in God and know his wondrous ways, I would be like a lost puppy having no place to go. I feel His presence around me, and I know that my life does not have to be like a tidal wave that comes crashing down. God uplifts me and keeps me stable. This is all I ask for, to be like that beautiful calm sea."

Conservation in Times of Grief

Special mention must be made of conservation in times of grief and loss. It may seem odd to talk about helping clients "hold on" to a loved one following a death. Psychotherapy with people who are grieving, however, involves not only assistance in accepting loss but also help in maintaining a connection with the essence of the life of the loved one (Klass, 1988). Here, the task is one of integrating the cherished memories of the deceased or, from a spiritual perspective, the essence of their spirit or soul.

Secularly minded therapists may find reports of continued attachment with a loved one who has died as abnormal or as a sign of psychopathology (see Exline, in press, for a discussion). There is, however, nothing unusual about these experiences. Although estimates vary widely, a review suggested that roughly one-third of people may have these experiences (Streit-Horn, 2011; see also *www.after-death.com*). In their follow-up study of caregiving partners of men with AIDS, Richards et al. (1999) found that 70% reported an ongoing relationship with the deceased 3–4 years later. All the more remarkable is that these reports emerged unsolicited through open-ended interviews with the survivors. The continued relationships took several different forms: active-living memories, communications with the departed person, a feeling that the loved one is present, and the sense that the loved one has become a part of the self. Although systematic research studies are still in relatively short supply (see Streit-Horn, 2011), Benore and Park (2004) assert that loved ones can sustain a relationship with the deceased without getting lost in a sea of grief. Moreover, a continued relationship with the loved one may benefit the survivor by affording a source of guidance, continuity in values and the sense of purpose, reduced feelings of isolation and distress, and an identity strengthened by memories of the deceased.

Therapists can help clients sustain a connection with loved ones who have died in a few ways. Simply talking about the deceased is a way of keeping memories and experiences alive. Consider the example of one client, Jane, who was feeling terribly isolated and depressed while undergoing treatment in a hospital for cancer. Her isolation was magnified by the death of both of her parents in the past year. Asked about how her parents had touched her life, Jane spoke movingly about their constant support and encouragement over the years. "I always knew they were with me," she said, "but now I feel so alone in the world." This conversation may have triggered an important experience that night:

> "I couldn't sleep and I was lying awake in the dark. And then I had the sense that someone had entered my room. When I turned to look, I saw it was both of my parents standing next to my bed. My mother didn't say anything. She just held my hand. She was always the quiet one. But my father told me that they loved me and that they'd always be by my side. I felt so comforted and I fell right to sleep. And I can still feel their presence."

Clients can also be encouraged to draw on rituals from their own religious traditions that have been designed to facilitate a continued attachment to the loved one. These rituals include memorials to keep the names of loved ones alive, sacred offerings on behalf of the deceased, or household shrines in honor of dead parents. For example, recognizing that altar-making is commonplace among many Spanish-speaking regions of the world, Bermúdez and Bermúdez (2002) encourage their Hispanic clients who are struggling with grief to construct homemade shrines. Clients fill their altars with personal artifacts, letters, toys, poems, prayers, photographs, and symbols of those who have died. These objects offer tangible memories and stories of the deceased that trigger recollections and reexperiences of the presence of the loved one more fully in their daily lives. The altar also functions similarly to a telephone through which clients can share thoughts and feelings with the deceased. These may range from expressions of love and caring to those of anger, regret, or estrangement. Any of these feelings, however, can help clients find greater peace with the memories of their loved ones.

Finally, the recollection of sacred moments with a loved one may be an especially powerful way to sustain an ongoing relationship with someone who has died. Recall that sacred moments are times of deep interconnectedness and strong spiritual emotion. These moments are experienced as transcendent, sources of ultimate truth, and unforgettable (Pargament, Lomax, McGee, & Fang, 2014), and they have been associated with mental health benefits, such as lower depression and anxiety, greater meaning and purpose, spiritual well-being, and resolution of spiritual struggles (Magyar-Russell, Pargament, Grubbs, Wilt, & Exline, 2020; Pargament et al., 2014; Wilt et al., 2018). Wong (2020) has developed a promising sacred moments reflection/meditation that can be used to help clients reconnect with their most treasured memories, including memories of those who have died (see Table 9.1).

TABLE 9.1. Treasure Chest Meditation

Breathe. Settle into your chair, with your hands resting comfortably and your feet touching the floor. Close your eyes if you feel comfortable doing so. Otherwise, settle your gaze on a space that's close to you.

Allow your attention to begin to turn inward. You can always return to your breath when you feel lost or when your mind wanders. Let your breath be your anchor. In. Out. Remember, there is no right or wrong way of doing this exercise. Breathe.

Picture a treasure chest in your mind. See if you can envision this sealed chest that contains your most precious memories. Consider the size of your chest—How big is it? How heavy? Perhaps your chest is made out of wood, wicker, or lined with fabric. Notice its colors and the finish.

Now imagine opening your treasure chest. Inside this box are your memories. Here are your life's sacred moments, collected in one place—as snapshots or moving pictures. You begin sifting through your chest of memories.

As you move through your memories, see if you can find one sacred moment that you experienced with your loved one. Maybe you experienced it with your loved one at home, maybe outdoors, maybe at a special event, or maybe in something seemingly ordinary. In any case, it is a moment in time that feels set apart from the others. Perhaps it's a moment that lifted you up. A moment that feels timeless. A moment that opened your heart to something really real. A moment of deep connection. Perhaps, as you hold this moment, the edges of it even glow.

With your eyes still closed or set downward, lift one finger when you have chosen your moment. You may have many sacred moments, but pick only one. Sit with this moment in your lap. Now allow your finger to come down, making contact with your chosen moment.

Imagine the essence of this moment wash over you and into you. Warmly enveloping you into this sacred memory. Drawing you into your sacred moment. Perhaps you are wholly absorbed into this scene. Notice what's ahead of you, behind you, around you. Recall the sounds of this moment. The temperature. Any tastes, smells, or movements that you made. Breathe in this sacred moment and draw what you need from it. Whether it be comfort, gratefulness, or love from this moment. Take in all that you need. Continue to be in this sacred space for the next couple of minutes.

Now that you have been filled by this moment, allow yourself to let go of it until next time. It will always be there for you. You can return to your treasure chest at any time. Now gently turn your attention outward, into the room, into the present, and all through your body. When you feel ready, open your eyes.

Note. From Wong (2020).

Transformation: Letting Go and Discovering New Ultimate Meaning

Letting go of the things we care about may be the hardest thing in the world to do (Pargament, 2007). Loving relationships, careers, cherished beliefs and values, dreams for the future—these are some of the sources of significance that lend stability, organization, purpose, and direction to our lives. The very idea of giving them up may seem unimaginable and resisted at all costs. This is especially the case when our purposes in life are imbued with sacred value. Our natural inclination is to conserve, to hold on and sustain what gives us meaning and purpose. Life, however, can insist on change. When old sources of meaning are lost or no longer viable, when long-held aspirations fail to meet changing times and needs, when the things we invest energy in no longer offer a sense of significance, it may be time to let go. The failure to do so can lead to the problems that clients bring to therapy. In these instances, clients often need help dealing with the two key processes underlying transformation: letting go and discovering new sources of ultimate meaning.

Letting Go

Returning to the case of Joseph, over the course of therapy it became apparent that he had never confronted the terrible pain of the loss of his dream of becoming a concert pianist, a dream that had held deep spiritual meaning for him. Instead, he had numbed himself through a job that had consumed much of his time but none of his passion and, more recently, time wasted on online gambling. And in doing so, he had turned into an invisible father and perhaps an invisible man as well, with little zest for living. In his refusal to mourn, he had become, in the words of Frankel (2005), "emotionally and spiritually frozen" (p. 48). This therapeutic understanding led to an important moment in treatment that occurred when Joseph's therapist noticed that he was humming softly to himself as he was walking into the office.

THERAPIST: What are you humming? It's a nice melody.

JOSEPH: Oh, I hadn't noticed. I think it's one of Béla Bartók's Romanian Folk Dances. I used to play it.

THERAPIST: Really! Could you pull it up on YouTube? I'd love to hear it.

JOSEPH: I don't know. I haven't played it in so many years.

THERAPIST: Even so, it's still very much alive in your mind. I'd love to hear it along with you.

JOSEPH: I don't know. [*Long pause*]. Okay [*with a great deal of hesitation*]. [*We listen to Bartók's Romanian Folk Dances on piano and Joseph starts to cry softly.*]

THERAPIST: Can you share a little about how you're feeling?

JOSEPH: I played that piece myself. I was so good . . . when I played it, I felt like God was inside of me. . . . I had so much potential . . . then it was gone—just like that. [*Breaks into sobs.*]

THERAPIST: [*Long silence*] You lost something that was a part of your soul.

JOSEPH: Yes, but it happened so many years ago.

THERAPIST: Maybe in years, but it sounds like you're continuing to grieve even now. [*Long pause*] You know, Joseph—I think it might help if you were able to grieve more openly. Airing out that wound could help it to heal more cleanly.

JOSEPH: How would I do that?

THERAPIST: Well, let's take it one step at a time. Could you bring in some other music that you loved as a child?

JOSEPH: I guess I could. Actually, I still have some old recordings of my own playing. I don't know why I held on to them—I haven't listened to them for many, many years.

THERAPIST: I'd love to hear some of your old recordings. Why not bring one in?

JOSEPH: [*Long pause*] Okay.

Over the next few sessions, Joseph brought in some of his old recordings and together he and his therapist listened. Coming face-to-face with the power and depth of his loss was a painful process for Joseph. But, with the help of his therapist, who normalized Joseph's grieving and supported his strength, Joseph began to face the reality of what he had to let go.

Therapists can draw on other resources to assist clients through the process of giving up old dreams. Of these, spiritual resources may be especially potent. Prayer, for example, can help reduce the power of destructive cravings and yearnings that have become a centerpiece of life. As one member of Narcotics Anonymous described it:

> I could get angry inside or upset inside and that stupid thinking will come back to me and say "yeah, I need a hit now" then I have to pray and I say the serenity prayer, "Lord grant me the serenity" . . . I have to let that go. I can't always have that with me (Green, Fullilove, & Fullilove, 1998, p. 327).

Ritual represents another valuable resource for letting go. Many of the most painful of transitions people experience today—infertility, miscarriage, divorce, illness, unemployment, retirement, moving into a nursing home— are "under-ritualized," leaving people without a way to fully express their sense of grief and loss (Lerner, 1994). Most recently, the pandemic of COVID-19 has forced many families to grieve the loss of loved ones without the benefit of rituals, such as funerals, that are designed to shepherd mourners through this time of anguish, supported by the love and care of family and friends. Therapists can help clients construct and engage in exercises and rituals that acknowledge the reality of their losses and give voice to their emotional pain. Consider the "Breath of God" exercise developed by Brenda Cole to help women with cancer let go of aspects of their lives that are no longer under their control and ability to attain (Cole & Pargament, 1999). Women begin by relaxing through deep breathing as they imagine a restful scene. They are then asked to imagine being surrounded by God's presence as a white light and inhaling the white light with each breath. Next, the women are encouraged to ask God what they most need to surrender and then listen for an answer. In the last part of the exercise, they visualize letting go of what can no longer be a meaningful part of their lives. As a group, participants found this exercise quite helpful.

Discovering New Sources of Ultimate Meaning

Letting go is only one part of the process of transformation. New sources of significant purpose must also be identified and nurtured to fill the gap left by old sources of meaning. Therapists have an important role to play in helping clients who may be struggling with lost meaning find new purpose. Support and encouragement are a necessary part of guiding clients through the often confusing process of discovery. Spiritually oriented clients can also find support from their personal faith. Here is one such prayer:

> My Lord God, I have no idea where I am going . . . and the fact that I think I am following your will does not mean that I am actually doing so. . . . I will trust you always though I may seem to be lost and in the shadow of death. I will not fear, for you are ever with me, and you will never leave me to face my perils alone. (Martin, 2006, pp. 64–65)

Meaning and purpose can be facilitated in therapy through dialogue, experience, and experimentation. Dialogue is one central component of Paul Wong's (2015) meaning therapy, an extension of Viktor Frankl's logotherapy, which is designed to help clients discover and foster greater meaning and purpose. Wong engages people in Socratic dialogue that centers around existential questions, such as "What is the point of all my striving? How do I know my true calling? What would make my life more meaningful and significant? What special mission or goals have all my experiences and gifts prepared me for?" (p. 161). He also asks clients to "fast-forward" and "Imagine yourself on your deathbed. What would be your biggest regrets?" (p. 161). Some evidence points to the effectiveness of this kind of approach. For instance, one study evaluated the impact of a group meaning-oriented therapy on Iranian students who reported elevated levels of depression and meaninglessness (Robatmili et al., 2015). The 10-session program focused on encouraging participants to identify their core values and goals and then create an action plan to realize their aspirations. Students in the treatment group showed significantly lower levels of depression and greater purpose in life than those in a control group immediately after therapy and 1-month posttreatment.

Also notable here are legacy programs for people at the end of life who may struggle to find a reason for going on in the face of the loss of many of the activities and attachments that had given their lives a sense a deep significance. Legacy programs are designed to foster meaning and purpose by capturing the accumulated wisdom of those who are dying and passing it on to their loved ones (e.g., Chochinov, 2002; Piderman, Breitkopf, et al., 2017). Interviews with patients are transcribed, shaped into narrative form, and shared with the patients to make sure they accurately reflect their legacies. The narratives are then assembled into legacy documents that are distributed to loved ones. Here is the distilled legacy of the wisdom of one woman: "Life's too short, life's too precious. Really pay attention to what you are doing. Don't take it for granted. Go out there and have a good time and enjoy life and make happy, fun memories, but don't take it for granted. Don't live it stupidly" (Piderman, Egginton, et al., 2017). In one evaluation of Piderman's spiritual legacy program, participants showed increases in quality of life, spiritual well-being, and positive religious coping (Piderman, Breitkopf, et al., 2017).

Some clients, however, may find it hard to articulate what it is that gives or has given them meaning. Purpose for them may be best revealed not through words but through moving personal experiences. After all, the things that matter most can take many forms, but they are never boring. They can be unveiled through stories that "touch the soul" (Elkins, 1995), periods of introspection that help locate an "inner mentor" (Kass, 2017), sacred moments from the past that continue to resonate (Pargament et al., 2014), or dreams that reveal hidden longings. Consider one 50-year-old client who had been struggling with a sense of emptiness in her life for many years. In one key session, she described a dream in which she saw herself sitting by a stream reading to children outside of an African village. As she talked about her dream in therapy, she began to cry. When her therapist asked her about her tears, she said she was crying because the dream both frightened her—she had never traveled outside of the Midwest—and strangely moved and excited her. Although she was hesitant, with the encouragement of her therapist, she started to explore the possibility of making her dream a reality. Eventually, she went on an educational mission to Africa through a local church. Her dream set in motion a new journey that led ultimately to a fulfilling, late-life career as a teacher.

As this clinical example also highlights, encouraging clients to experiment, try things out, and see what sparks their interest is another important way meaning and purpose can be fostered in therapy. Meaning in this sense comes from doing. Recall that with the gentle prodding of his therapist, Joseph had begun to babysit for his young grandchildren. This became an important source of meaning and satisfaction for Joseph. It didn't stop there though, as we hear in the following exchange:

JOSEPH: It's been a while since I've seen you but I have something interesting to report.

THERAPIST: What's that?

JOSEPH: Well, my 4-year-old grandson, Jimmy, was messing around on the floor with a toy xylophone. I sat next to him and played a little tune. He copied me almost perfectly. I played a little harder tune and he copied that, too. It blew me away.

THERAPIST: That does sound amazing. It sounds like he's naturally talented.

JOSEPH: Well, I wondered about that. So I went out, bought a little keyboard, and brought it over. Darned if he wasn't able to play some simple tunes right away. He seemed to really enjoy it—I couldn't get him away from the keyboard. So I asked my son and daughter-in-law whether they would mind if I gave him a few lessons. They were fine with it. I gave him a few lessons and we had a ball. I think he's really got a gift. He's learning to read music and he's only begun to read English!

THERAPIST: Jimmy reminds me in some ways of another child prodigy: you! But I know music for you became a source of terrible pain and loss. What's it like now for you to be teaching Jimmy keyboard?

JOSEPH: I'm in a different place now. You've helped me put a lot of that pain behind me. I always thought that God had turned his back on me, but now I see that I had turned my back on other possibilities for my life. And now I am so excited that I might be able to help Jimmy develop his own gift. I don't care what he does with it. I just want him to find some of the joy that I was able to find in music.

THERAPIST: Sounds like you have a new mission.

JOSEPH: Yeah, it's not what I had dreamt of earlier in my life. It may sound a little corny, but maybe my real purpose now is to make sure that God's gift of music gets passed on to someone else. I don't know. All I know is it resonates with me now.

THERAPIST: Music to your ears! [*Laughter*]

Joseph had discovered a new source of deep significance and, in the process, his life was transformed.

CONCLUSIONS

Psychotherapy is designed in large part to help people realize their aspirations. Yet some people come to therapy struggling to articulate their aspirations or grappling with lost or unfulfilled dreams. These struggles of ultimate meaning may be embedded within many other clinical problems. In these cases, therapists face the challenge of helping clients find an authentic guiding vision.

Clinical work of this kind is neither simple nor straightforward for at least a few reasons. First, generic meanings in life cannot be imposed. Rather, they must be discovered or created by each individual. As Buber (1950) wrote, "Every man's foremost task is the actualization of his unique, unprecedented, and never-recurring possibilities and not the repetition of something that another, be it even the greatest, has already achieved" (p. 149). Therapists can help guide clients through the process of identifying and realizing their significant purposes in life. Second, it takes a great deal of strength, wisdom, and courage, as well as time and patience, to grapple with questions of ultimate meaning—to know when to hold on and when to let go, to confront the pain of lost dreams, and to face the anxiety of finding a new guiding vision. Clients need considerable support to move toward greater meaning and purpose. Finally, the therapeutic pathway toward ultimate meaning requires sensitive attention to both the client's personal needs and desires, and the client's sense of deeper meaning, higher calling, or divine spark within the self. Helping clients find a way to harmonize these very human and very spiritual strivings to achieve an authentic guiding vision is part of the art of therapy.

Clinical work involving questions of ultimate meaning can certainly be challenging. It is, however, vital work because an authentic guiding vision is an essential ingredient of what it means to be whole. We turn now to a related form of struggle that centers around the challenge of making meaning and sense of the world: struggles with doubt.

CHAPTER 10

Struggles with Doubt

When [the eclipse] came to pass . . . there were a tumult and disorder.
All were disquieted, unnerved, frightened. Then there was weeping.
The common folk, raised a cup, lifting their voices, making a great din,
calling out, shrieking. There was shouting everywhere.
—Response of the Aztecs to the 16th-century eclipse reported by
BERNARDO DE SAHUGAN, cited in Aveni (2017, p. 251)

Throughout history, eclipses and other unusual celestial events have shaken and disturbed people, raising unsettling questions about how the universe works. These questions highlight the need to make sense of the cosmos, particularly what is most uncanny, strange, and mysterious. Anthropologist Clifford Geertz (1966) maintained that meaning-making is a primary concern of all people within all cultures. To function effectively, humans must be able to understand their world.

Of course, efforts to achieve understanding apply not only to the physical universe but also to the social and personal world. For thousands of years, people have sought answers to life's most fundamental existential questions: How did we get here? Who are we and how should we live our lives? How should we relate to one another? Why is there pain, violence, and suffering in the world? What becomes of us when we die?

The religions of the world are designed, in part, to offer compelling answers to baffling questions and to provide reassurance that what may seem incomprehensible is in fact comprehensible, that there is a larger order lying beneath what may seem chaotic (Geertz, 1966). Religiously based answers are intended to be deeply felt, utterly convincing understandings that speak to what is true, what is "really, real" (Geertz, 1966). In theistic traditions, God is said to hold the key to truth; in fact, God may be defined as the truth, as we hear in the autobiography of Gandhi (1968): "I worship God as Truth only. I have not yet found Him, but I am seeking after Him" (p. 11). It is important to add that, more and more today, people are seeking their own answers to life's great existential questions through personal spiritualities that revolve around nontheistic understandings of the sacred or develop outside the boundaries of traditional religious institutions (Russo-Netzer & Mayseless, 2014). Whether the answers people arrive at are institutionally based or more personally constructed, they reflect the same human need to make sense of the world.

There are times, though, when the most basic beliefs and assumptions about the world—religious, spiritual, and nonreligious—are shaken. Listen, for example, to the words of a Nicaraguan adolescent: "[I] sometimes doubt whether God really exists . . . I don't understand why He lets little children in Third World countries die of starvation and diseases. . . . It seems like He just doesn't care. Does He?" (Kooistra, 1990, pp. 91–92). In these times, what had once seemed convincing and true makes less sense and people begin to struggle with doubt. There is a lot at stake when worldviews that were supposed to answer deep questions become sources of question and confusion in themselves, not only because seeking answers to questions is of intrinsic value but because meaning-making frameworks help ground and orient people as they seek out many other forms of significance, including a sense of emotional security in the world, personal identity, connectedness with others, a sense of ultimate purpose in life, and a closer bond with what people hold sacred. It should not be altogether surprising then that the effects of doubt may be strong and far-reaching. In this chapter, we take up the topic of doubt-related struggles. Our focus is on religious and spiritual doubts in particular because we believe that these are among the deepest and most troubling of all doubts.

We define struggles with religious and spiritual doubts as confusion, tension, and strain about fundamental beliefs regarding matters related to the sacred (to save space we often refer to these struggles with doubt as "doubt struggles," or, in some cases, simply as doubts, although we recognize that not all doubts necessarily involve struggles). Doubts are not the same as unbelief. Unbelief, like belief, involves a level of certainty and conviction, but in the case of unbelief, the certainty focuses on what one doesn't believe. Doubt, marked as it is by uncertainty and confusion, occupies a place of its own between belief and unbelief (cf. Pruyser, 1974). Doubt could conceivably lead in several directions: Those who doubt might eventually make a firm decision to believe or not believe. In contrast, some people might find themselves struggling chronically with doubts. Others might intentionally adopt a doubting or skeptical attitude as a stable approach to religious and spiritual matters or other beliefs.

Understood this way, struggles related to doubt are not necessarily inconsistent with belief or faith. The Nicaraguan adolescent above was simultaneously expressing both doubts about God and beliefs in God. Some religious thinkers go further and assert that doubt is an integral part of faith. Tillich (1975) emphasized that, because religious language and symbols cannot adequately capture what is of ultimate truth, questions and doubt provide an important check against the risks of a kind of idolatry that freezes people into the worship of concrete or literal religious symbols and expressions rather than the deeper truths they represent. Summing it up, he wrote, "Doubt is not the opposite of faith; it is an element of faith. Therefore there is not faith without risk" (p. 116). In some religions, such as Zen Buddhism, doubt is an explicit part of the tradition. "Great doubt: great awakening. Little doubt: little awakening. No doubt: no awakening" is the way 16th-century Zen Master Boshan (2016, p. 4) put it. And doubting is an integral part of American civil religion. In a letter to his nephew, Thomas Jefferson encouraged him to "Question with boldness even the existence of a God, because, if there be one, he must more approve of the homage of reason than that of blind faith" (cited in Seldes, 1985, p. 207).

Doubts can vary in breadth. Some people experience a general and diffuse sense of confusion about life, a "puzzlement about how things are going" in the world (Holley, 2011, p. 757) or about religion in general. In contrast, others experience specific questions and doubts about more particular beliefs commonly associated with religious faith. Is there a God (or gods), a spirit world, or an afterlife? Have they selected the "true" religion? Do their religious teachings about the origins of the universe and life, sexuality, morality, and suffering make sense? Of course, one doubt may lead to another, and eventually the entire edifice of belief may begin to teeter. Although doubts may be singular, research on religious doubting by a leader in this area, Bruce Hunsberger, suggests there may be a "doubt syndrome" with various types of doubt clustering together (Hunsberger, McKenzie, Pratt, & Pancer, 1993).

There is certainly nothing new about doubts. In her book *Doubt: A History*, Jennifer Hecht (2003) considers how, throughout history, doubt has coexisted with religion. In England, for example, the 19th century was labeled the Age of Doubt, a time when scientific advances threw into question the most fundamental assumptions by which people had lived (Lane, 2011). This was an "epoch of incredulity," as well as an "epoch of belief," as Charles Dickens (1902, p. 3) famously introduced in his book *A Tale of Two Cities*. In Russia in 1880, Fyodor Dostoevsky published *The Brothers Karamazov*, in which we hear "God sets us nothing but riddles. . . . Too many riddles weigh men down on earth" (2017, p. 128).

If statistics are any guide, we continue to live in an age of doubt. In our large sample of adults (Exline, Pargament, & Grubbs, 2014), 45.4% experienced some level of religious or spiritual doubt-related struggles over the past few weeks, such as feeling confused about their religious or spiritual beliefs. Among patients with advanced cancer, 20.0% reported some level of doubt about their faith or belief in God (Winkelman et al., 2011). A survey of Christian high school adolescents revealed that 77.0% were currently having some doubts about religion (Kooistra, 1990).

Tied as they are to sacred matters that involve both core beliefs and basic emotions, doubt-related struggles can be embedded in many of the problems people bring to therapy, including depression, anxiety, anger, and interpersonal conflicts. In short, struggles with doubt deserve more explicit attention in the practice of psychology.

WHAT WE KNOW ABOUT STRUGGLES WITH DOUBT

In this chapter, we review what we are learning from emerging research on the struggles that surround doubt. First, we focus on the roots of struggles with doubt. Then we consider the consequences of these struggles. We will see that they can lead to disorientation, distress, and decline. There is, however, another potentially more positive side to doubt. Writings by theologians and psychologists, supplemented by many narrative accounts, speak to the key role doubting can play in growth, including spiritual maturation. As with other spiritual struggles, doubt struggles can lead to greater brokenness and decline and/or greater wholeness and growth. We then examine how we can apply this knowledge to help clients struggling with doubt move toward greater wholeness in their lives.

Sources of Struggles with Doubt

From the perspective of our model, doubt struggles, like other spiritual struggles, grow out of the interplay between the individual's life experiences, orienting system, and significant purposes.

Life Experiences

In her Pulitzer Prize-winning work of nonfiction *Pilgrim at Tinker Creek*, Annie Dillard (1974), watches in horror as a frog dies in a pond after it had been poisoned and paralyzed by a water bug: "The spirit vanished from him as if snuffed. His skin emptied and dropped; his very skull seemed to collapse and settle like a kicked tent. He was shrinking before my eyes like a deflating football" (pp. 7–8). Dillard struggles to square her beliefs in a knowing and loving Creator with the gruesome examples of violence she witnessed in nature. This confrontation between belief and experience is one of the primary sources of struggles with doubt.

Even though the orienting system can help people make sense or meaning (cf. Park, 2005) out of challenging events, some life experiences are of such magnitude that they are difficult, if not impossible, to assimilate. These experiences create what Hecht (2003) called "meaning ruptures" (p. xii), a shaken system of beliefs and an orientation to the world that no longer offers understanding of suffering and loss or clear guidance in the search for significance.

One study revealed that a staggering 90% of mothers who had given birth to a child with profound intellectual disability expressed some doubts about God's existence (Childs, 1985). In an interview study of survivors of the suicide of a loved one, the majority (most of whom were religious believers at the time of the suicide) voiced deep questions about their faith (Dransart, 2018). Krause and Hayward (2012a) surveyed a sample of older African Americans and found that those who had accumulated more lifetime traumas were more likely to report religious doubts.

Life experiences do not have to be heart wrenching to trigger struggles with doubt. A variety of experiences can elicit these struggles. For example, Kooistra (1990) interviewed a group of Roman Catholic and Dutch Reformed high school students and identified several primary sources of struggles with doubt:

- *The problem of evil.* Doubts elicited by cruelty and injustice in the world.
- *Violations of self-interest.* Doubts triggered by personal losses and disappointments.
- *The problem of hypocrisy.* Doubts fostered by the hypocrisy of religious individuals, leaders, and institutions.
- *The human creator.* Doubts resulting from exposure to beliefs that people created the idea of God only to serve their own emotional and social needs.
- *Conflicting evidence.* Doubts growing out of evidence that challenges religious teachings.
- *The problem of relativism.* Doubts rooted in exposure to diverse religions that also claim to be true.
- *Failure of ritual.* Doubts following the failure of rituals (e.g., prayers, faith healing) that were believed to reveal the power of God.

In one of the few studies of American Muslims on this topic, Chouhoud (2018) surveyed a sample about their doubts regarding Islam and found a similar set of major triggers.

Doubt can also grow out of other spiritual struggles. Studies have shown that people who struggle spiritually with God, with the demonic, with moral issues, with questions of ultimate meaning, and with other people are also more likely to experience doubts about religion and spirituality as a whole (Exline, Pargament, Grubbs, & Yali, 2014). In short, many experiences are capable of triggering fundamental doubts about religious and spiritual claims.

Certain transitional periods in life are also particularly ripe times for struggles with doubt. Doubts occur among all age groups. Even so, a small but significant inverse relationship has been reported between doubting and age, with doubts reaching their highest points during adolescence and early adulthood and then declining (Galek, Krause, Ellison, Kudler, & Flannely, 2007; Stauner et al., 2015). Doubting during this time of life, Fowler (1981) and Erikson (1968) have written, is a natural part of the process of transition from the faith of childhood and family to a more autonomous point of view and, ultimately, faith of greater wholeness and maturity later in life. Doubting can also be understood as a key part of identity formation in adolescence and early adulthood (Marcia, 1966), particularly among those in the status of "moratorium"—a time of actively exploring religious and spiritual alternatives without making religious commitments. Hunsberger, Pratt, and Pancer (2001) found that adolescents in moratorium status did indeed report more struggles with doubt than those who were not actively exploring spiritual issues or had formed their identity.

We should note that much of the research above focuses on triggers of doubt among traditionally religious groups of people. However, secular individuals, including atheists, are not immune to these struggles. Their struggles with doubt may be elicited by different kinds of life experiences—namely, unusual events, such as out-of-body experiences, mystical experiences, near-death experiences, encounters with God, or visitations by the spirit of someone who has died. Unusual experiences of these kinds might throw more secularized worldviews into question and doubt. For example, in a study of undergraduates who did not believe in God (Exline, Uzdavines, & Bradley, 2015), a prompt was given to ask them to imagine how they would feel if they suddenly received strong evidence that God existed. The most endorsed response, by a large margin, was confusion.

Psychiatrist James Lomax presented an apt illustration through the case of a cardiologist he was seeing for major depression (Lomax & Pargament, 2011). In the course of treatment, the client admitted to an experience that made her feel "strange" and "uncomfortable." She and her fiancé had planned a trip to Alaska. Unfortunately, her beloved mentor was dying, so before she left, she visited him to tell him how much he meant to her. In Alaska, while dog sledding on a glacier, she heard the voice of her mentor say, "Yes, I've died, but I love you. I will always love you, and you will do well" (p. 81). When she returned to her hotel, she learned that her teacher had indeed died while she was on the glacier. The experience was, on the one hand, very moving; on the other hand, it was also confusing, disturbing, and even embarrassing to her as a secularized physician working in a mainstream secular context.

Many religious people would respond to a visitation from the spirit of a loved one with excitement and gratitude. However, the very same experience could become a source of distress, disorientation, and struggle to someone with a more secularized worldview or a religious individual who is wary of reports of encounters with spirits. It follows that to understand the roots of doubting, we also have to consider the character of the individual's orienting system and significant purposes in life.

Orienting System and Significant Purposes

Let's consider three factors that set the stage for struggles with doubts.

Asking Questions as a Way of Life. As we noted above, doubts can arise at any point over the lifespan. In fact, for some people, raising questions can be part of an ongoing search for truth and a preferred way of being, an approach that is central to the individual's life pathway and destination. This is the essence of the quest orientation defined by Batson et al. (1993). In Chapter 3, quest was described as an approach that "involves honestly facing existential questions in all their complexity, while at the same time resisting clear-cut, pat answers" (p. 167). Although the final truths may never be known, "still, the questions are deemed important, and however tentative and subject to change, answers are sought" (p. 167).

Even though the quest orientation includes doubt as a core element, quest does not necessarily imply struggle around one's doubts. Delving into difficult questions about life is not inevitably accompanied by conflict, tension, and disruption, but neither is it a purely intellectual pursuit. Instead, we might think of struggles with doubt as one of the natural, common, but disquieting, by-products of general inquisitiveness. In this vein, struggles with doubt have been tied to higher scores on the measure of quest orientation (Kojetin et al., 1987) and a tendency to think in more complex analytical ways (Hunsberger et al., 1993).

Doubt struggles may also grow out of encounters with new ideas and diverse people and practices. In his study of religious apostasy, Zuckerman (2012) comments that "Experiencing, witnessing, or learning about other people who do things differently, believe different things, and/or hold different outlooks on life can stir up a process of critical self-reflection" (p. 156). One apostate's religious doubts were triggered by a conversation with the first atheist she had ever met:

> I remember asking him: do you believe in God? And he was like, "I don't know, I don't think so, really" . . . It was a shock to me that this could happen. He was somebody that I thought was really, really smart. He was a good person. . . . It kind of opened the door . . . where it's possible to doubt it. (p. 115)

Social settings that expose people to diverse groups, beliefs, and practices may be especially fertile ground for struggles over doubt. One such context is college, where students are likely to meet people who come from very different backgrounds and hold very different spiritual values and beliefs. In their longitudinal study of college students, Small and Bowman (2011) found that doubt struggles were more commonplace among students who attended colleges with a more ecumenical worldview that embraced the goodness of all people and found value in all the great religions. Moreover, struggles with doubt were higher in colleges where faculty provided more support for engaging religious and spiritual issues.

Some evidence suggests that college students who are more religious may be more vulnerable to doubt struggles, perhaps because they may be especially likely to have their worldview shaken by encounters with diverse people, beliefs, and practices. In support of this notion, Stauner, Wilt, Exline, and Pargament (2017) examined the relationship between the salience of religious beliefs of college students and their struggles with doubt over four points of time in college. They found that greater religious belief salience was predictive of more doubt struggles over time. As we are about to see, however, this finding may be specific to the college context.

Commitment to Religious and Spiritual Beliefs. Not long ago, the Most Revd Justin Welby, archbishop of Canterbury, made the controversial admission that he had some occasional doubts about God: "Is there a God? Where is God? . . . The other day I was praying over something as I was running, and I ended up saying to God, 'Look, this is all very well, but isn't it about time you did something, if you're there?' " (Baird, 2014). The comments of the archbishop serve as a reminder that faith and doubt are not necessarily inconsistent with each other. Having said that, it remains the case that people who are firmly committed to a set of religious and spiritual beliefs are generally less likely to report struggles with doubts. To this point, Flannelly (2017) reviewed the research literature on this topic and found that religious and spiritual doubt was less common among people who held stronger religious and spiritual beliefs, and greater religious commitment. It is important to add that some people who are ostensibly committed to their beliefs may in fact have a fragile hold on their worldview. They adhere to their beliefs not because they are intrinsically meaningful but in response to extrinsic social pressure, fears of the consequences of not believing, or the promise of external rewards. Those who hold this kind of extrinsic belief orientation are more prone to struggles with doubt (Puffer et al., 2008). Taken as a whole, with a few exceptions (e.g., Exline, Pargament, Grubbs, & Yali, 2014; Stauner et al., 2017), these findings suggest that struggles with doubt are less frequent among those more personally and deeply committed to a set of spiritual and religious beliefs.

This overall result makes good sense when we consider the critical role of the core set of beliefs, especially religious and spiritual beliefs, in orienting, stabilizing, and guiding the individual toward significant purpose in life (McIntosh, 1995). When these beliefs are shaken, people face threats to their worldview, identity, security, and sense of control. Perhaps for this reason, core beliefs tend to be resistant to question, challenge, and change.

Batson (1975) conducted an important study that illustrated this point. He had Presbyterian high school students complete a measure of their beliefs in the divinity of Jesus and the infallibility of the Bible. Next, the students read a presumably accurate, but in fact contrived, article from the *New York Times* reporting on recently discovered evidence "proving" that Jesus was not the son of God. As Batson predicted, those students who expressed religious belief and accepted the disconfirming information from the article as true showed a significant increase in the strength of their religious convictions. These core beliefs were clearly of deep value to many of the students, and when confronted with material that represented a potential threat to these valued beliefs, they responded not with questions and doubt but with greater commitment that served to preserve and protect the tenets they hold sacred.

Embeddedness in Secure Relationships. Beliefs serve not only the need for comprehension and understanding but also desires for affirmation, social identity, and belonging. When they are shared, systems of belief become part of the glue that bonds people together as families, institutions, and cultures. In contrast, raising questions and doubts could be socially, as well as personally, disturbing. This may help to explain why those who are more embedded in social networks and religious networks in particular are less likely to experience doubt struggles. In this vein, Krause and Ellison (2009), two key figures in research on doubt, worked with a sample of older adults and found that spiritual support from congregation members and involvement in Bible-study groups reduced the likelihood of struggles around doubt over time. Greater involvement in religious institutions, past and present, has also been associated with less doubt (Flannelly, 2017; Hunsberger et al., 1993).

A vivid example comes from the classic work in the psychology of religion, *When Prophesy Fails* (Festinger, Riecken, & Schachter, 1956). Leon Festinger and his colleagues studied a religious cult that was convinced that the world was about to experience a cataclysmic flood that would wipe out most of humanity. Cult members, however, were to be spared, taken in a spaceship to another planet for purification and returned to Earth, where they would bring light to a world repopulated by those who had been saved. The failure of the spaceship to appear on the predicted date, Festinger and colleagues assert, led to a state of dissonance in which deeply held beliefs were undeniably disconfirmed by the facts. As the researchers predicted, however, this disconfirmation did not result in the demise of the cult. Instead, members essentially doubled down on their beliefs, in part by rationalizing (e.g., the Earth had been spared as a result of the cult's activities), and in part by intensified efforts to convince others of the truth of their beliefs and bring them into the fold. None of this would have been possible, however, without the mutual affirmation and encouragement of cult members for their shared worldview. Most of the members had disconnected themselves from other relationships and invested all of their resources into the cult. The cost of doubting, social and personal, then would have been impossibly high. As one member put it, "I've given up just about everything. I've cut every tie: I've burned every bridge. I've turned my back on the world. I can't afford to doubt" (p. 168).

When social and spiritual connections are less strong and secure, the value of adhering to a common set of beliefs may diminish and questions and doubts may become more likely, perhaps in part to spur independence from more troubled relationships. Studies of various relationships support this idea. Kooistra and Pargament (1999) found that struggles surrounding doubt were higher among parochial high school students who saw their parents as more conflicted, authoritarian, and insincere about religion. Similarly, higher levels of doubt over time were linked to more problematic family environments in another investigation of high school students (Hunsberger, Pratt, & Pancer, 2002). Relevant, too, are findings by Exline, Grubbs, et al. (2015) that linked doubt struggles to perceptions of God as distant. Overall, these findings suggest that doubts tend to emerge from less secure social and spiritual connections.

In sum, like other spiritual struggles, struggles with doubt grow out of the interplay between life experiences and transitions, the orienting system, and significance. Specifically, struggle with doubts are more likely following difficult life experiences or transitions, such as adolescence. These struggles are also more common among those who take an inquisitive orientation to life in the search for truth, have less of a hold on core religious and spiritual beliefs, and feel less embedded in secure relationships. Shortly, we will see that an understanding of these roots can help guide practitioners in their efforts to help clients struggling with doubt. First, however, we turn our attention to another practically important body of knowledge concerning the consequences of doubt struggles.

Doubt Struggles Can Lead to Growth and Decline

From the perspective of our framework, struggles with doubt, like other struggles, represent potentially important crossroads leading to distress, disorientation, and decline, to greater wholeness and growth, or to both. We also assume that doubt-related struggles have important implications for the religious and spiritual life of the individual. What does the research literature have to say about these ideas?

Negative Implications of Struggles with Doubt

As we have noted, doubt struggles involve disconcerting questions about fundamental beliefs that orient people and guide them toward their significant purposes in living. As one adolescent put it, "[Doubting] makes me feel really scared and nervous. If I can't be sure of a religion, how can I be sure of anything?" (Kooistra, 1990, p. 105). Struggles with doubt can leave people uncertain about who they are, where they are going in life, and how to get there. No wonder then that doubt struggles have been consistently associated with signs of distress, disorientation, and decline.

Doubt-related struggles have been tied to greater anxiety and depressed mood in studies involving a variety of samples (e.g., Ellison & Lee, 2010; Krause & Wulff, 2004; Pargament, Zinnbauer, et al., 1998; Zarzycka & Zietek, 2019). Struggles have also been linked to lower levels of indicators of well-being, such as life satisfaction and happiness (see Flannelly, 2017, for a review).

Struggles with doubt may have more serious implications for mental and physical health. In research with a large national representative sample of adults in the United States, Galek, Krause, Ellison, Kudler, and Flannelly (2007) examined the relationship between religious doubts and several types of psychiatric symptoms, including paranoid ideation, hostility, obsessive–compulsiveness, phobic anxiety, and somatization. Higher levels of doubt were associated with each type of symptomatology. In addition, struggles with doubt have been related to lower self-rated health (Krause & Wulff, 2004), PTSD symptoms among Vietnam veterans (Berg, 2011), and depressive symptoms among Mexican Americans (Krause & Hayward, 2012b).

The majority of this literature is cross-sectional in design. This leaves unanswered the question of whether doubts lead to disorder (primary struggle model), disorder leads to doubts (secondary struggles model), or doubts are both a cause and effect of disorder (complex model). In support of a primary struggle model, Krause (2006) found that higher levels of doubt among practicing Christians predicted declines in self-esteem, life satisfaction, and optimism over a 3-year period. Wilt, Grubbs, Lindberg, Exline, and Pargament (2017) provided some evidence in support of secondary and complex struggle models. Working with three samples over the times of 2 weeks, 3 months, and 1 year, they compared the struggle models in terms of how well they fit the data. Both secondary and complex struggle models fit the data better than the primary struggle model, as well as a model in which anxiety and doubt simply accompany each other without affecting each other. Clearly, more research is needed on these thorny questions, but these initial findings suggest that doubt-related struggles have the potential to be both a cause and effect of distress and disorder. More longitudinal research is also needed to determine just how long-lasting the effects of doubt struggles may be.

One other set of findings is important to highlight. They address the question, Are people who are more religious and spiritual more likely or less likely to experience the costs of doubt-related struggles? Theoretically, a case could be made for both possibilities. Doubting, to those more deeply involved in spiritual life, may represent a greater threat to their identity, worldview, commitments, and values. As a result, the doubts of these individuals may be more strongly tied to disorientation and decline than the doubts of their less religious and spiritual counterparts. On the other hand, to the extent that greater religious and spiritual involvement is accompanied by stronger resources for coping with doubt, then we might expect the opposite pattern, with doubting among the more spiritually oriented associated with less distress and decline. Several studies speak to this question and they consistently indicate that doubting is more disturbing for people who are more religious and spiritual or within contexts that are less tolerant of doubts (e.g., Gauthier, Christopher, Walter, Mourad, & Marek, 2006; Kézdy, Martos, Boland, & Horváth-Szabó, 2011; Krause & Wulff, 2004).

Overall, struggles with doubt often appear to be accompanied by signs of distress, disorientation, and to some extent decline. Doubting also appears to be generally more disturbing to more religious and spiritual people, perhaps because their doubts represent more of a risk to their most fundamental beliefs. At first glance, this general pattern of findings seems to suggest that doubt struggles are another class of psychological problems or disorders. In fact, according to the most recent diagnostic system of the American Psychiatric Association, "loss or questioning of faith" can be diagnosed as a "religious or spiritual problem" (V62.89; Prusak, 2016). There are some reasons, however, to question whether struggles with doubt deserve this psychiatric label.

Positive Implications of Struggles with Doubt

A number of psychological theorists dissent from the idea that questions and doubts are problematic or pathological. Instead, they speak to the vital role of questions and doubts in fostering growth. As we noted earlier, developmental psychologists, such as Piaget and Erikson, described the ways tensions, questions, and conflicts push people toward the resolution of cognitive and emotional conundrums and challenges, and propel them toward higher levels of maturity. Similarly, doubts with respect to spiritual and religious matters have been said to foster the achievement of a strong identity, creativity, wisdom, humility, life transformation, and a broader and deeper orientation to the world (e.g., Baltazar & Coffen, 2011; Batson et al., 1993). Recall the title of Frankel's (2017) book *The Wisdom of Not Knowing: Discovering a Life of Wonder by Embracing Uncertainty*. Baltazar and Coffen speak to this point in a similar fashion: "The presence of doubt forces the individual to question past knowledge, and to develop new ways to integrate previous and newly acquired knowledge into an harmonious and consistent new discovery" (p. 189).

These are strong sentiments. Can they be supported? Hecht (2003), for one, points out that many of the world's greatest accomplishments were achieved by people whose questions about religion may have been part of the impetus for their discoveries. These figures include Socrates, Thomas Edison, Elizabeth Stanton, and Sigmund Freud. We can also find narrative accounts of growth-enhancing changes that occur following times of doubt-related struggle (e.g., Done, 2019; Ortberg, 2008). These writings would suggest that it may be helpful, literally, to "give people the benefit of the doubt" (Lane, 2011).

Theoretical writings and narrative accounts, however, have not been consistently supported by research findings. Only a few investigations have directly examined the relationships between doubt-related struggles and growth. In one study, the two processes were not significantly related to each other (Calhoun et al., 2000), and in another, struggles with doubt were associated with lower levels of growth (Pargament, Zinnbauer, et al., 1998).

Other lines of research, though, hint at more positive implications of doubt struggle. For example, we saw earlier that college students who attended colleges with a more ecumenical worldview and faculty who were more supportive of engaging in religious and spiritual issues were more likely to experience struggles with doubt (Small & Bowman, 2011). Conceivably, the questions that arise from this exposure to diversity could lead in the long run to a more personally owned stance toward spirituality.

Recent studies have also raised some questions about findings linking doubt-related struggles to distress and lower well-being. Some of these studies have also shown that, when the effects of the other forms of spiritual struggle are controlled, doubt struggles are no longer significantly linked to distress and poorer well-being. In fact, they sometimes become associated with signs of less distress and greater well-being (Exline, Pargament, Grubbs, & Yali, 2014; Stauner, Exline, & Pargament, 2016; Wong & Pargament, 2019).

How do we make sense of these puzzling findings? Perhaps by controlling for the other forms of spiritual struggles we are removing some of the general emotional pain that is part and parcel of questions and doubts in the spiritual domain. What is left in doubt struggles, then, may be a purer spirit of inquiry, exploration, and quest that holds more positive implications for growth and well-being. In support of what is admittedly a lot of conjecture, studies have shown that doubt struggles appear to go hand in hand with a questing orientation (e.g., Kojetin et al., 1987). However, while struggles over doubt are associated with lower levels of well-being, quest is generally more predictive of growth, creativity, and complex thinking (Batson et al., 1993; Calhoun et al., 2000; Hart et al., 2020).

Before we try to reach any definitive conclusions about the potentially positive implications of doubt struggles, it is important to stress that research in this area is still relatively new and developing. Longitudinal studies are needed because, as with other struggles, it may take quite a while for signs of growth and transformation to emerge following periods of doubt. Studies should also try to identify those factors that may lead to growth, including markers of wholeness, such as virtues, a guiding vision, wisdom, and cohesiveness.

Even though work in this area is still emerging, it seems safe to say that struggles with doubt do not inevitably lead to growth, at least in the short term. On the contrary, there is a clearer connection between struggling with doubt and distress, disorientation, and decline than with wholeness and growth. Nevertheless, it does not follow that doubt struggles should be treated as pathologies. If we take the theoretical writings, personal accounts, and initial research findings seriously, then it also seems safe to say that struggles with doubt have the potential to foster growth. Of course, given the ties between doubt and distress, any growth that takes place is unlikely to be pain-free. The term *growing pains* may be especially apt when it comes to struggling with doubt.

Religious and Spiritual Implications of Struggles with Doubt. Before turning to the more practical side, it is important to consider one more question: Is there a place for doubt in the individual's spiritual journey? This is one of the most contentious questions within religious and spiritual circles, and the answers have varied, sometimes dramatically. On one side, doubting has been viewed as, at best, an impediment to a life of faith and, at worst, a sure path to the loss of one's soul. For example, in the New Testament, readers are instructed to "believe and not doubt, because the one who doubts is like a wave of the sea, blown and tossed by the wind. That person should not expect to receive anything from the Lord. Such a person is double-minded and unstable in all they do" (James 1:6-8). Within the Quran, a terrifying fate is said to await those who doubt, especially those whose doubts have become fixed or led to disbelief: "Throw into Hell every stubborn disbeliever, Preventer of good, aggressor, doubter" (Quran 50:24-25). Harsh views of doubters are also articulated in modern times. For instance, one minister asserted that because all independent thought came from the devil, anyone who raises religious questions must be possessed (Jones, 2002).

Severe sentiments such as these help explain why struggles with doubt may be so threatening to people. Doubt can be experienced as a sin, a challenge to God's authority, and a failure to trust in God. These harsh views may also help to explain research findings tying doubt struggles to spiritual distress and decline. In one particularly well-done study, Van Tongeren, Sanders, et al. (2019) examined the effects of spiritual struggles on the ways college students experienced and understood God over 1 year. They found that struggles, especially doubt struggles, led to experiences of God as more punishing and less good. These feelings led, in turn, to changes in doctrinal beliefs about God as a less loving and good being. Focusing on adults who had lost a grandparent within the last 2 years, Patrick and Henrie (2015) found that those who experienced more struggles with doubt were less likely to report a deepening of their faith and spiritual understanding.

There is, however, another stream of thought about the place of doubt in the spiritual life of the individual. According to a number of writers, it is unquestioning certainty rather than doubt that impedes a deeper faith. As Allport (1950a) wrote, "Unless the individual doubts he cannot use his full intelligence and unless he uses his full intelligence he cannot develop a mature [religious] sentiment. . . . The mature religious sentiment is ordinarily fashioned in the workshop of doubt" (pp. 102, 294).

Many people do, in fact, appear to value their struggles with doubt, according to Krause and Ellison (2009). In their survey of older adults who reported religious doubts, the majority agreed that their doubts had helped them understand their faith better. Stories of people who experienced spiritual growth and transformation through their process of doubting are also available in the literature. Done (2019), for example, described how his struggles with doubt led him to make matters simpler rather than more complex: "Doubt, like shears, began to prune my faith," he writes. "It was an exhilarating, challenging, and exhausting process. But if I wanted to grow, I first had to cut back" (p. 186). Ultimately, he realizes, the search for certainty could never be successful. What he could attain, however, was a loving relationship with God, and in that relationship, he concludes, "You can still pursue the unknown, but you won't do it alone. You'll still have doubts, but you'll also have love. . . . And love lives in the hope that someday, somehow, all our tension, angst, worries, wonders, and doubts will be resolved" (p. 192).

Struggles with doubt may lead some in a different direction: to a withdrawal or complete exit from religious and spiritual life. Hunsberger and colleagues (2002) reported that, on average, high school students who experienced more doubts about religion declined in their religiousness over the next 2 years. Doubts about religion, even in childhood, also appear to play an important role in apostasy or the leaving of one's faith community (Altemeyer & Hunsberger, 1997). Whether apostasy is a good or bad thing depends on one's attitude toward organized religion. In fact, some research suggests that leaving the fold may be accompanied by both distress and relief. Apostates, in one study, reported several signs of distress: loss of friends, alienation from family, and a sense of having thrown away an entire orientation and guide for living (Altemeyer & Hunsberger, 1997). These same apostates, however, also talked about their newfound sense of freedom, open-mindedness, and personal strength and power.

In this section, we reviewed a wide body of literature that revealed many roots of struggles with doubt and then many potential outcomes. We saw that doubt struggles are sources of distress, disorientation, and decline. However, a more limited body of work also hints at possibilities for growth and positive transformation through doubts. Struggles with doubt could conceivably lead in many spiritual directions as well, including darker views of God, an enriched spiritual orientation, or a partial or total withdrawal from religious and spiritual life (Exline, 2002b; Fisher, 2017). The key question for practitioners is how to help clients struggling with doubt move away from brokenness and decline, and toward greater wholeness and growth. We shift our focus now to this question.

HOW TO ADDRESS STRUGGLES WITH DOUBT IN PRACTICE

Jamal, a 20-year-old bright and articulate college sophomore, came to therapy complaining of anxiety, insomnia, and ruminations. His symptoms had begun shortly after he entered college. The son of traditional Muslim immigrants from

Syria living in a close-knit, homogeneous community in Detroit, Jamal was the first of his extended family to go to college. His parents were very proud of him and the scholarship he had won. However, they were also concerned that he would turn away from Islam and had asked him to promise to be a good Muslim in college. Jamal had made that promise, even though he didn't really know what it meant to be a good Muslim.

Jamal had been a dutiful son, fulfilling his religious obligations regularly but without deep personal conviction or motivation. He said, "I did what Muslims do, and didn't give it more thought than that." In college, though, Jamal found himself immersed in a whole new world of ideas and experience. His major, physics, he found to be especially exciting, but also very troubling. "With all that I'm learning," he said, "I have a hard time seeing a God above pulling all of the strings." He also found himself bewildered and amazed by the wide array of religious attitudes of his friends on campus, including those who were atheists. "So many different ideas. How could they all be right?" he wondered.

Jamal had briefly raised some of his questions to his parents who, for the first time he could remember, responded angrily. They told him he must stop thinking that way and fight against this dark side of himself through prayer and study of the Quran. Jamal felt similar pressure from his imam to whom he admitted having some doubts. However, Jamal wasn't able to make his doubts go away. Quite the opposite, they had become stronger over time and were causing anxiety and sleeplessness. Antianxiolytic medication had not been helpful. Jamal didn't know where else to turn. He had to talk to someone, but he feared any further conversation with his parents or religious community would result in disappointment and even rejection. He came to the counseling center because he wanted a more objective point of view on his problems in a place that offered the safety of anonymity.

How can therapists aid clients, like Jamal, whose struggles with doubt are one important source of their psychological problems? In this section, we offer a multimodal approach that is designed to help therapists who see people caught up in painful times of spiritual and religious doubt find greater psychological well-being and wholeness. Many of the tools and resources that we have already presented in the context of other spiritual struggles can be applied here. Rather than repeat ourselves, however, we focus below on the clinical practices that are especially relevant to clients who struggle with doubt.

Being Transparent about the Methods and Values of Psychotherapy

People wrestling with doubts can be swayed toward or away from different religious points of view depending on the advice they are given, as research has shown (Hunsberger et al., 2002). That is not the job of the therapist, however. Practitioners are not arbiters of absolute truth or ultimate reality. As Allport (1950a) put it, "It is not the function of the psychologist to pass on the legitimacy or illegitimacy of any doubt" (p. 102). What therapists can do is provide clients with a safe place to explore and understand their doubts more fully so they can make their own informed choices about how to realize the lives they envision for themselves. Whatever insights and decisions the clients may come to, practitioners are ethically bound to respect those perspectives and choices, unless those choices pose a danger to themselves or others.

Of course, clients who struggle with doubts may not fully understand what therapists can and cannot do. Consciously or unconsciously, they may look to their helpers for answers to their painful questions. In response, therapists must be transparent about the methods and values that define the psychotherapy process. Consider, for example, the following conversation that took place early in therapy between Jamal and his therapist:

JAMAL: All of these questions and doubts are driving me crazy.

THERAPIST: How are they driving you crazy, Jamal?

JAMAL: I can't stop thinking about them. Why are we here? How did life begin? How will it all end? Is there really a God? The questions keep me up at night and make me very nervous.

THERAPIST: These are some very deep and profound questions, but it sounds like they're also very hard to live with for you. How have you been trying to do that?

JAMAL: I try to think about other things. I try to exercise a lot. I pray to God, who I'm not even sure exists, to take them away. But nothing works. That's why I was hoping you could give me some answers or help me get all of these damned questions out of my mind.

THERAPIST: I'm sorry you're going through such a painful time, Jamal. But I want to be clear with you about what we do in psychotherapy, so you can decide whether this is the kind of help you're looking for. This place is really about helping people understand themselves better; that includes their thoughts, their feelings, their relationships, and especially their conflicts, questions, and doubts. The idea is that with greater understanding (and some other tools as well), people will be better equipped to sort out some of their questions, make clearer decisions about how to handle their doubts, and come closer to realizing their hopes and dreams. Through that process, we believe, you should start to feel better. Here's the thing, though. I can't and wouldn't want to try to give you answers to your questions. Even if I had them, those would be my answers, not yours. Instead, I want you to try to make sense out of your questions for yourself. In here, my role is to serve as a guide who can help you find your own way through this thicket. And one of the most important things I can do as a guide is to ask you questions that may illuminate the pathway for you. Does any of this make sense?

JAMAL: So you're saying your job is to raise questions about my questions so I can reach my own answers.

THERAPIST: Right. How does that sound to you?

JAMAL: There you go again with your questions. [*Both laugh and then pause*] That's kind of ironic. I'm having trouble because of my questions, but you're saying the way out is through more questions.

THERAPIST: Yes, but maybe questions that shed more light than darkness.

JAMAL: What makes this really hard is that everyone I've talked to—my family, my imam, my teachers—have told me to stop asking questions.

THERAPIST: I hear you and I want you to know that my goal in working with you is not to be in any way disrespectful of Islam, your family, or your teachers. My job is not to convince you to be a Muslim, or not to be a Muslim, to have questions, or not to have questions. But having said that, therapists, including me, do value both questions and the importance of you finding your own answers, wherever that may lead you.

JAMAL: I take it that you're not a religious person yourself?

THERAPIST: No, I'm not. But I enjoy working with people who come from many religious backgrounds. You're one of my first Muslim clients, so I look forward to learning more about Islam as I get to know you.

JAMAL: Hey, I'm no expert myself.

THERAPIST: Well, maybe we could do some learning together. It may take some time and you may need to be patient, but I'm really hopeful that you'll be able to sort through these challenging questions. Before we go ahead though, I want to make sure you've had a chance to think about whether this is the right place and whether I'm the right person for you. Will you do that before I see you next week?

JAMAL: Good question. [*Laughs*] I'll think about it and let you know next week.

This kind of open discussion about the methods and values of therapy is an important prelude to effective clinical work with those struggling with doubt. Knowing how practitioners are likely to approach doubts in therapy allows clients to make a more informed choice about whether they want to continue in mental health treatment. Jamal decided to return to therapy with a better idea of what to expect.

Normalizing, Accepting, and Supporting Struggles with Doubt

Clients can be reluctant to talk about their doubts in therapy because the topic often raises feelings of guilt, worries about critical reactions from others, or fears of divine retribution. These concerns may be well-grounded in responses from family, friends, or religious communities when doubts about matters of faith have been raised. Baird (1980), for example, recounts the experience of a student who came back home from college and opened up about the spiritual questions she was having. A family member responded, "If you just wouldn't think about these kinds of questions, you would be so much happier" (p. 176). Attempts to suppress struggles with doubt though are not likely to be very effective, as Jamal discovered. To this point, Krause and Ellison (2009) found that struggles with doubt had more negative effects over time on the self-rated health of older adults who coped by suppressing their doubts. Clients then may need encouragement if they are to open up about their struggles surrounding doubt in therapy. Therapists can foster a welcoming climate for this kind of dialogue in a few ways.

First, it is important to normalize struggles with doubt. Earlier in the chapter, we noted survey findings that show that doubt struggles are not unusual. This point holds true for Muslims as well. In one study of Turkish Muslim theology students, small but notable percentages indicated that they experienced faith-related questions (39%), confusion (14%), uncertainty (14%), and contradiction (11%; Ok, 2004). As with tensions that arise within the realms of intellect, emotion, and relationships, doubts about sacred matters can be framed as a natural and normal part of human development and spiritual development more specifically. Questions about the universe, indeed questions about God, from this perspective often arise out of a larger sacred quest for enlightenment. Notable examples highlight this point. No less than eminent physicist Stephen Hawking (1988) ends his classic book *A Brief History of Time* with a quote reflecting some of his own spiritual questions and doubts:

> Why does the universe go to all the bother of existing? Is the unified theory so compelling that it brings about its own existence? Or does it need a creator, and if so, does he have any other effect on the universe? And who created him? . . . If we find the answer to that, it would be the ultimate triumph of human reason—for then we would know the mind of God. (pp. 174–175)

Second, clients can be cautioned against two extremes in their approach to struggles with doubt: attempts to suppress their doubts on one side and losing themselves in their doubts on the other. Mindful acceptance as we have discussed in terms of other spiritual struggles can be a useful stance toward doubts, too. Rainer Maria Rilke (2001) captured this attitude:

> Have patience with everything unresolved in your heart and to try to love the questions themselves as if they were locked rooms or books written in a very foreign language. Don't search for the answers, which could not be given to you now, because you would not be able to live them. And the point is, to live everything. Live the questions now. Perhaps then, someday far in the future, you will gradually, without even noticing it, live your way into the answer. (p. 14)

Finally, therapists can encourage clients to find support as they struggle with their doubts. The support may come from the religious world of the client. In this regard, clients can be asked to identify and reach out to supportive people within or outside of their tradition who have encountered similar questions (Jones, 2019). Some clients may seek out support from the very God they are questioning. This is just what we hear in part of Anne Brontë's (1920) powerful poem "The Doubter's Prayer":

> Oh help me, God! For thou alone
> Canst my distracted soul relieve;
> Forsake it not; it is thine own,
> Though weak, yet longing to believe.
>
> Oh, drive these cruel doubts away;
> And make me know, that Thou art God!
> A faith, that shines by night and day,
> Will lighten every earthly load. (pp. 39–40)

Therapists, too, can offer clients support for their doubts that might be hard to find elsewhere. Simply acknowledging the strength and courage it takes to grapple with doubts about matters as central as faith can be affirming to clients. And "accompaniment instead of answers," as the client journeys into unknown territory (Jones, 2019, p. 2), may be the greater source of support and antidote to the sense of alienation that can come with doubt.

Most of the examples above have focused on the doubt struggles of more religiously or spiritually oriented people. However, agnostics or atheists may need similar support for their own struggles with doubt. Recall our earlier account of the secular physician who encountered the spirit of her beloved mentor while dogsledding on a glacier in Alaska (Lomax & Pargament, 2011). Her doubts centered not around her spiritual and religious belief system but around a spiritual experience that challenged her *non*spiritual and religious belief system. Fearful that she might be losing her mind, she asked her psychiatrist, James Lomax, whether other people also have visitations by people who have died. "Only if they are lucky," Lomax replied, a response that was both normalizing and affirming (p. 81). Consider how Jamal's therapist helped normalize his client's struggles.

When Jamal's therapist shared findings from surveys of Muslims on their spiritual questions and doubts, Jamal was surprised to hear that he was not alone in his struggles. He had never met another Muslim who voiced the kinds of questions he was wrestling with. Jamal's therapist also encouraged him to keep an eye out for Muslims he might feel comfortable talking to, and over the next few months, Jamal was able to become friendly with two other Muslim students who were physics majors and, it turned out, also grappling with religious tensions. In addition, Jamal found himself heartened by the words of other scientists who saw no conflict between a life of faith, reason, and doubt. In one session, he brought in a quote by Galileo (Galilei, 1988), who had said, "I do not feel obliged to believe that that same God who has endowed us with sense, reason, and intellect has intended to forego their use" (p. 20).

Exploring the Doubts

When struggles with doubt are met with clinical understanding and support, clients become more willing to explore these spiritual tensions and how they might address them in their lives. There are two key parts of this process of exploration.

Specifying the Doubts

For many clients, doubts may be cloudy and hard to put into words. In addition, it may be difficult for clients to separate what others want them to believe from what they believe themselves. Therapists can assist clients in finding their own voice and sharpening the questions they are confronting, how these questions are a source of tension and strain, and what's at stake in the conflict. This is how Jamal's therapist helped Jamal delve more deeply into his doubts:

THERAPIST: Jamal, I've heard you question whether you're a good Muslim several times in here. I wonder if you could tell me more about what it means to you to be a good Muslim?

JAMAL: I'm not sure I even know. I know what my parents, imam, and Sunday school teachers would say: they'd tell me I need to believe in God, the angels, God's prophets, the holy scriptures as God's revelation, the afterlife, and God's will.

THERAPIST: And where do you stand on those beliefs?

JAMAL: [*clasps his head*] I don't know. I don't know. I don't know. Just thinking about what I believe makes me feel anxious and sweaty.

THERAPIST: I'm sorry this is so painful for you. The doubts you are experiencing can be very troubling. Are you willing to keep going with our conversation?

JAMAL: [*deep breath*] Yes, let's keep going.

THERAPIST: Okay. Let me ask you a question that may sound like it's off the topic, but I'm wondering about it right now. I know you really enjoy physics. My guess is you must have a lot of questions about all of the new information that is flooding into the field. Do those questions also make you nervous?

JAMAL: No, I love those questions! It's like we're starting to uncover all of the mysteries in the universe!

THERAPIST: I hear that enthusiasm. What's the difference between the exciting questions you have in physics and the questions that keep you awake at night about being a good Muslim?

JAMAL: [*long pause*] I'm not frightened about the answers that may come from physics, but I am worried about where my religious questions may take me. What if I discover that I'm not a good Muslim and really don't believe in God or Islam? Then I'm going to lose my family, my friends, my community, even my identity and soul. And then what? Who am I, if I'm not a Muslim?

THERAPIST: So there's a lot at stake here for you.

JAMAL: Yeah, I feel trapped. If I keep all of my questions to myself, I may be living a lie. But if I express my doubts, I'll lose everything.

THERAPIST: You know, Jamal. I wonder if you're not jumping the gun here. It seems like you're so concerned about how your family and your community might respond to your doubts, that you haven't given yourself the chance to sort out where *you* stand on these important religious questions. What if we start by trying to put other people to the side for the time being, and explore more about what you believe, what you doubt, and what you don't believe? Then, we can take it from there.

JAMAL: Okay, that makes some sense, but it does make me a little nervous.

THERAPIST: Well, keep me posted on that. Remember to focus on breathing regularly if it gets intense for you. And remember, too, that being a little nervous can be a good thing if it helps us figure things out.

Broadening and Deepening Understandings of Doubt and Spirituality

Struggles with doubt can be grounded in orienting systems that lack breadth and depth. For example, Jamal was taking his readings of the Quran at face value without exploring their deeper meanings. In addition, he was not making a distinction between doubts and disbelief. Furthermore, his questions about whether he was a good Muslim emphasized his uncertainty about core beliefs within Islam to the exclusion of other important aspects of the tradition, such as living by a set of moral values and engagement in religious practices and rituals. Therapists can help clients struggling with doubt by encouraging broader and deeper spiritual perspectives that offer new possibilities for living with and perhaps resolving doubts.

One way clients can explore their doubts with greater depth and breadth is by reading about others who have struggled with similar tensions (see Table 10.1). In this vein, Fowler (1981) has written that "Stories, symbols, myths, and paradoxes from one's own or other traditions may insist on breaking in upon the neatness of the previous faith and press one toward a more dialectical and multileveled approach to life truth" (p. 183). Similarly, clients who are open to the experience can learn by sharing their doubts with family, friends, and strangers

TABLE 10.1. Illustrative Readings about People Who Experience Struggles with Doubt

Altemeyer, B., & Hunsberger, B. (1997). *Amazing conversions: Why some turn to faith and others abandon religion.* Amherst, NY: Prometheus Books. (General)

Chodron, P. (1997). *When things fall apart: Heart advice for difficult times.* Boston: Shambhala. (Buddhist)

Done, D. (2019). *When faith fails: Finding God in the shadow of doubt.* Nashville: Nelson Books. (Christian)

Fowler, J. W. (1981). *Stages of faith: The psychology of human development and the quest for meaning.* San Francisco: Harper & Row. (General)

Frankel, E. (2017). *The wisdom of not knowing: Discovering a life of wonder by embracing uncertainty.* Boulder, CO: Shambhala. (Jewish)

Humphreys, J. (2007). *In God we doubt.* London: Hodder & Stoughton. (Christian)

Kornfield, J. (1993). *A path with heart: A guide through the perils and promises of spiritual life.* New York: Bantam Books. (Buddhist)

Ortberg, J. (2008). *Know doubt: Embracing uncertainty in your faith.* Grand Rapids, MI: Zondervan. (Christian)

Taylor, D. (2013). *The skeptical believer: Telling stories to your inner atheist.* St. Paul, MN: Bog Walk Press. (Christian)

---

from the same or different religious traditions. Genia (1990) described interreligious encounter groups in which people revealed their own spiritual doubts and concerns with one another and then found new meanings that were enriched by the perspectives of other faiths.

Some people come to terms with their doubts by broadening and shifting their focus from matters of faith-related beliefs and truths to other dimensions of religion and spirituality. Regardless of one's beliefs, questions, or doubts about creed or dogma, people can still experience a sense of connectedness to the sacred in many ways, including acts of altruism to others, hiking, music, practices such as meditation and yoga, or simply a decision to take a leap of faith. Listen to the way one woman framed her leap of faith in the language of hope rather than reason:

> Life is, after all, a series of leaps of faith. Falling in love and believing that I will grow old with my husband is a leap. Losing a parent and believing I will recover is a leap. Giving birth to children and letting go as they grow, hoping they will lead safe, happy lives is a leap. Living in a world of chaos, believing good will prevail over evil, is a leap. (Idliby, Oliver, & Warner, 2007, p. 108)

Jamal was helped by a few of these approaches. He began to explore readings about Islam, from both classic and contemporary sources, and from faithful, doubtful, and former Muslims. He would bring some of his insights into therapy. Jamal was relieved to discover distinctions in the Quran between doubting and disbelieving. Doubting that led people away from the life of faith, he found, was strongly condemned. Not so much, though, for doubts that resulted in a deepened faith. At the suggestion of his therapist, who was doing her own exploration of Islam through readings and conversations with Muslim colleagues, Jamal also read the report of a large national survey showing that Muslims expressed a variety of ways to be a Muslim (Pew Research Center, 2017b). Much to his surprise, he learned that a significant minority of Muslims (15%) did not feel that believing in God or loving the Prophet Muhammad (28%) were essential to what it means to be a Muslim. Asked in therapy about aspects of Islam that he did find compelling, Jamal talked about the mystical feelings he occasionally experienced through prayer; his appreciation for the values of Islam, such as charity, modesty, humility, family, hospitality, and forgiveness; and the sense of connectedness and closeness he felt in his family and community. Gradually, it became clearer to Jamal that he did not want to turn away from his faith.

At the same time, his questions and doubts about core Islamic beliefs remained very much alive. As his orientation to his doubts broadened and deepened, Jamal started to consider the possibility that he might be able to live as a Muslim with some doubts, at least for now. And in this process, Jamal's symptoms of anxiety and sleeplessness began to diminish, though he continued to be preoccupied with religious and spiritual issues.

Integrating Doubts into a Cohesive Approach to Life

It is difficult to imagine how people could possibly grow intellectually, emotionally, socially, and spiritually without the growing pains of doubt. Encounters with doubt along with mystery, contradiction, paradox, limitations, and imperfections are all parts of the human experience. The challenge lies in weaving these strands into the fabric of a cohesive life of greater wholeness. Therapists themselves must be able to arrive at a treatment orientation that is sufficiently broad, deep, and cohesive to manage the diversity and complexity of people and their struggles. In words that may well apply to both therapists and clients, Frankel (2017) notes, "We heal into wholeness . . . by making ourselves into vessels that can contain opposites" (p. 213). Helping clients make room for doubts in their lives is an important therapeutic task, one that may call for gentle prods to think about questions, doubts, beliefs, and truth in a different light. By way of illustration, consider one snippet from a fictional conversation between two priests:

> FATHER JUDE: Black is black and white is white.
>
> FATHER DAMIEN: The mixture is gray.
>
> "There are not gray areas in my philosophy," said Father Jude.
>
> "I have never seen the truth," said Damien, "without crossing my eyes. Life is crazy." (Erdrich, 2001, p. 135)

To foster greater cohesiveness, clients may also find value in a larger metaphor that places doubting within the larger scope of their lives, a unifying metaphor that provides an alternative to thinking about doubts as signs of pathology, weakness, or failure. Our framework of spiritual struggles points to one such useful metaphor: life as a journey. This is, of course, not a new idea. Far from it, according to virtually every religious tradition, each of us is engaged in a lifelong journey. Doubts and spiritual struggles are simply a natural part of this journey.

Let's take a look at one program for college students wrestling with doubts and other spiritual struggles that builds explicitly on this metaphor.

Winding Road

Developed by Pargament's research group at Bowling Green State University, the Winding Road program is a 9-week group spiritually integrated intervention based on the unifying metaphor of spirituality as a journey (Dworsky et al., 2013). Bumps, obstacles, detours, dead ends, and getting totally lost are only to be expected along this winding road. These are times of struggle and no spiritual journey would be complete without them. Winding Road was designed to help college students who are experiencing distress and disorientation related to their doubts integrate their struggles more fully into their lives by (1) accepting spiritual questions, doubts, and conflicts; (2) exploring spiritual struggles; (3) reducing stigma and facilitating group support for struggles; (4) broadening and deepening their orientations to spirituality; and (5) enhancing emotional, behavioral, and spiritual well-being. Over the course of the 9 weeks, students from diverse religious and spiritual backgrounds share stories of their spiritual journeys and their experience of struggles along the way. They visualize the spiritual destinations they are striving to attain, in part, by imagining an encounter with the future spiritual self they would like to become. They describe the diverse ways they understand and connect with what they hold sacred. And they engage in a surrender ritual in which they identify and let go of uncontrollable aspects of their struggles.

Although the program was relatively short, students showed a number of significant changes: less shame and alienation related to struggles, a more positive and accepting image of God, greater ability to manage feelings of distress associated with their struggles, and less psychological distress generally. Some students came to greater peace through greater acceptance of their struggles. As one student put it, "I'm okay with that fact that I have struggle now. It's okay to not have the answer right now. That's a little scary, but that's okay. It's okay to be scared. It's okay to be confused" (Dworsky et al., 2013, p. 329). Students as a group, however, manifested significant declines in their levels of spiritual struggle over the course of Winding Road, in some cases by reaching a new spiritual perspective. One student wrote of her transformation:

> I used to not know what I believe and felt I had to decide. . . . Now I feel like there is a kind, divine force. . . . I don't know if it's a God or whatever, it might be just a force, but I believe that now versus one divine being . . . it's more like it's everywhere. (p. 327)

Winding Road has since been replicated in work with adults with mental illness (Reist Gibbel et al., 2019).

The metaphor of life as a journey was also familiar and helpful to Jamal. Later in therapy, Jamal was asked to take a step back and reflect on the progress he had been making over the past year. Consider the signs of change and greater wholeness in Jamal's life:

JAMAL: Well, it's not been easy and I still feel anxious sometimes. But I'm learning more about myself. I realize now that I've always been a curious person. As a child my parents used to ask me: "Why so many questions?" When I left the shelter of my home and family for college, it's like a strange new universe opened up for me—new places, new people, new ideas. And my head started to spin.

THERAPIST: And what was that head-spinning feeling like for you?

JAMAL: It was incredibly exhilarating at first, but it changed when my questions began to focus more on God and Islam. Then I felt like I was starting to spin out of control.

THERAPIST: That makes sense—a big part of the foundation you had built your life on was being shaken. Where do things stand now for you with your questions, doubts, and struggles?

JAMAL: I still have them, but now I can see them more as part of my overall life, you know, one part of my journey. I had thought that with all of my questions about God and Islam, I had failed a spiritual test and that my life was pretty much hopeless. Now, I see that I will continue to be challenged. That's an important idea within Islam and I like it—the Quran is filled with stories of tests and challenges and the good things that can come from them. Things are more complicated now, but more interesting, too.

THERAPIST: More complicated but more interesting?

JAMAL: Yeah, it's like trying to get your head around light being both waves and particles. That's really hard to grasp but what a fascinating idea! I am both a Muslim with doubts and an aspiring physicist. How crazy is that? But it's kind of intriguing, even though it's still a little disturbing. I'm no Einstein, but like him, I'm looking for a unified field theory, at least in my personal life.

THERAPIST: I'm really impressed with how deeply you've been thinking about your life and your struggles. Let me ask another question: Where do you stand now with your question about whether you're a good Muslim?

JAMAL: I can't say I'm a good Muslim yet. For now, I'm settling for just trying, and trying to be more patient with myself while I'm at it. I did register for a class on Islam this fall and I'm really looking forward to it.

THERAPIST: That's great! It sounds like you're making some good progress. What do you see as your unfinished business?

JAMAL: Well, we never really talked about my parents. The focus was more on me and I think that was a good way to start. But I still have to decide whether to open up to my parents about all of my questions and doubts. On top of that, I've been dating this non-Muslim woman and I haven't told them.

THERAPIST: What kinds of concerns do you have about opening up to your parents?

JAMAL: I know they love me and I used to think it was totally unconditional. I'm not so sure anymore. I don't know if they'll continue to love me if they knew more about what I'm going through. And I can hardly think about what they'll do if they find out I'm seeing a non-Muslim woman. Maybe they'll freeze me out? Maybe they'll cut me off?

THERAPIST: Is that something you want to talk about more in here?

JAMAL: Let me think about it. Part of me doesn't want to rock the boat with my parents. I just want to appreciate them as they are. But part of me feels like it's time for me to speak up. I'm thinking that may be the next step on my journey.

THERAPIST: That's an important decision and deserves some careful thought. I'm here if you'd like to talk with me about it.

Through therapy, Jamal was able to find some relief for his symptoms and grow in some important directions. He described a number of signs of greater wholeness: more awareness of himself, his doubts, and his faith; a deeper appreciation for life's complexities and paradoxes; greater affirmation of himself and what he was going through; and a more cohesive emerging vision of his life, one that contains room for both faith and doubts within his larger "unified field theory." Of course, Jamal's journey is still a work in progress. As we have stressed, struggles in one domain may have a cascading effect, leading to struggles with other aspects of spiritual life. This point may be especially relevant to struggles around a foundational religious belief that upholds the entire religious edifice. Jamal's struggles with doubt, for instance, have brought him face-to-face with potentially powerful, unresolved interpersonal struggles with his family and perhaps larger religious community. Jamal may or may not be ready to wrestle with this new set of issues, in or outside of therapy. In any case, Jamal is in a stronger position to take on new challenges and struggles as he continues on his path.

CONCLUSIONS

Doubt occupies an important and distinctive place between belief and unbelief. Although it has received less attention than its more "certain relatives," struggling with doubt deserves greater attention, especially in the context of therapy. In this chapter, we considered how therapists can understand and address struggles with doubt in clinical practice. This can be challenging work. Doubting is a natural part of life. Yet, because doubt struggles involve core beliefs that orient and guide people, these conflicts can be deeply disturbing. How then do people come to terms with their doubts in ways that facilitate growth? This is the key question for treatment. Understandably, clients may look to their therapists for quick and easy answers to their dilemmas to relieve their distress and confusion. As we have stressed, however, practitioners are in no position to offer ultimate truths or answers to the profound questions about religious and spiritual matters that arise as people progress through life. There are a few things therapists can do, though. First, they can provide tools to help clients manage the distress that comes with doubts. Second, they can create a receptive space in which clients' most troubling doubts are met with acceptance, interest, and understanding rather than judgment or criticism. Third, therapists can accompany and guide clients on their journey, shedding some light occasionally to help them find their way through these dark times. Whatever way the client may choose to go, the life journey will continue and, as part of that journey, the client's search for the sacred will continue, evolving in perhaps new and surprising directions. The end result may be doubts that are resolved or doubts that remain. But in either case, clients can move toward a broader, deeper, more affirming, and more cohesive orientation to life—in short, a life of greater wholeness.

In the next chapter, we shift our focus from doubting to a related form of struggle: moral struggles.

CHAPTER 11

Moral Struggles

"I am, you see, two men," Charles Dickens purportedly told Fyodor Dostoyevsky in a face-to-face conversation. "Only two?" Dostoyevsky replied.

—cited in SLATER (2009, p. 502)

The potential for inner conflict is embedded in the human condition, as Dickens and Dostoevsky were well aware. The pieces of ourselves—thoughts, feelings, impulses, values, morals, and connections—can grind, clash, and collide, leading us to feel at war within. How we reconcile our different aspects and move toward lives of greater integration is one of the fundamental challenges we all face. At best, we are able to create some degree of wholeness out of what William James (1902) called our "divided selves." We are not always successful, though; no one is ever a fully finished product.

This chapter focuses on how to understand and address one particularly challenging intrapsychic spiritual conflict: moral struggles. This is not a new topic. Accounts of people struggling in their efforts to live up to their highest spiritual values lie at the heart of religious literature. The story of the very first man and woman in the Bible—Adam and Eve—centers around a moral failure, the eating of the forbidden fruit from the Tree of Knowledge of Good and Evil and the powerful consequences of this act. Moral struggles also loom large among figures in the New Testament, as we hear in the confession of the apostle Paul: "I do not what I want to do but I do the very thing I hate" (Romans 7:15). The Bhagavad Gita, a story central to Hindu scripture, focuses on a moral dilemma: Should Arjuna, the prince of his people, lead his army in a civil war against an enemy that includes loved ones, family, and friends? Before he attained Buddhahood, Siddartha Gautuma was said to have struggled with the temptations of thirst, desire, and delight sent by Mara, the Buddhist Lord of the Senses.

People continue to struggle with moral conflicts in this day and age in many contexts: the man grappling with guilt and shame after killing someone while driving under the influence of alcohol, the combat veteran trying to come to terms with actions committed against civilians in the war, the wife unable to reconcile her continued involvement in an extramarital affair with her sacred marital vows. At the time of this writing, many health care workers on the front lines of treating COVID-19 feel forced into the position of "playing God" as they struggle with the moral dilemmas of deciding who can have access to the inadequate supply of potentially life-saving ventilators and oxygen and who cannot.

Signs of moral struggle are commonplace, according to surveys. In our large-scale survey of over 18,000 adults (Exline, Pargament, & Grubbs, 2014), 57.5% indicated that, in the past few weeks, they had experienced some level of moral struggles, such as wrestling with attempts to follow their moral principles and feeling guilty about not living up to their moral standards. In a study of military veterans, moral struggles were the most frequently experienced of all spiritual struggles (Breuninger et al., 2019). According to an anonymous online survey of college students, of those who viewed Internet pornography, approximately two-thirds reported inconsistencies between their behavior and their spiritual beliefs, as well as feelings of guilt and shame (Twohig, Crosby, & Cox, 2009).

Moral struggles involve questions that can be very unsettling because they touch on matters of deepest significance. One set of questions revolves around personal identity and self-worth: Am I a good, decent, and moral person? Some questions deal with matters of responsibility: Where does my responsibility begin and end? How much of the fault is mine? Other questions are more relational in character: Can I still be loved by others? Can God still care for me? Can I ever be forgiven? Still other questions focus on personal strength and self-discipline: Do I have the inner strength, the "moral muscle," as Baumeister and Exline (1999) aptly put it, or am I too weak to master my impulses? These questions should not be shrugged off as abstract, philosophical, or intellectual musings. They are often deeply troubling.

Perhaps not surprisingly then, moral struggles can be a source of great pain. Consider the words of Peter Moen (1951), a Norwegian journalist who was imprisoned by the Gestapo for his role in the resistance movement against the Nazis. Under torture, Moen gave up the names of fellow members of the resistance, knowing this might well lead to their imprisonment and death. Using a thumbtack to punch out his story on toilet paper in his cell, Moen likened the intensity of his moral pain to that of his physical torture: "I write under the burning humiliation of these problems. It is a moral rack where a man is stretched out longer than he is. So here I lie under torture and can free neither arms nor legs" (p. 56).

Moral struggles can be deeply interwoven into many of the problems that bring people to therapy. In anxiety, we can find the fear of failing to live up to one's core beliefs and values. The guilt and shame associated with self-evaluations of a morally flawed character can be a central feature of depression. Addiction has been called a spiritual disease because the individual has become disconnected from his or her higher self (Decker, 1993). Moral injury has been identified as a salient aspect of PTSD (Koenig, 2018b). Beneath the surface of marital conflicts can often be found moral violations, such as infidelity and lying. The moral struggles associated with psychological problems may also be part of the motivation that brings people into treatment. In a large-scale study of Vietnam veterans, Fontana and Rosenheck (2004) found that engagement in treatment was predicted not by PTSD symptoms but by the guilt and loss of religious faith associated with killing others or failing to prevent the killing of others. Similarly, in a study of military veterans in a residential treatment program for gambling disorder, among all of the spiritual struggles they were experiencing, moral struggles were the most prevalent at both baseline and the end of treatment (Gutierrez, Chapman, Grubbs, & Grant, 2020).

Drawing on the empirical and theoretical literature, and our framework of spiritual struggles, in this chapter we focus on ways to understand moral struggles. Building on this knowledge, we describe a spiritually integrated approach to moral struggles in treatment, tapping into the wisdom of religious traditions and of diverse therapeutic orientations, including psychodynamic, trauma-oriented, cognitive-behavioral, interpersonal, and humanistic therapies. We will see that while moral struggles can be wrapped in pain, distress, and disorder, they also contain the potential for greater wholeness and growth.

WHAT WE KNOW ABOUT MORAL STRUGGLES

Let's begin with a definition. Moral struggles involve tension, conflicts, and strains around the incongruity between one's own values or moral standards and one's own actions. Moral struggles may focus on acts of commission, such as criminal acts of violence, or acts of omission, such as remaining passive or silent while witnessing violence. From an external vantage point, moral struggles may appear to be appropriate and deserved in some instances, as in the case of an adolescent who struggles with guilt after stealing from his or her parents. In other instances, they may seem unjustified and unwarranted, as in the case of a woman who feels responsible for abuse at the hands of her husband. In still other cases, the struggles may be morally ambiguous, as in Moen's (1951) terrible guilt after revealing the names of his fellow resistance fighters, but only under torture. The strain of moral struggles can be marked by several emotions, but guilt and shame loom most large.

What makes these struggles spiritual in nature, readers may wonder? After all, people who do not believe in God or perceive the sacred in their lives are not immune to moral struggles. However, the reality is that moral values and practices are often explicitly or tacitly shaped by religious institutions and/or imbued with sacred meaning. Every religious tradition teaches its adherents concepts of vice and virtue, albeit with some differences and some commonalities among them. For example, the world's religions generally espouse some version of the Golden Rule, the sacred duty to extend the same kindness and compassion to others that we would hope to experience for ourselves. Other animating principles and virtues can also be sanctified not only by religious institutions but also by secular institutions and individuals. The document perhaps most central to the founding of the United States, the Declaration of Independence, embeds fundamental human rights in a divine context: "We hold these truths to be self-evident, that all men are created equal, that they are endowed by their Creator with certain unalienable Rights, that among these are Life, Liberty and the pursuit of Happiness." This document is one of the underpinnings of what has been called American civil religion. Individuals can also be perceived as manifestations of divinity and sacredness, as we hear in the words of Kushner (1989):

> Where is God? God is found in the incredible resiliency of the human soul, in our willingness to love though we understand how vulnerable love makes us, in our determination to go on affirming the value of life even when events in the world would seem to teach us that life is cheap. (p. 178)

Because moral values and virtues are often replete with a deeper sacred meaning, they take on special importance in peoples' lives. Likewise, the failure to live in accord with these sacred values has special significance. More than a mistake or an error, it can become a sin, a transgression, a desecration eliciting feelings of guilt and shame (Pargament, Magyar, et al., 2005). It becomes, in short, a source of moral struggle.

We now look more closely at what we are learning about these struggles from theory and research.

Moral Struggles Can Lead to Both Growth and Decline

Moral struggles can threaten to shake or shatter an individual's orienting system and significant purposes in living (Pargament, 2007). Nevertheless, while they are fraught with the possibility of psychological, social, and spiritual harm, they also carry the potential for wholeness and growth.

Moral Struggles and Growth

We have stressed throughout this book that spiritual struggles are neither pathological nor a sign of weak faith. This point certainly holds true for moral struggles. No one can fully or consistently live according to his or her highest values. We all fall short at times, and the struggles that follow can be understood as a sign of our spiritual, moral, and ethical character, what Karff (1979) described as a badge of our humanity. In this vein, one set of experimental studies showed that people who do the right thing after overcoming moral conflict are viewed by adults as morally superior to those who are unconflicted (Starmans & Bloom, 2016). Conversely, the lack of moral struggle surrounding immoral actions may signal serious problems rather than strength. In fact, therapists may very well want to foster moral struggles among clients with a weak conscience, such as those who have committed crimes against others without remorse or guilt (Grand, 2000).

Moral struggles may result in greater self-control and personal growth more generally. By anticipating the moral struggles likely to follow their offenses, people may be more likely to avoid these mistakes and keep their destructive impulses at bay. This kind of "struggle anticipation" may be especially common among more religious and spiritual people, and explain in part why religion and spirituality have often proven to be effective in regulating impulsive behaviors, such as crime, drug use, and delinquency (McCullough & Carter, 2013). Furthermore, moral struggles can prompt soul-searching about the most fundamental questions of identity, ultimate purpose, and the pathways the individual wants to follow in life. "Guilt," Baumeister and Exline (1999) asserted, can push people "to act in virtuous ways" (p. 1183). Empirical evidence backs up this idea, suggesting that remorse about one's offenses is often linked with more attempts to repair relationships (e.g., Fisher & Exline, 2006).

With the help of resources (e.g., forgiveness, confession, making amends) well designed to meet the challenges of moral struggles, people may be able to experience not only a sense of redemption but also changes and transformations that have far-reaching consequences. For example, in an experimental study of Roman Catholics, McKay, Herold, and Whitehouse (2013) found that, in comparison to those who recalled a transgression not followed by religious absolution, those who recalled a time when they received absolution through confession engaged in more prosocial behavior (e.g., donating money to the church). In another study of patients with HIV in the midstage of their disease, those who reported that they were able to overcome their spiritual guilt also described shifts away from drugs and promiscuous sex, and shifts toward a more benevolent view of God and religious involvement (Ironson et al., 2016). Not only that, reports of overcoming spiritual guilt were predictive of greater rates of survival over the following 17 years. Of note, long-term survival was tied to overcoming spiritual guilt but not to guilt measured more broadly. Popular literature is filled with inspirational stories of people who committed moral violations—crime, drug and alcohol use, family neglect, bullying—and were successful in turning their lives around.

An empirical study by Saritoprak and colleagues (2018) lends some credence to these stories. Their study focused on the role of "spiritual jihad" as a pathway to transformation and growth among Muslims dealing with moral struggles. Although the term *jihad* has often been associated with acts of violence and terrorism committed in the name of Islam, the authors note that jihad actually refers to "struggle" or "hardship" that can be of two types: greater and lesser. The greater jihad has to do with an internal spiritual struggle: Much like a moral struggle, the greater jihad involves a battle to master internal destructive impulses. (Saritoprak et al., 2018, also note that the lesser jihad, external struggles for the sake of Islam, takes many forms, the majority of which are nonviolent.) To test the hypothesis that a spiritual jihad mindset fosters growth and transformation, the researchers created a spiritual jihad measure, with items such as "I believe the struggle is a way in which I can understand my imperfect nature" (p. 11). Working with two samples of adult Muslims who had recently experienced a moral struggle, Saritoprak et al. found that a spiritual jihad mindset toward moral struggles was associated with reports of significantly greater spiritual growth, posttraumatic growth, and positive religious coping in both samples. The Saritoprak et al. study suggests that there may be positive implications of moral struggles for well-being and growth.

Moral Struggles and Decline

Researchers and practitioners have paid more attention to the potential downside of moral struggles than their upside. Of particular relevance here is recent work on the topic of *moral injury*. This term grows out of the experiences of military veterans returning from the Middle East conflict. Moral injury describes, in part, the negative consequences suffered by people as a result of their participation in or passive witnessing of acts that violate their moral code (Drescher et al., 2011; Litz et al., 2009). These consequences range from depression, anxiety, and alcohol and drug use to aggression, symptoms of PTSD, suicidality, and poorer physical health (Held et al., 2019; Koenig, 2018b).

Theory and research on moral injury is still relatively new and questions arise about how best to define and operationalize moral injury. Our theoretical framework of spirituality and spiritual struggle, we believe, adds further refinement to the meaning of moral injury and its relationship to spiritual struggle. From our perspective, it is important to differentiate among three related processes that lie beneath the umbrella of moral injury: (1) morally injurious events, (2) moral struggle, and (3) morally injurious consequences. Just as stressful events of all kinds do not necessarily lead to poorer mental and physical health, morally injurious experiences do not necessarily result in morally injurious consequences. How these experiences are understood and handled plays an important role in determining whether the experiences lead to injury. Especially important is the question of whether a morally injurious event throws the individual into a moral struggle. If so, then drawing from our model of spiritual struggles (see Chapter 2) we would propose that it is the moral struggle rather than the experience of a morally injurious event that most directly affects the likelihood of morally injurious consequences and other subsequent problems.

Some research supports this point. Two studies involve military veterans. In one such study, spiritual struggles of all kinds, including moral struggles, fully or partially explained the relationship between the exposure to morally injurious events and PTSD symptoms, anxiety, and depression (Evans et al., 2018). Similarly, another study of veterans revealed that guilt related to the exposure to combat accounted for the connection between combat exposure and PTSD (Henning & Frueh, 1997).

Several empirical studies have tied moral struggles to a variety of problems. Among war zone veterans, those who reported higher levels of moral struggles also described greater morally injurious consequences, such as feeling unworthy of being loved and desires for revenge (Currier, Foster, & Isaak, 2019). In addition, moral struggles and struggle-related phenomena have been associated with higher levels of depression among Buddhists (Falb & Pargament, 2013), pornography users (Perry, 2018), and adults in a national sample (Abu-Raiya, Pargament, Krause, et al., 2015). Moral struggles have also been linked to greater signs of anxiety (Abu-Raiya, Pargament, Krause, et al., 2015), and obsessive–compulsive disorder (OCD; Olatunji, Abramowitz, Williams, Connolly, & Lohr, 2007). With respect to other health concerns, moral struggles have been predictive of alcohol use (Stauner, Exline, Kusina, & Pargament, 2019), the severity of problematic gambling (Gutierrez et al., 2020), and more intense suicidal ideation among people being treated for anxiety and depression (Exline et al., 2000).

Overall, these findings demonstrate clear connections between moral struggles with markers of moral injury, including distress, disorientation, and decline. Even so, questions remain about this literature. The majority of research in this area has been cross-sectional, so we cannot tell whether moral struggles are leading to mental health problems (primary struggles), the result of mental health problems (secondary struggles), or both (complex struggles). In addition, it is unknown whether moral struggles and their possible effects are long-lasting. We suspect they may be. It is difficult, for example, to imagine COVID-19 medical workers quickly resolving their moral struggles over who and who does not receive potentially life-saving ventilators and oxygen. Anecdotal reports also suggest that moral struggles can be enduring, at least in some cases. Recently, the *New York Times* asked readers to reflect on their high school experiences and then respond to the question of whether they had ever acted toward girls or women in ways they now regret (Wittmeyer, 2018). Seven hundred fifty responses came in and a "remarkable number" of readers described incidents in which they had mistreated women, in some instances, many years earlier. As a rule, these men felt that their misbehavior continued to be a source of pain and regret for them. One 81-year-old man recalled one such experience when he was 16:

My most vivid recollection is of kissing Diane in the back seat of a car on a double date. . . . She obviously didn't even want to kiss. I tried again and again. She didn't say no or stop. She just sat there frozen. To this day, I think of that experience with shame and regret. Those feelings come over me at unexpected times. And I'm nearly 82 years old now. I should have stopped. And I'm sure I should have apologized. I did neither. I'm sorry, Diane.

Finally, research has largely neglected the implications of moral struggles for the individual's relationship to religious institutions and the sacred. One study did find moral struggles to be a motivating force for apostasy, according to analyses of extensive interviews with those who had left organized religion (Zuckerman, 2012). Having violated religiously based teachings, many individuals left their congregations, feeling it was not possible to live up to its moral standards. It is also important to recall that moral struggles are often intertwined with other types of spiritual struggle. For example, wrestling with moral shortcomings could lead to fears of punishment from God or concerns about evil or the demonic.

Taken as a whole, this emerging body of study underscores a point we have made about spiritual struggles in general: We have to be careful not to sentimentalize moral struggles. While they may potentially foster growth, positive change is not inevitable. In fact, empirical studies point more consistently to signs of distress, disorientation, and decline accompanying moral struggles. However, these findings are not so strong as to suggest that moral struggles inevitably result in decline, either. Adding further complexity here are some findings that suggest moral struggles may be tied to higher levels of *both* growth and decline (Zarzycka & Zietek, 2019). We return then to the metaphor of a fork in the road. Which direction people take, growth and/or decline, may depend on their ability to create greater wholeness out of the incongruity they feel between their higher and impulsive selves. As we will see shortly, therapists can play an important role in this regard.

Roots of Moral Struggles

Few, if any of us, go through life without facing some questions about right and wrong, good and bad, and our own essential decency. These questions and conflicts are likely to grow out of a particular set of religious, situational, sociocultural, and personal factors. For example, a central task for Hindus is to harmonize personal desires, behaviors, and values with dharma, a set of key unifying principles representing the eternal moral order and sacred reality (Hodge, 2004). This process is not easy, however, and at times can involve considerable struggle, particularly among second- and third-generation Hindu immigrants who must try to reconcile dharma with the more individualistic and material values in the United States.

Major life crises can also set the stage for moral struggles. Times of war, perhaps most notably, expose people to a variety of morally challenging actions that might involve killings, harm to noncombatants, guerilla warfare, and imprisonment and torture, as in the case of Peter Moen (1951). In the context of war, many combatants feel they have committed fundamentally irreligious acts, such as the breaking of divine commandments and the usurpation of divine responsibilities (Tick, 2014). And military veterans who report more distressing military experiences are also more likely to voice moral struggles, according to a study by Breuninger et al. (2019). There is, however, no one-to-one correspondence between any life event, even war, and moral struggles. Not all soldiers struggle with moral issues. On the other hand, ostensibly less morally relevant events— unemployment, illness, death, accidents, marital and family conflict—can be sources of moral struggle.

Moral struggles also grow out of the challenge of accommodating two existential realities built into the human condition: the fact that we are moral beings motivated to varying degrees to live by a set of higher-value principles that define what it means to be a good person, and the reality that we are containers of impulses, appetites, and imperfections that require attention. Both our higher selves and impulsive selves are critical parts of the search for significance. Without a sense of higher purpose many people would experience their lives as empty and meaningless. Our survival is also dependent on the orientation we take to our human limitations, appetites, and drives, including hunger, sex, and aggression. Moral struggles occur when difficulties arise in regulating each of these sides of ourselves and reconciling the two with each other. Fueling these potentially troubling tensions may be moral overcontrol on the one hand and impulse undercontrol on the other.

Moral Overcontrol

Overcontrol in the moral realm is marked by two related problems: a lack of moral redemptive resources for coming to terms with human limitations and error, and moral perfectionism grounded in the fear of falling short.

Insufficient Moral Redemptive Resources for Dealing with Human Limitations and Error. Fallibility and flaws are an inherent part of being human. Kurtz and Ketcham (1992) capture this point in their articulation of a "spirituality of imperfection." They write, "Spirituality begins with the acceptance that our fractured being, our imperfection, simply is" (p. 2). Nevertheless, infractions can raise disturbing questions and disrupt peoples' most fundamental beliefs and values about themselves and the world. Why did I do such a thing? Those who answer this basic question through attributions of self-blame are especially likely to experience moral struggles (Wilt, Evans, et al., 2019).

There is, however, an important finer distinction to be made between guilt-related self-attributions, those that focus on errors that were made in a particular situation (e.g., "I made a mistake"), and shame-related self-attributions toward the self, those that go beyond the particular situation (e.g., "I am a bad person"). Guilt-related attributions appear to be less disruptive and disturbing because they allow for the possibilities that the individual may not be solely responsible for the offense and that the guilt could be alleviated through atonement and purification (Tangney, Stuewig, & Masheg, 2007). Shame-related attributions, on the other hand, are more problematic because they place exclusive responsibility for the mistake on enduring, difficult-to-change qualities of the person that go beyond the specific situation.

Shame intensified the moral struggles of Peter Moen (1951). Recall that the immediate trigger of his struggles was his failure to protect the names of fellow members of the Nazi resistance. However, his diary makes clear that he was experiencing a deep sense of shame that went well beyond his recent behavior. He wrote, "I must recognize with bitter and painful regret how inexpressibly badly I have lived. . . . I pray with all my heart for my future—that I may be otherwise than the worthless thing I have been all my life" (pp. 26–27).

Shame-related appraisals are decontextualized explanations; they neglect the contributions of other forces to morally difficult situations. That Moen's (1951) offense took place under torture did not appear to diffuse the total responsibility he took for his behavior. By overlooking the part that other forces play in negative events and the moral complexity they create, shame-based appraisals oversimplify life situations and may well lead to moral struggles and subsequent disorientation, distress, and decline.

These harsh appraisals could be mitigated by redemptive resources, religious and nonreligious, that enable people to reduce the intensity of moral struggles and their consequences. Religious traditions, as a rule, do not expect flawless performance. As Kurtz and Ketcham (1992) have written, "Spirituality helps us . . . accept the imperfection that lies at the very core of our human being. Spirituality accepts that 'If a thing is worth doing, it is worth doing badly'" (p. 2). Many of the key figures in religious literature were quite human, suffering from shortcomings that ranged from irritability and lustfulness to shyness and speech impediments. In the world's religions we can find an abundance of redemptive resources—forgiveness, grace, compassion, confession, atonement, making amends—that appear to be tailor-made to the challenge of redeeming people from their offenses and limitations. Taking a "fearless moral inventory" of themselves and making amends to those who have been harmed are also key ingredients of 12-step programs.

Moral Perfectionism and the Fear of Falling Short. The likelihood of moral struggles is also magnified by a moral perfectionism based on fears of falling short. By that we mean the fear of not living up to moral and spiritual standards as a result of human error or a focus on satisfying human needs and appetites. These fears can be stoked by a moral code in which anything less than perfection signifies a grievous failing. John Henry Newman, a 19th-century Catholic cardinal, captured this kind of fearful moral perfectionism:

> It would be better for sun and moon to drop from heaven, for the earth to fall, and for all the many millions who are upon it to die of starvation in the extremist agony . . . than that one soul . . . should commit one single venial sin. (Seldes, 1985, p. 307)

There are other authoritative religious writings that, on the face of it, would seem to insist on error-free perfectionism in the moral realm (e.g., "You therefore must be perfect, as your heavenly Father is perfect"; Matthew 5:48). Anxieties about committing offenses leading to divine disapproval, punishment, or rejection may account, in part, for research findings that show that people who are more religious are generally more prone to moral struggles (Exline, Pargament, Grubbs, & Yali, 2014; Grubbs, Perry, Wilt, & Reid, 2019; Sawai et al., 2017; Wilt, Evans, et al., 2019). Before we judge religion too harshly, it is important to add here that religious traditions as a rule do not expect the attainment of perfection.

Moral perfectionism and the fear of falling short have several other non-religious underpinnings. These include worries about disapproval and rejection from others, fears that a single misstep will lead to a total loss of control, and the threat moral offenses pose to the sense of purpose and identity people can gain from pursuing elevated moral goals (Lynch, 2018). Regardless of its causes, however, the fear of making mistakes is problematic because perfection is not a possibility. The devotion to avoiding mistakes only sets the stage for moral struggles when errors do occur. Moreover, the pursuit of perfection can take needed time and energy away from the realistic challenge of coming to terms with human frailties and needs.

Later in this chapter, we explore how therapists can help clients counter moral overcontrol by building their resources to find redemption when they come face-to-face with human limitations and error, and by developing a more sustainable, humane, moral vision.

Impulse Undercontrol

Moral struggles are also rooted in the challenge of moderating human impulses. This can be a stressful task, requiring a lot of time and effort. One interesting study of German adults spoke to this point (Hofmann, Vohs, & Baumeister, 2012). Over the course of 1 week, people were contacted by cell phone and asked to describe their immediate experiences, specifically, their desires and their efforts to regulate these desires. Over 7,000 desires were reported. Participants also commonly described attempts to resist these desires, particularly the impulses for sleep, sex, leisure, eating, and spending. However, not uncommonly, their efforts at self-control failed.

Giving in to impulses is often viewed negatively, particularly when these appetites are indulged excessively. From a religious vantage point, each of the Seven Deadly Sins—gluttony, sloth, greed, lust, envy, anger, pride—can be understood as a failure of self-control (Baumeister & Exline, 1999; Schimmel, 1992). In the mental health field, problems in regulating impulses, appetites, and desires are also said to lie at the root of a variety of psychological disorders, most notably impulse-control disorders, compulsive disorders, and addiction disorders. Failures in self-control have also been implicated in many other psychological and social problems, including borderline personality disorder, family violence, sexually transmitted diseases, and unwanted pregnancy (Vanderbleek & Gilbert, 2018). All of these disorders and problems, we suspect, increase vulnerability to moral struggles, though research in this area is lacking.

Impulse undercontrol emerges out of both large-scale social and individual factors. Cultural forces can create a context that encourages this kind of impulse dysregulation in obvious and not-so-obvious ways. American culture is filled with open invitations to give in to any number of temptations: inducements to buy lottery tickets or visit a casino, advertisements for liquor on television and the physical presence of bars that thrive in virtually every neighborhood and town, or online pornography that makes enactments of almost any sexual fantasy only a few clicks away. Culture can also foster impulse undercontrol more subtly. Research suggests that a shift in American culture has occurred over the last century away from the moral virtues that provide some measure of constraint and control over self-centered appetites and desires. Using a Google search program, Kesebir and Kesebir (2012) examined American books in the 20th century and tracked the frequency with which terms related to morality and virtues appeared. Over this time span, they found a significant and often steep decline in the appearance of morality terms (e.g., conscience, dignity, righteousness, uprightness, and virtue) and in the appearance of specific virtues (e.g., kindness, mercy, love, gratitude, humility, patience, and wisdom). These findings are consistent with what has been described as the movement toward a culture of individualism and narcissism in the United States (Putnam, 2000; Twenge & Campbell, 2009).

As important as larger social and cultural forces are, there is clearly more to problems with impulse control. After all, not everyone responds to cultural inducements to indulge or overindulge their appetites. People vary in their ability to control themselves, in their "moral muscle" (cf. Baumeister & Exline, 1999). Like other muscles, the strength of the moral muscle varies across individuals— simply put, some people have greater moral discipline than others. Many factors, such as self-awareness and the motivation to live morally, appear to contribute to the individual's degree of self-discipline (Vohs, Baumeister, & Schmeichel, 2012). Like other muscles, the strength of the moral muscle also varies according to the demands that are placed on it. When the ego is depleted by life's stresses and strains, the moral muscle may also become fatigued. Numerous studies have shown that ego depletion makes people more likely to give in to temptations, such as drinking, cheating, and stealing (Baumeister & Vonasch, 2015; Haggar, Wood, Stiff, & Chatzisarantis, 2010; Mead, Baumeister, Gino, Schweitzer, & Ariely, 2009). Finally, on a more positive note, like other muscles, the moral muscle can be strengthened through exercise, such as self-monitoring and physical exercise (Baumeister, Gailliot, DeWall, & Oaten, 2006). Religious and spiritual resources have an important role here as well, as we discuss shortly.

Conclusions

We have explored what we know about moral struggles, both its implications for growth and decline, and its underlying roots. As is true of other spiritual struggles, moral struggles are tied to signs of distress, disorientation, and significant problems. However, as is the case with other struggles, they may also result in growth and greater well-being, though the evidence is less well established here. All in all, the fork-in-the-road metaphor seems to apply to moral struggles; along the path to significance, they can lead to growth or decline (and sometimes both).

We also described how moral struggles are rooted in morally charged life situations and the existential challenges of living with our moral values and our basic human desires and limitations. People are generally able to find ways to integrate these twin parts into a cohesive whole. Not always, though. People can become imbalanced by pursuing elevated ends in ways that leave no room for missteps on the one hand, or by trying to satisfy human needs to the exclusion of higher values on the other. As Frankel (2005) succinctly put it, people can be enslaved by their morality or by their impulses. Both moral overcontrol and impulse undercontrol increase the individual's vulnerability to tension, strain, and conflict in the moral realm. As we note later, these two contributors to moral struggle can feed into each other.

Theory and research on moral struggles is still relatively young. Even so, it offers a basic foundation for practical efforts to help moral strugglers move toward greater wholeness and growth.

We turn now to the ways practitioners can address moral struggles in psychotherapy.

HOW TO ADDRESS MORAL STRUGGLES IN PRACTICE

In our experience, relatively few clients say they are coming to therapy for help with moral struggles. More often, moral struggles reveal themselves within other presenting problems. Thus, it is important to be sensitive to the moral questions and conflicts that can go hand in hand with a host of psychological concerns.

Therapists should listen carefully for the red flags of moral struggles—guilt, shame, embarrassment, self-contempt, sin, feeling unforgivable—and respond by encouraging clients to talk about moral matters in therapy.

This is not to say therapists can or should be arbiters of what is good and bad in life. Judgmentalism is not an appropriate part of the therapist's role. Therapists must be able to empathize with and support morally struggling clients who fear criticism and condemnation. Even so, therapists cannot afford to ignore moral issues either. At times, it is the responsibility of the therapist to offer the client a "reality check," such as the risks of continuing to engage in impulsive behaviors. Most importantly, however, the therapist's role is to help clients explore their moral conflicts, clarify their ultimate values, and consider how they might live more consistently by what they hold to be of greatest significance.

In the remainder of this chapter, we present a multimodal approach to moral struggles that makes use of a variety of resources drawn from different therapeutic models and applied with clinical discernment. Although we take up the problems of moral overcontrol and impulse undercontrol separately, we will also see that the two problems can feed into each other. The challenge for therapists is to help strugglers achieve greater integration and wholeness in the realms of both morality and impulse.

Moving beyond Moral Overcontrol

Nadine, a 45-year-old Roman Catholic woman, day care worker, and mother of three, came to therapy after a car accident in which she struck a young deaf child who had run out into the street between parked cars. The boy had suffered a broken collarbone. "It's all my fault," she said right away. "I had worked overtime and had only a few hours of sleep, but I needed to get back to work and was running late. So I was groggy." Although Nadine was not charged with a traffic violation, her judgment of herself was unsparing: "What I've done is absolutely unforgivable." She stopped attending her parish and withdrew into herself. The scenario of the accident played itself over and over again in her mind. Nadine complained of her fatigue, depression, and guilt. But feelings of guilt were nothing new to her. "Even before the accident, I carried around this feeling of failure and guilt," Nadine said.

> "All I ever wanted out of life was to be a good caring person. My parents were strong, socially conscious Catholics who passed on the importance of giving to other people. I tried to be like them, but instead, I've let everyone down in my life—my children, people at work, and my church. And now I've injured a deaf child."

Apart from her role in the accident, it was hard to find a realistic basis for Nadine's overarching sense of guilt. She had raised her children single-handedly after her divorce. She had juggled child rearing with work at her low-paying job. In addition, Nadine was the primary caregiver to her older mother who was trying to remain in her home despite increasing infirmities. On top of these heavy burdens, she was involved in visiting sick shut-in members of her church. When asked how she managed all of these caring activities, she laughed ruefully and said, "I don't. They manage me. I just try to put out the fires." Asked about how she tried to replenish herself, Nadine said:

> "Well, as my father used to say, 'don't coddle yourself; there'll be plenty of time to rest in the hereafter.' But I'm not as strong as he was. I almost never show it, but I feel weak. I don't do nearly enough and I feel ashamed of myself. Sometimes I just want to run away."

Though the car accident had brought Nadine into therapy, her moral struggle appeared to be longer-standing, deeply rooted in a harsh moral code that brooked nothing less than perfection, offered no room for human frailty or need, provided no resources for her own renewal when she made a mistake, and left her unable to reconcile the accident with her vision of herself and significant purpose in life. Nadine would need help creating a more sustainable moral vision. The first priority, however, was attending to her sense that she fell outside the realm of redemption.

Drawing on Redemptive Resources

Like Nadine, many clients run into problems because they are unable to balance their moral aspirations with compassion and forgiveness for themselves when they fall short of their vision. While the therapist's job here is not to judge or offer absolution of responsibility for moral offenses, problems of moral overcontrol cannot be overlooked. Instead, clients can be encouraged to explore and possibly access redemptive resources. Redemption does not mean overlooking or condoning transgressions, but rather involves finding some compassion and forgiveness for oneself to balance or soften the harshness of personal judgments and responses to these offenses.

In their work with morally overcontrolling strugglers, therapists can help clients along three pathways toward greater forgiveness for themselves (Fisher & Exline, 2010): (1) accepting appropriate responsibility, (2) repentance and making apologies and amends, and (3) finding greater self-compassion.

Accepting Appropriate Responsibility. Forgiveness and compassion rest in part on the ability of clients to judge themselves fairly in response to questions about whether they committed an offense and their degree of responsibility for the infraction. For instance, replaying the situation in her own mind, Nadine focused solely on her own blame for the encounter and overlooked extenuating circumstances, such as the fact that the child had run into the street without look-ing out for traffic. Therapy with clients like Nadine should not discourage them from their own painful soul-searching but rather try to broaden and deepen their reflective process to place difficult situations in a larger context. In Nadine's case, this context included the ceaseless demands on her time, the heavy burden of raising her children and caring for her mother on her own, the role of chance in the coming together of all the factors that led to the accidental injury to the child, and the fact that she was cleared of any legal violation in the accident. A more nuanced, contextualized appraisal would also consider the good intentions of the client and the moral complexities of many situations.

Deeply conscientious clients steeped in a culture of individualism and per-sonal responsibility may resist efforts to reach a fairer appraisal of their actions. More contextualized explanations may sound like excuses for misbehavior or raise fears of loss of purpose, identity, control, and esteem in the eyes of oneself, others, and God. Further exploration into the roots of personal overresponsibil-ity may be necessary. There are, however, morally complex, ambiguous situa-tions that simply defy any kind of objective appraisal. As Wortmann et al. (2017) point out, even if the explanation may seem harsh from the outside, "The patient is typically the expert about objective guilt vis-à-vis their own ethical system" (p. 256). At times, shifting the focus to reparation may be a more effective path-way to compassion and forgiveness.

Making Apologies and Amends. Clients whose image of themselves as moral and decent beings has been shaken or broken by their own offenses may be in need of what Litz et al. (2009) described as "an equally intense real-time encounter with a countervailing experience" (p. 701). To repair the sense of bro-kenness, the world's religious traditions offer their adherents a variety of coun-tervailing experiences that involve repentance, making amends, and atonement (or "at-onement"): the sacrament of reconciliation within Catholicism; the annual Yom Kippur service of atonement within Judaism; *tawba*, the act of repenting and seeking forgiveness from God for one's sins within Islam; repentance verses used in periods of self-reflection within Buddhism; and counseling from reli-gious leaders (see Wortmann et al., 2017, for a review). For example, Mahatma Gandhi reportedly met a Hindu man who confessed: "I am going to Hell. I mur-dered two Muslim children after the Muslim murdered my family." Gandhi's advice was to change his karma by making reparations: "You may indeed go to Hell. But there may be a way out. Find two orphaned Hindu children and raise them as Muslims" (Decker, 1993, p. 42). Therapists can encourage their clients to explore redemptive resources from their own traditions. Clients who are not a part of a religious community can explore other ways to make apologies and amends. Nadine, for example, decided to meet the child she had injured and help with the expense of his physical therapy. Through these redemptive processes,

clients have a chance to move beyond a potentially overwhelming and debili-
tating sense of guilt, and weave mistakes from their past into a new and more
benevolent story of their lives.

Again, clients may resist these attempts at apology and reparation for a number of reasons: feelings that the damage done is irreparable, fears of rejection and
judgment from others and God, or feelings that the costs of making apologies and
amends are too high (Exline, Deshea, & Holeman, 2007). Each of these concerns
will need the sensitive attention of practitioners, for repentance and reparation
can be a valuable pathway to a regained sense of moral purpose.

Finding Compassion for Oneself. Even after making amends to those who
have been hurt, clients may continue to struggle with guilt, shame, and self-punitiveness. Finding compassion and forgiveness for oneself is another important
ingredient of redemption. Self-compassion, according to Kristin Neff (2003),
involves three components: being able to soothe oneself with loving kindness and
compassion in times of struggle; being able to recognize and accept that imperfection is a characteristic of all human beings; and being able to take a balanced,
mindful approach to uncomfortable feelings about oneself that neither magnifies
nor suppresses the negative emotions. Self-compassion is neither self-indulgence
nor self-pity; it does not let the individual off the hook for making amends or
self-improvement, Neff stresses. In fact, self-compassion has been associated
with greater motivation to learn from, repair, and avoid repeating past offenses
(Breines & Chen, 2012). More generally, meta-analyses have shown that self-
compassion is tied to less psychopathology, greater well-being, and resilience to
stressors (see Neff & Knox, 2017, for a summary). A meta-analysis of emerging
research on forgiving the self has yielded similar results (Davis et al., 2015).

Several effective methods for fostering self-compassion have been developed (e.g., Gilbert, 2010; Neff & Germer, 2013; Smeets, Neff, Alberts, & Peters,
2014). These include attending to one's own self-critical language and replac-
ing it with kinder phrases, writing a letter to oneself from the perspective of a
compassionate friend, and meditating on prayer-like phrases of loving kindness
before bed, such as "May you be at peace," "May you be kind to yourself," and
"May you be free from suffering."

Religion and spirituality are also important sources of compassion and forgiveness for many people. The sacred literature of most traditions contains a
number of passages that offer divine compassion and love for people who have
committed transgressions. Portrayals of a God who loves and embraces rather
than condemns people who have sinned are also available in more current writings, as in the following example:

> God in heaven holds each person by a string. When you sin, you cut the string. Then
> God ties it up again, making a knot—and thereby bringing you a little closer to him.

Again and again your sins cut the string—and with each further knot God keeps drawing you closer and closer. (Kurtz & Ketcham, 1992, p. 29)

Several studies have pointed to mental health benefits for people who experience compassion and forgiveness from God (see Exline, Wilt, Stauner, Harriott, & Saritoprak, 2017, for a review). These include greater purpose in life, lower levels of suicidality, greater life satisfaction, less death anxiety, fewer alcohol problems, and more unconditional forgiveness of others.

To foster spiritual compassion among clients, therapists have used a variety of techniques, such as empty-chair exercises in which clients imagine sharing their moral struggles with God and receiving divine love and forgiveness in return (e.g., Sherman, Harris, & Erbes, 2015). Group interventions have also shown promise as a vehicle for spiritual support and compassion among military veterans dealing with trauma, such as moral injury (Harris, Park, Currier, Usset, & Voecks, 2015). The kind of caring shared in groups, Kurtz (2007) maintains, is essential to healing and wholeness among those struggling with shame: "Because we share hurt, we can share healing. . . . Caring makes whole from within: it reconciles me to myself-as-I-am. . . . Caring enables me to touch the joy of living, that is the other side of my shame" (p. 53).

Some religiously based obstacles can make it hard for clients to access spiritual compassion. Among them, the feeling that an unforgivable sin was committed deserves special attention. Nadine, for example, resisted efforts to find compassion for herself. Her actions, she believed, represented a desecration that had created an irreparable breach with God and her religious community. Though this may seem to be a harsh judgment from the outside, psychotherapists are in no position to determine whether a sin is truly forgivable. It is important for therapists to address the sense of falling beyond the pale of redemption in ways that are respectful of the client's orienting frame of reference. In this vein, Nadine was asked to consider and discuss stories of compassion and forgiveness within Catholicism, such as the parable of the Prodigal Son in which the father welcomes back his son who had returned home destitute after squandering his inheritance. With encouragement in therapy, Nadine also spoke to her priest about her feeling that she was unforgivable. The priest helped Nadine move toward absolution through the sacrament of reconciliation, which provided an important benefit that could not be achieved through psychotherapy alone. In cases such as Nadine's, collaboration between clergy and mental health professionals may be the most effective way of addressing religiously based obstacles to redemptive resources.

Important as redemption can be, for some clients, the problem of moral overcontrol calls for more than these resources. This was certainly true for Nadine, whose moral struggles predated her car accident and grew out of an unsustainable vision of moral perfection for herself and her life.

Creating a Sustainable Moral Vision

Moral perfectionism is problematic not because of the individual's exceptionally high moral standards but because so little space is given to the inevitable missteps that will occur in the pursuit of a higher moral purpose. This leaves the individual vulnerable to emotional exhaustion and breakdown. Therapy then should be directed not to lowering the client's moral code but to helping the client develop a more viable approach to morality, one accepting of human needs and limitations.

On the face of it, helping clients like Nadine create a more balanced life should be relatively straightforward. It can be in some instances. It may be sufficient to point out that everyone faces tough choices about competing moral demands, the inevitable mistakes that are part and parcel of living, and the need to attend to our basic needs if we are going to reach our goals. Nadine's therapist noted that the competitive swimmer who tries to save time by refusing to turn her head to breathe will not go very far. However, that simple appeal to reason may not be enough. Nadine responded by pointing out that she had read about competitive swimmers who trained themselves not to have to come up for air as often. With Nadine and other clients, several more basic fears may need to be addressed before a more sustainable, humane moral vision can be realized.

Allaying Fears of the Loss of Significant Purpose. Among individuals who organize their lives around elevated moral goals with little regard for their own needs or limitations, unsparing devotion to moral principles can become a fundamental source of esteem from others, closeness with God, and identity and self-worth. With good reason, clients will fight to hold on to this central, often sacred, life-defining purpose. Therapists must make clear that they are not asking their clients to compromise on their moral purpose or turn their backs on its many benefits. Certainly, the world needs more people committed to elevated values and goals. But clients can be encouraged to explore a key question: By minimizing or neglecting their own human needs and requirements, have they been helped or hindered in realizing their uplifting goals? Nadine, for example, came to realize that in her commitment to caring for others to the neglect of herself, she had become so emotionally depleted that she was a less effective mother, daughter, worker, and church volunteer. As importantly, she recognized that her physical and emotional fatigue likely contributed to the car accident. That realization allowed her to consider some ways to care for herself as she cares for others and, in doing so, become better able to live out her moral vision over the long haul.

Allaying Fears of a Life Out of Control. A perfectionistic morality can provide some measure of reassurance that the world of the individual, both internal and external, is in fact controllable. However, moral perfectionism can also be accompanied by fears that an offense will lead to consequences so dire that recovery will be impossible, that life will fall apart. With so much at stake, people, like Nadine, experience an impossible burden of responsibility.

How can clients continue to move toward morally responsible lives while accepting the limits of their personal control? Helping struggling clients grapple with this challenge is an important therapeutic task, one that calls for a great deal of sensitivity and support. Nadine, for example, needed reassurance that she could in fact indulge her fantasy of running away (for at least a few days now and then) to relax, exercise, and socialize without catastrophic results for her and for the people in her world. With the help of her therapist, Nadine started to challenge her fear that attention to her own needs would result in their overindulgence. She also began to remind herself that self-care does not equal selfishness.

Without the illusion of complete control and total responsibility, clients are also more likely to need help in facing competing moral demands and complicated, morally ambiguous problems that do not permit a perfect solution. How, for example, could Nadine manage the situation when both her children and her parents are ill and need her attention? Difficult as these times are, they can also become turning points. Nadine was able find some relief as she came to accept that her control is in fact limited; that she is not solely responsible for all of the problems that come up; that life throws each us wicked moral curve balls tough for even the best batters to hit; and that while perfect clarity and perfect solutions are not possible for human beings (especially in the moral realm), greater clarity and better solutions are.

Allaying Fears of Rejection by Others. For people who have devoted themselves to uplifting moral ends that place the needs of others consistently ahead of their own, the idea of making more room for personal needs may raise fears about the reactions of others. Will they be disappointed, angered, or rejecting? In many cases, the worst fears of clients in this regard are not realized; friends, family, and coworkers can be understanding and supportive when clients try to find greater balance between the needs of others and themselves. Not everyone in the client's network of relationships may react so kindly, though. Used to being well-taken care of, they may respond with critical feedback and pressure to return to old patterns of caregiving. To forestall these reactions, clients can let others know about the changes to come. Although taking off the mask of being in full control and having limitless strength may elicit a lot of anxiety for clients, it may also be freeing. Nadine, for example, discovered that in the process of disclosing her own needs for support, she started to feel less like a fraud, while creating opportunities for deeper, more reciprocal relationships. There were others in her world who were able to support her as she had supported them.

It is important to recognize that fears of rejection tied to being less than perfect can be more deeply rooted in childhood experiences, particularly those involving critical parents and authority figures, including God. In these cases, longer-term depth-oriented therapy may be needed to help people develop greater mastery over the critical voices from the past. Nadine, for instance, began to learn how to respond assertively to the voice of her demanding father whose approval was contingent on her caring for others.

Allaying Fears of a Damaged Relationship with God. As we noted earlier, theists often imbue their offenses with sacred meaning. More than mistakes or errors, they become sins, desecrations, or transgressions that raise the threat of separation from God and the potential for divine punishment (Pargament, Magyar, et al., 2005). While remaining respectful of the client's perspective, therapists could point out that, according to most traditions, only the divine has absolute perfection. Even the most devout will commit moral breaches. Nevertheless, most religious traditions teach that people can still pick themselves up and continue along a path to moral improvement, learning from misdeeds that in fact spur spiritual growth.

Relevant here is work by Richards, Owen, and Stein (1993), who developed and evaluated an intervention for devout Mormon college students struggling with self-defeating perfectionism. Their eight-session group program consisted of reflections on perfectionism, religious readings, and examining distorted thoughts about goals and expectations, all designed to foster a more balanced approach to living a spiritual life. Over the course of the program, participants improved on measures of depression, perfectionism, self-esteem, and well-being.

In more extreme cases, anything less than scrupulous attention to moral behavior may raise fears of sin and separation from God. Scrupulosity, often tied to OCD, can become immobilizing because avoiding any possibility of committing a sin becomes a central goal, though it severely limits the individual's ability to engage fully in life. In work with scrupulosity, the goal is not to encourage people to accept their sin but to accept the risk of sinning (Greenberg & Huppert, 2010). In this regard, Huppert and Siev (2010) described their clinical work with an ultra-orthodox Jewish woman, Sara, who presented with scrupulosity and OCD. Her fears of committing a sin, specifically the fears of violating Jewish dietary laws about keeping kosher, had led her to a variety of avoidant and preventive activities—excessive hand washing, mental reviewing, cleaning—that had damaged her relationships with her husband and children. Working from a cognitive-behavioral orientation, the therapists helped Sara recognize that her preoccupation with sinning was in fact disrupting her ability to realize important spiritual goals, including caring for her family and maintaining a close relationship with God based on awe and respect rather than fear of punishment. They then helped Sara create a hierarchy of fearful situations and gradually exposed her to these risks while reminding herself that "I want to live my life with peace and happiness, raising my family, relating to my family, teaching and serving

God without OCD. Therefore, I will take the risk" (p. 391). Sara was able to make significant improvements that she maintained over the course of a year.

In short, the process of creating a sustainable moral vision does not mean that clients must give up the pursuit of higher ends—rather, they can develop a more fully dimensional vision that allows for the realization of moral values, while accepting human limitations and needs. However, to lighten the burden of moral overcontrol, clients must also be able to access resources that help them recover and move forward from their errors. Having reviewed how therapists can help clients move beyond moral overcontrol, we now turn to the problem of impulse undercontrol.

Moving Beyond Impulse Undercontrol

Bob, a 40-year-old accountant, came to psychotherapy complaining of generalized anxiety. Bob had worked for several years in the accounting department of a large religious denomination. However, he had never advanced in his job and salary increases had been minimal. The father of two middle school-age daughters, Bob admitted to feeling a great deal of financial pressure, compounded by his wife's insistence that he ask for a raise. Therapy with Bob focused on helping him explore his feelings, identify and respond to some of his catastrophic thoughts, and develop more assertiveness skills at work and at home. Bob became somewhat less anxious and decided to terminate therapy.

In what was to be the final session, Bob hesitantly mentioned that he had something else on his mind that had been bothering him for a while. He had gotten into the habit of viewing pornography on his computer at home fairly regularly. At the end of the day, after his children had gone to bed, Bob would go down to his computer in the family room and masturbate to online pornography. It gave him something to look forward to, he said, and took his mind off of his problems. On top of that, his wife had never been very affectionate and Bob felt some justification in taking care of his own needs.

One late evening, Bob was about to start watching porn, when one of his daughters surprised him by entering the family room, saying she couldn't get to sleep. Bob realized how close he had come to committing an act that would have damaged his family. Since that close call, Bob had been feeling ashamed of himself. What kind of man was he, he wondered? A total loser, he felt, a father and a husband who worked for a major church and snuck around at night masturbating to images of people having sex.

Bob had tried to put an end to viewing pornography on his own, but hadn't been successful. "I try," he said, "but I can't stop thinking about it, and the pressure builds up until I don't know what else to do." Bob often slipped up at home and had even begun to stay late at work so he could look at pornography on his office computer. Admitting his porn use in therapy, Bob said, was a last resort. "I've been afraid you'll think I'm a real loser, too," he said. Bob's therapist replied, "Actually, I think it's taken a lot of courage for you to share your feelings with me about such a sensitive issue. It sounds like your pornography use has become a problem for you. Would you like to explore it further here?" Bob made another appointment.

Clients who have difficulty controlling their own impulses are rarely devoid of moral values. Rather, like Bob, they cannot consistently inhibit their immediate desires in favor of more abstract though elevated goals, such as being a good person, that may not be realized so quickly. Researchers and practitioners have identified and developed many ways to help people resist the temptation to overindulge.

In the next section, we focus on three approaches that have particular spiritual relevance: behavioral control, mindful acceptance of impulses, and activating the higher self.

Behavioral Control

Many people, like Bob, try to suppress their impulses on their own through sheer willpower, or "moral muscle." And yet, as we noted earlier, the moral muscle can become fatigued by stressors and demands, and weaken the individual's moral resolve. This was the case with Bob who, in spite of his desire to put an end to pornography use, found himself slipping when he became preoccupied with his dissatisfaction at work, his feelings of frustration with his wife, and paradoxically, the shame and guilt he felt for using pornography. Willpower alone may not be sufficient for many people facing the challenge of moderating their impulses and, in fact, may be counterproductive at times. In one study of college students who were viewing pornography, those who made greater efforts to suppress their sexual thoughts and urges experienced more negative consequences as a result of their online behavior (Twohig et al., 2009). Similarly, in a study of Israeli Jewish adolescents, Efrati (2019) found that boys and girl who were more religious were more likely to try to suppress their sexual-related thoughts and behaviors. However, these efforts to suppress were associated with higher levels of compulsive sexual behavior and lower well-being, in turn.

Self-control training can help increase the moral muscle of clients like Bob. This kind of training involves a number of elements, including education about self-control, keeping a diary to monitor failures and success in self-control, setting realistic goals to create successful control experiences, rewarding achievement of goals, and expressing positive rather than suppressing negative emotions (Berkman, 2017). However, many clients may also need to draw on external resources to facilitate greater self-control. Bob, for instance, found that he needed help from his wife. With encouragement in therapy, he eventually disclosed his pornography use to his wife and more general dissatisfaction in the marriage. This created another mini-crisis for Bob, his wife, and his marriage, but with conjoint counseling, the couple weathered this storm and reached a new level of honesty in their marriage. Bob's wife became a source of support to him in his desire to stop using pornography. She was agreeable to bringing the computer into the bedroom to help Bob monitor his use, which had an immediate positive result.

Religious and spiritual support are also important resources in achieving greater self-control (McCullough & Carter, 2013). Almost every religious tradition provides its members with a number of methods for managing urges and appetites that could interfere with the goal of ultimate spiritual significance: realizing a connection with the divine. Adhering to regular religious practices generally may facilitate self-discipline. Bob, for instance, became a regular attendee at religious services and a men's group at church; it helped take his mind off his urges and reminded him of who he was trying to become.

Religious traditions also offer more specific techniques to foster self-control. Consider a few examples. Within one of the six major schools of Hinduism, hatha yoga, individuals learn a variety of self-control methods. Though Western practitioners tend to emphasize the yoga positions, yoga encompasses a wider array of practical ideas, including breathing exercises, proper diet, cleansing, meditation, ethics, and an entire system for spiritual growth and liberation (Burley, 2000). Initial studies suggest that yoga holds promise for better physical and mental health (Büssing, Michalsen, Khalsa, Telles, & Sherman, 2012; Park, Groessi, et al., 2014), and control of addictions in particular (e.g., Posadski, Choi, Lee, & Ernst, 2014). Within Islam, Muslims can follow teachings of the Prophet Muhammad on taking regular account of one's cravings, and keep a detailed daily self-reflection log on their urges, behaviors, and triggers (Haque & Keshavarzi, 2014). And across the theistic traditions, people can look to God for strength and support in resisting their urges through prayers devoted to just this purpose. Consider, for example, this 12th-century prayer from Hildegard of Bingen, a German Benedictine: "Let me recognize that the hunger I feel is a hunger of my soul that only you can satisfy. Let me not dull that hunger with a thousand sweet substitutes for the nourishment that only you can give" (Kirvan, 1999, p. 165).

Mindful Acceptance of Impulses

Although we can find strong ascetic elements within faith traditions, most religions recognize that human urges and impulses have some value and, rather than attempt to eliminate desires, try instead to encourage moderation. One such moderating approach to cravings and desires is mindful acceptance; this resource is grounded in, but not limited in, its application to Buddhism and the contemplative traditions. Mindful acceptance, one of the centerpieces of acceptance and commitment therapy (ACT), rests on the premise that thoughts and feelings cannot be controlled (Hayes et al., 2016). Not only that, attempts to eliminate undesirable thoughts and urges are likely to backfire, strengthening rather than weakening the individual's ability to pursue significant value and purpose in life. Rather than overindulge in undesirable thoughts and cravings or attempt to suppress them, mindful acceptance offers a third alternative: accepting all thoughts and feelings that enter consciousness, observing these emotions and urges nonjudgmentally, and then allowing them to pass as new thoughts and feelings emerge. Paradoxically, in accepting the undesirable urges without dwelling on them, they begin to recede in power and intensity.

Mindful acceptance is potentially applicable to the problems of impulse undercontrol. For example, Bob was helped by learning about and adopting a mindful acceptance approach to his desires to use pornography. He practiced the following exercise drawn from Gateway to Wholeness (2020), an eight-module online spiritually integrated educational program for people experiencing pornography-related problems (*gatewaytowholeness.com*):

> As you are sitting quietly, you may have a sexual urge or desire to use porn. If you experience this urge, gently but firmly resist giving in to it, keep your posture the same. See if you can become curious about your experience, watching what it is like for you to experience this urge and not give into it. What exactly are the physical sensations? What thoughts come up? Just keep watching, observing all the thoughts, feelings and sensations associated with it. You may find that after one urge fades another one arises. If it helps, you may visualize these urges as waves, starting as a small swell in the water, growing in size steadily, until they finally break and diminish. Take a minute or two more watching these urges and exploring what they are like for you.

Empirical studies have shown mental health benefits of mindful acceptance treatment (Keng, Smoski, & Robins, 2011; Lindsay, Young, Smyth, Brown, & Creswell, 2018), including studies of clients who experience problems of OCD, impulse control, and addiction (Öst, 2014).

Activating the Higher Self

With the loss of impulse control often comes the sense that all decency has been lost, too, as if the excessive behaviors have totally eliminated the potential for any goodness. As Bob put it, "I'm a total loser." To regain greater mastery over their appetites and desires, clients must also be able to reclaim the better angels in their human nature, what has been variously called the moral compass, the inner heart, the soul, the true self, the inner voice, or the higher self (Kass, 2017; Palmer, 2004). Here we are speaking of people at their best, the good and wise parts of themselves, and their most elevated reasons for living. Therapists have identified several ways to activate the higher self so it can serve as a stronger guiding force in the pursuit of significant purpose.

Palmer (2004) has emphasized the importance of providing a caring and compassionate space for clients to locate and amplify their own inner voice. The soul is shy, Palmer says, "we may see it only briefly and only out of the corner of any eye" (p. 59). What is needed then is a sensitive nondirective approach that allows people to "come to life in their own way and time" (p. 63). Palmer holds that the role of the helper is to guide this process by allowing for silences, asking questions that expand rather than restrict exploration, bearing witness to the client's experience, and speaking one's own truth.

Visualization exercises can also help clients reconnect with their better side. The following visualization, taken from the online Gateway to Wholeness (2020) program for problematic pornography proved valuable to Bob (*gatewaytowholeness.com*):

> Now I want you to try to remember a time in your life . . . maybe a specific day or a particular situation . . . when you felt like you were at your personal best. A time when you were acting in accordance with your core values and most important priorities for the person you want to be deep down inside.
>
> Maybe this was a time that you responded selflessly . . . helped another person through a tough situation in life . . . apologized for a wrong-doing to repair a relationship . . . resisted a tempting situation . . . or simply avoided retaliating.
>
> Try to bring yourself back to that moment and remember what it felt like to be inspired, and not just impulsively self-centered. Recall the emotions you felt as this scenario unfolded. Recognize that real and powerful dimension of yourself that is still very much a part of who you are.

Another way to strengthen the higher self is by doing virtuous deeds that shift the client's motivational focus from satisfying appetites to attaining elevated ends. In this vein, DeSteno (2018) summarizes research showing that self-control is enhanced by acts of compassion, altruism, and gratitude to others.

More direct cognitive-behavioral methods can activate the higher self. A good example comes from the work of Arthur Margolin, Kelly Avants, and their colleagues, who developed spiritual self-schema (3-S+) therapy (Avants, Beitel, & Margolin, 2005). This manualized eight- to 12-session treatment grows out of cognitive psychology and Buddhist philosophy, though it is tailored to the religious and spiritual orientation of each client. The therapy rests on the assumption that addictive behaviors are an automatic response to a habitually activated self-schema, known as the "addict self," made up of cognitive labels, such as impulsive, aggressive, selfish, and irresponsible. The goal of 3-S+ therapy is to replace the addict self-schema with a spiritual self-schema marked by compassion (doing no harm to oneself or others) and mindfulness. Clients are taught that the spiritual self rather than the addict self is the more accurate reflection of the client's true nature. Several techniques are used to facilitate the shift from addict self to spiritual self, including (1) mindful meditation to recognize when and how the addict self is activated; (2) observing the impermanence of cravings; (3) identifying thoughts that trigger cravings and sabotage spiritual progress; (4)

spiritual self-affirmations; and (5) reflecting on spiritual values, including generosity, morality, equanimity, wisdom, and renunciation.

The empirical findings of 3-S+ are quite promising, particularly when we keep in mind that their clients who are HIV+ opiate dependent are generally resistant to treatment. In one study (Avants et al., 2005), clients demonstrated a significant shift in their schemas as measured by a computerized reaction time task. Participants also reported significant declines in illicit drug use according to their self-reports and the percentage of heroin- and cocaine-free urine screens. When asked what was most helpful about the treatment, one client said, "The freedom. The freedom of knowing that my true self is my spiritual [self] not the addict [self]. That's a freedom itself" (p. 176).

Finally, it is important to note that, from some spiritual and religious perspectives, the higher self may be activated not by direct efforts at control but rather through a recognition of the limits of personal control and a willingness to defer control to a higher power. This is a hallmark of the 12-step approach to addiction. The first three of the 12 steps involve admitting powerlessness over addiction, recognizing that only a greater power can heal the individual, and deciding to turn one's life over to the care of God. Many narrative accounts of recovering addicts describe experiences in which God has touched their lives, leading to a dramatic transformational shift away from an identity oriented around addiction to one that centers around a higher power (Sremac & Ganzevoort, 2013, p. 416).

In short, therapists can take a variety of approaches to help clients achieve better impulse control so they can strive toward lives of significant purpose, lives more consistent with their higher selves. Litz et al. (2009) reach an optimistic conclusion from their work with service members and veterans that "[Those] who earnestly seek care are struggling, but still capable of reclaiming goodness and moral directedness, and forgiveness and repair is possible in all cases" (p. 701).

Breaking the Undercontrol/Overcontrol Cycle

We have drawn from a variety of therapeutic modalities and spiritual resources to offer ways to address the problems of moral overcontrol and impulse undercontrol that can interfere with the well-being and growth of moral strugglers. Although we treated these two forms of dysregulation separately, they can be interrelated (Vanderbleek & Gilbert, 2018). Feeling the burden of a harsh, perfectionistic moral framework, clients may try to break out from those shackles or find immediate emotional gratification by impulsive overindulgence. Overdoing it, however, only prompts further guilt and shame that leads back once again to a commitment to a morality that has no space for human error and needs, and so on. Life for these clients has the feel of a roller coaster at times, with unnerving oscillations between the extremes of moral domination and impulse excess. Bob, for example, had begun to experience this cycle of impulsive pornography use followed by tremendous guilt and shame that triggered further risky behavior. Practitioners working with clients caught up in the out-of-control/overcontrol cycle will need to deal with both problems.

In this regard, Ano, Pargament, Wong, and Pomerleau (2017) developed a promising, brief, manualized, group intervention ("From Vice to Virtue") for people facing both of the problematic sides of moral struggles. On the moral over-control side, the program challenges moral perfectionism, encourages more realistic and humane expectations, and facilitates greater use of redemptive resources, such as apologies and, when appropriate, reconciliation. On the impulse under-control side, participants identify a specific vice to resist and a specific virtue to cultivate, and then implement a concrete plan for self-monitoring and change that draws on spiritual resources for strength, motivation, and sustenance. Ano et al. evaluated the effectiveness of this program in a nondenominational Christian church. Compared to a wait-list control group, participants in the From Vice to Virtue program reported significantly greater ability to resist their vice and express their virtue. Group participants also showed significant improvements in stress and spiritual development over the course of the program. These gains were maintained at a 4-week follow-up.

CONCLUSIONS

We began this chapter by noting that moral struggles are embedded in the human condition. There is a natural tension that arises by virtue of the reality that we are both moral beings and beings of impulse and appetite. This tension cannot be resolved by attempts to eliminate one or the other of these two sides of human nature. Indeed, that will only inflame the problem. Blaise Pascal, 17th-century French theologian and scientist, wrote, "He who should be angel becomes a beast"(Kurtz, 2007, p. 15). Progress along the pathway to wholeness and growth requires an acceptance of these two fundamental aspects of ourselves. As Kurtz and Ketcham (1992) wrote, "It is the embrace of the both-and-ness, both saint and sinner, both beast and angel, that constitutes our very being as human" (p. 186). Progress toward wholeness and growth also rests on the wisdom to make more informed choices about our double sidedness, life direction, and goals. This brings to mind Chittister's (2003) story of the Native American elder who felt as if two wolves were fighting in his heart, one filled with anger and desires for vengeance and the other filled with love and caring. His disciple asked, "But which wolf will win the fight in your heart?" The elder answered, "It depends on which one I feed" (p. 103). Of course, people must find a way to feed both morality and impulse without falling into the traps of sating or starving one or the other. Therapists can help clients engage in the process of balancing and reconciling the imperatives of morality and impulse. The ultimate goal of this process is not an uneasy truce between these two sides of ourselves but rather the discovery of ways that body and soul can work in synergy with each other. Rosmarin (2018) captures the spirit of this kind of complementarity: The "body–soul connection," he says, occurs "when the soul provides for the body's material needs and comforts and encourages it to achieve for its own (the body's) benefit, while the body receives the gifts of support and guidance from the soul and pushes itself to follow its (the soul's) directive" (p. 25). With help, clients who are struggling morally can use the spiritual tensions within themselves as a springboard to greater unity, coherence, and wholeness.

In the next chapter, we shift our focus to a type of struggle often connected to moral struggles: struggles with the demonic.

CHAPTER 12

Demonic Struggles

> I was doing all those wrong things because I was under the influence of the bad spirits of my father. . . . Satan was destroying my life and I never understood why.
>
> —SREMAC AND GANZEVOORT (2013, p. 423)

In daily life, people sometimes encounter adversaries: those who oppose their interests and might even try to harm or attack them. But what if these adversaries are believed to come from the supernatural realm, imbued with mysterious powers and abilities far beyond those of mere mortals? Although fictional clashes between superheroes and villains might come to mind, people can also experience real-life struggles of this type if they believe in supernatural evil. For them, life might become a locus of an epic battle, one in which powerful antagonists strive to harm or even destroy human beings. Granted, some might see such a battle as purely metaphorical in nature, akin to moral struggles—perhaps a battle between higher and lower parts of the self (Saritoprak et al., 2018), or a struggle against an evil inclination that all humans share, as captured by the *yetzer hara* concept in Judaism (Luzzatto, 1997). But others may see their adversaries as actual supernatural entities, whether these be personal (the devil, demons, evil spirits) or impersonal (dark energies or an evil force).

For many reasons, this is an extraordinarily confusing and difficult area. One issue is that psychologists and scientists, who on average tend to be much less religious than the general population (Delaney, Miller, & Bisonó, 2013; Ecklund, 2010), are unlikely to believe in supernatural evil (Leavey, 2010). They may find themselves puzzled or frustrated about whether and why modern adults "still believe" in such things.

But the fact remains that many people in the United States do believe in supernatural evil. In the 2005 Baylor Religion Survey (as reviewed in Baker, 2008), a majority of Americans (75.1%) reported that they absolutely (57.8%) or probably (17.3%) believed in Satan, and many also reported belief in demons

(47.7% absolutely, 21.9% probably) and hell (55.6% absolutely, 17.9% probably). Beliefs in human-mediated evil are also quite common: 31.0% in a 2008 Harris Interactive Poll reported belief in witches, and 16.0% of U.S. participants in a 2009 survey reported belief in witchcraft, curses, and/or the evil eye (Pew Research Center, 2009).

Believing in supernatural evil is one thing; *wanting* to believe in it is another. For instance, in a large survey of undergraduates, most reported that they did not want to believe in the devil, although they did want to believe in God (Wilt, Stauner, & Exline, 2020). And this brings up another reason why research and clinical work on this topic is challenging: The idea that supernatural evil exists—or might possibly exist—is unsettling to consider. It can make the world seem like a hostile, dangerous place. Further, people who believe in supernatural adversaries may not feel confident that they can avoid the dangers. Given the fear factor, both clinicians and clients may prefer to steer away from these disturbing topics. And researchers have, for the most part, taken the same tactic; there is less research on demonic struggles than on other struggles covered in this book.

Despite these challenges, we believe demonic struggles are vital to understand. Belief in supernatural evil is a foundational, non-negotiable part of some worldviews, and struggles around such beliefs can be a major source of strain for people who experience them.

MAP FOR THIS CHAPTER

The first half of this chapter provides a conceptual framework for understanding demonic struggles, referring to relevant research where possible. We begin by considering several different forms that demonic struggles could take. Next, we highlight a wide variety of factors that could lead to demonic struggles, including both background and situational factors, before laying out some potential consequences of these struggles. The second half of the chapter offers some tentative clinical suggestions, keeping in mind that there is little research or psychotherapy-focused writing on this challenging topic.

UNDERSTANDING DEMONIC STRUGGLES

To be able to assist people struggling with the demonic or evil in their lives, it is important to first have some understanding of demonic struggles. We give a broad overview in this section.

The Meaning of Demonic Struggles

Although demonic struggle can take diverse forms, we suggest that a core idea underlies them: a sense of being opposed by a supernatural adversary. This adversary would be assumed to have malevolent intentions, wanting to cause harm. To get a mental picture of the types of strategies such an adversary might use, it is not necessary to limit ourselves to supernatural entities. Instead, it might be helpful to envision not only how human adversaries behave but also what predatory animals do when hunting down their prey. (Along these lines, the New Testament actually does speak of the devil as "a roaring lion, seeking whom he may devour"; I Peter 5:8.) To illustrate, here are some examples of strategies that adversaries could use to cause harm:

- *An adversary could intentionally cause pain and suffering,* using a "direct attack" strategy to harm others by causing stressful, painful, or damaging events.

- *An adversary could trick, deceive, or manipulate others* into making damaging choices. Even things that appear, on the surface, to be positive (e.g., beautiful, pleasant, or helpful) could be weaponized to lure people into danger.

- *An adversary could try to stir up fear,* intimidating others with displays of dominance and aggression, and causing them to lose confidence, thus preventing counterattacks.

- *An adversary could strive to weaken others,* perhaps oppressing them by wearing them down mentally, emotionally, or physically—or by separating them from crucial allies and resources in a "divide-and-conquer" strategy.

- *An adversary could try to block others from reaching their goals,* rendering them ineffective in their most vital pursuits. They might directly plant obstacles or traps to obstruct progress, or they might use subtler means to divert energy, such as discouragement, distraction, or lulling others into a sense of complacency and security.

We propose that, generally speaking, the types of situations that bring supernatural evil to mind usually involve one or more of these adversarial themes. As we explore below, people could see these adversaries as actual supernatural entities (the devil; evil spirits or forces) or as metaphorical, psychological constructs. Let's take a closer look at both of these ideas.

Actions Initiated by Supernatural Evil Agents

When people think about what an encounter with supernatural evil would look like, many will think of personal supernatural agents (e.g., the devil, demons, evil spirits) that intentionally cause problems or harm. Along these lines, the four demonic struggle items in our Religious and Spiritual Struggles (RSS) Scale (Exline, Pargament, Grubbs, & Yali, 2014) tap the idea of harmful actions by the devil or evil spirits: "felt tormented by the devil or evil spirits," "worried that the problems I was facing were the work of the devil or evil spirits," "felt attacked by the devil or evil spirits," and "felt as though the devil (or an evil spirit) was trying to turn me away from what was good."

But how, exactly, would the devil or evil spirits try to harm people? Before turning to the more common, psychologically focused forms of demonic struggles, let's briefly take up the supernatural lens and consider a few more dramatic, attention-grabbing examples.

Dramatic Experiences. Some of the most extreme events that people might attribute to supernatural evil involve claims of *demonic possession*, in which an evil spirit is believed to have entered a person and taken (at least partial) control. Although popularized in modern movies such as *The Exorcist*, possession beliefs have been widespread throughout human history and across cultures (Begelman, 1993; Laycock, 2015; McNamara, 2011). In a landmark study of 488 societies in the 1960s, anthropologist Erika Bourguignon (1976) found that about 75% of these societies showed beliefs in possession.

People may also accuse others of worshiping evil entities, such as the devil. For example, the 1980s witnessed a moral panic around widespread, highly controversial reports of Satanic ritual abuse (Fraser, 1997; Rogers, 1992). And even now, at the time of this writing, the QAnon movement, which alleges that a cabal of Satan-worshiping pedophiles secretly rules the world, has gained considerable traction in the United States (Roose, 2020).

Dramatic claims about the demonic are not limited to possession and Satan worship. People might also claim to see, hear, or otherwise sense the presence of evil spirits, but without having the spirits enter and take control (Brocas, 2018; Earl et al., 2015). For example, many people throughout history have reported encounters with malevolent ghosts (Fleischhack & Schenkel, 2016), which some believe to be demons (Driscoll, 2015). Some people may also try to harness supernatural forces to harm others, as reported in accounts of witchcraft and black magic (Collins, 2015; Rio, MacCarthy, & Blanes, 2017).

Everyday Events. In some cases, then, people perceive demonic entities engaging with people in direct, dramatic ways that seem to violate natural laws. But more typically, people who believe in supernatural entities see them operating in the world in subtle, indirect ways that may be difficult to detect or prove. For example, many people see the devil as having some ability to affect people's thoughts and emotions, or to operate through other people or life events (Exline, Wilt, et al., in press; Jensen, 2009; Ray, Lockman, Jones, & Kelly, 2015). If this is true, then the devil could use any of these strategies to harm people.

C. S. Lewis (1942/1982) provided a superb example of this type of reasoning in his classic book *The Screwtape Letters*. Screwtape, a demon in training, tries a wide array of techniques to torment, tempt, and deceive people, often using subtle manipulations. To sabotage his victim's faith, Screwtape learns how to plant (or encourage) certain thoughts and feelings: pride, confusion, self-absorption, discouragement in response to spiritual dryness, and a focus on the annoying qualities of fellow church members, to name just a few.

Granted, these subtle types of events would be unlikely to convince skeptics of demonic activity, as obvious natural explanations do exist. Instead, the key ideas here center on multiple levels of causality: Supernatural and natural explanations can coexist, because supernatural entities (including evil ones) can work through natural mechanisms (Weeks & Lupfer, 2000). Along these lines, studies have shown that some people make demonic attributions for events ranging from physical illness (Pargament, Koenig, et al., 2001) to mental health conditions (Hartog & Gow, 2005; Nguyen, Yamada, & Dinh, 2012) and divorce (Krumrei et al., 2011), even when natural explanations exist. Human spirits and magic may also be blamed for negative events, including mental illness (Collins, 2015).

These last few examples illustrate that people do not always view supernatural evil in terms of personal, intentional beings, such as a devil or demons; instead, they might view evil as a force—perhaps a dark energy or a "dark side." But the more impersonal such a force seems, the more likely it is to be seen as something metaphorical or symbolic, rather than something that actually exists as an entity. We turn to this possibility next.

An Evil Inclination within Human Nature

Regardless of whether people believe in supernatural adversaries, they may see evil as a part of human nature: something located within individuals, with psychological underpinnings. When evil is framed in purely natural terms, without invoking any sort of supernatural activity, demonic struggles show substantial overlap with the broader category of moral struggle.

Sometimes people reserve the category of evil for extremely serious moral transgressions, things so terrible that they deserve a category of their own. Genocide would be a ready example here. By labeling genocide as evil, people are effectively drawing a moral boundary around it, using it as a prototype that illustrates the very worst of human behavior. In fact, the atrociousness of some human behaviors may raise the possibility of a supernatural evil source underlying them: What else could explain how people could behave so abominably? Yet some would argue that in externalizing evil as ultimately demonic, sinful, and depraved, people may underestimate its banality, its everyday nature. Hannah Arendt (1963) made this point when referring to Adolf Eichmann, the Nazi doctor responsible for horrific medical experiments on people in concentration camps, but some people reacted strongly against her framing (Benhabib, 2014), preferring interpretations that emphasized Eichmann's evilness—his otherness. They wanted to reserve the category of evil for extreme, almost unthinkable moral horrors: things that they could presumably keep at a safe distance from themselves.

Arendt's (1963) emphasis on the banality of evil points toward the idea of an evil inclination (Luzzatto, 1997) that all human beings share, rather than being reserved for extreme cases (see also Baumeister, 1997; Mikulincer & Shaver, 2012). Within a naturalistic frame, evil might be seen as a metaphorical "demon on the shoulder" that tempts us to do wrong, or our own "inner demons" that can lead us in destructive directions. Jung (1954/1985) also took a psychological approach, framing evil as a result of repressed destructive feelings that create a "shadow." As Russell (1975) wrote, the devil could be said to personify "meaningless, senseless, malicious, destructiveness: in essence, annihilation" (p. 81). Writing in the aftermath of Nazism and the Holocaust, Jung was sensitive to the atrocities that can occur when people refuse to acknowledge their own personal capacities for evil, instead projecting them onto other people.

Although the idea of evil is likely to bring up thoughts of destructive behaviors, other forms of evil could be subtle and passive: laziness, avoidance, or carrying on with things that no longer have life. In other words, evil could reflect sins of omission, not just sins of commission. Along these lines, Erich Fromm (1973) spoke of "life turning against itself" (p. 31) and an "attraction to what is dead, decaying, lifeless, and purely mechanical" (p. 27). Another idea that we have found useful is to frame evil as "live" spelled backward: Anything that goes against life, in all of its fullness—anything that deadens the soul—could be seen as evil.

Prevalence of Demonic Struggles

Earlier we showed that belief in the devil, ghosts, and hell are common in the United States today. But simply believing in these entities isn't enough to cause demonic struggle; in fact, such beliefs might be a normative—even central—part of religious teachings. Given this important caveat, what do we know about the prevalence of demonic struggles?

In our broad study of U.S. adults (Exline, Pargament, & Grubbs, 2014), 32% reported having demonic struggles in the last few weeks, and in our large undergraduate study, 50% of students reported demonic struggle in the past few months (Exline et al., 2014b). Although the average intensity of demonic struggles was low in those samples, moderate levels of demonic struggle have been found in samples of U.S. veterans (Breuninger et al., 2019) and Israeli Palestinian Muslim undergraduates (Abu-Raiya, Pargament, Exline, et al., 2015).

We have found that people rarely bring up demonic struggles when asked to focus on a specific spiritual struggle from their lives (Exline, Pargament, & Grubbs, 2014; Fletcher et al., 2020; Wilt, Takahashi, Jeong, Exline, & Pargament, 2020). Why do so few people mention demonic struggles? One possibility is that few people actually attribute problems to supernatural evil. Students in our studies report less belief in the devil than in God (Wilt, Stauner, & Exline, 2020), and they see the devil as less powerful than God (Exline, Wilt, et al., in press), so maybe most people do not see demonic activity as relevant in daily life. Or they might believe in the demonic, and even attribute some events to evil forces, without being troubled by these beliefs.

Another, more methodologically focused possibility is that our range of items is too limited. On the RSS, the RCOPE, and the Brief RCOPE, our items focus specifically on the devil and evil spirits, so they do not tap an internalized "evil inclination" or more general evil forces. We also do not ask specifically about ghosts or other types of spirits.

Spiritual struggles tend to correlate positively with one another (Exline, Pargament, Grubbs, & Yali, 2014). However, when people are asked to focus on important struggles, they might see demonic struggles as secondary parts of other overlapping struggles. Moral struggles are the clearest candidates for overlap with demonic struggles, and moral struggles are very common. There is also potential overlap with divine struggles, especially in terms of fear of divine punishment, and interpersonal struggles, particularly in cases in which people see God as being on their side and might tend to demonize outgroups. So, even though demonic attributions and some demonic struggle might be relevant in these cases, they may not take center stage.

People may also hesitate to mention demonic struggles because they fear that others will judge them negatively for holding such beliefs, which might be seen as antiquated, antiscience, or ultraconservative in religious terms. Along these lines, students have reported that they felt less positively about those who believed in the devil than those who believed in God (Exline, 2019). Similarly, they expected that others would view them less positively if they believed in the devil than if they believed in God. As such, concerns about stigma could lead to underreporting of demonic struggles.

Roots of Demonic Struggles

When are people most likely to experience demonic struggles? In this section, we consider a wide range of factors that could lead people to make *demonic attributions*: to decide that demonic entities are playing a role in a situation, either by causing or influencing events. We then highlight some factors that could increase the sense of threat in response to a demonic attribution, which we suggest is an important factor in moving from demonic attribution to demonic struggle. As we consider when, why, and for whom demonic struggle occurs, we look not only at features of the specific situation but also at background, orienting system factors that could play important roles. For example, we consider how certain religious and cultural beliefs, personal experiences, personality factors, and mental health conditions could affect the odds of demonic attributions and associated struggles.

We focus primarily on attributions to the devil, both to streamline the presentation and because most of the existing research focuses on the devil; however, most of the ideas that we present here could also be applied to other supernatural adversaries, such as demons, malevolent ghosts, evil spirits, or impersonal evil forces (e.g., black magic, curses, dark forces).

Demonic Beliefs as Part of Daily Life: Foundations of a Worldview

We suggest that certain background beliefs and behaviors can shape orientations to the world that foster demonic attributions and associated struggles. Of course, there are some chicken-and-egg issues here: People who believe strongly in supernatural evil are likely to interpret many experiences using this lens, and powerful or frequent experiences attributed to supernatural evil may, in turn, strengthen the belief that evil entities exist. We consider some worldview-level factors first, before getting into specific situations that might prompt demonic struggles.

Belief That a Supernatural Adversary (Such as the Devil) Exists. A first, obvious step toward demonic attributions is a strong belief that supernatural evil actually exists. Without such a belief—or at least some openness to the possibility—a person might wrestle with metaphorical "demons" or concerns about evil in the world, perhaps in the context of moral or interpersonal struggles, but this is not the same as seeing an actual supernatural entity as being involved. Since we have devoted the previous chapter to moral struggles, most of our discussion here focuses on attributions about evil that are more explicitly supernatural. Let's consider beliefs about the devil as an example. Our own work (Wilt, Stauner, & Exline, 2020) suggests that undergraduates are more likely to believe in supernatural entities, including the devil, if they have been *socialized* to believe in these entities (e.g., via religious, cultural, or parental teachings) and if they actually *want* to believe in them. Belief that these entities exist, in turn, strongly predicts perceived experiences with them.

See the Devil as Powerful, Personal, and Broad in Influence. In order to believe that the devil caused something, it is not enough to simply believe that the devil exists; a person must also believe that the devil intervenes in the world (see Wilt, Stauner, & Exline, 2020). As we suggest in our work on *supernatural operating rules* (Exline, Wilt, et al., in press), people should be more likely to attribute events to the devil if these events fit with their ideas about how the devil operates. For example, people would seem unlikely to attribute a tempting thought to the devil if they see the devil as a weak or disinterested figure, one with little power or motivation to affect their daily lives. On the other hand, people who believe that the devil has the ability to influence their physical health, thoughts, and behavior, combined with strong intentions to personally harm them, may live in a state of great vigilance against this threatening antagonist.

Consistent with this reasoning, our own research (Exline, Wilt, et al., in press) suggests that college students with some belief in the devil report more personal experiences with the devil if they see the devil as *powerful* (e.g., able to affect a person's life events, thoughts, and health; able to violate natural laws and work through natural events), *intentional* (e.g., being motivated to harm people), and *broad in influence* (i.e., intervening often, through many modes, and in the lives of many people vs. targeting just a few select people). On average, these students usually see the devil as having a moderate degree of power, influence, and intention to intervene in the world—more than ghosts and spirits, but less than God (Exline, Wilt, et al., in press).

Socialization and Religious Involvement Make Thoughts about the Devil Salient. If people strongly believe that the devil exists and intervenes frequently and broadly in the world, then thoughts of the devil should come easily to mind in daily life. Socialization and religious engagement play a large role here. Deep involvement in a faith tradition that focuses on the devil, such as Christianity or Islam (and perhaps especially the more fundamentalist sides of these traditions), should make thoughts of the devil more accessible in a few ways: by strengthening overall belief in the devil and by frequently mentioning the devil's involvement in the world, thereby making the devil into a more prominent adversary in people's worldviews. Religious conservatives are more likely than liberals to hold such views, as shown in an interview-based study of children, adolescents, and adults (Jensen, 2009). For example, the Christian Bible actually refers to Satan as "the ruler of this world" (John 14:30), essentially implying that everything on Earth could be influenced by the devil. It is unsurprising, then, that demonic struggles correlate so highly with religiousness in our initial studies, which typically have focused on Western Christian samples (e.g., Exline, Pargament, Grubbs, & Yali, 2014).

Although belief in the devil may be less prominent in other religious traditions, individuals from those traditions may still believe in evil entities. For example, Greenberg and Witztum (2001) describe their clinical work with haredi (strictly orthodox) Jews who are caught up in perceived struggles with satanic and demonic forces. In other cultures, beliefs in witchcraft (Collins, 2015), ancestral spirits (Bojuwoye, 2013; McCabe, 2008), or jinn (Dein & Illaiee, 2013; Lim, Hoek, & Blom, 2015) might be similarly salient in people's day-to-day lives.

Dispositions, Personal Experiences, or Psychological Disorders Foster Demonic Beliefs. Although social and religious factors play a major role, individuals differ greatly in their readiness to adopt a supernatural worldview that includes the demonic. Some people are more likely than others to believe in supernatural or paranormal phenomena in general (Aarnio & Lindeman, 2007; Bader, Mencken, & Baker, 2010). To give just a few examples: Some studies suggest that intuitive reasoning styles, as opposed to analytical ones, are linked with more paranormal and religious belief (Pennycook, Cheyne, Seli, Koehler, & Fugelsang, 2012; Shenhav, Rand, & Greene, 2012). Children, due to developmental limitations in reasoning ability, are more likely than adults to engage in magical thinking (Barrett, 2012), which could include thoughts about the devil, demons, or ghosts. Along the same lines, adults may believe in supernatural evil because of strong tendencies to search for meaning (Park, 2013) and agency (Barrett, 2011) behind negative events, especially when natural explanations seem elusive.

Looking past basic beliefs, people should find thoughts about the devil easier to access if they have a large "bank" of past experiences that they have attributed to the devil. Granted, anyone could conceivably have such an experience, and even a single powerful event (e.g., a terrifying vision of hell; genocide) might be enough to convince someone of the reality of evil. But people could also collect experiences over time, perhaps by putting themselves in situations that would increase the odds of such encounters. For example, they might engage in occult practices (magic, witchcraft, fortune-telling), spiritual healing (shamanism, deliverance ministry or exorcism, energy medicine), or attempts to interact with human spirits (ghost hunting, mediumship, ancestor worship). Some people may also be seen as having unique talents in these areas, such as prophetic or healing gifts or abilities to see, discern, or communicate with spirits. Due to their special abilities, these people might perceive demonic presences or messages that others might not perceive. Of course, some people may see these perceptions not as special abilities but as signs of psychopathology, which we consider next.

The mental illness lens can be important to consider when reflecting on potential causes of demonic attributions. Many cases of perceived demonic possession have been linked with dissociative states and associated traumas (Begelman, 1993; During, Elahi, Taieb, Moro, & Baubet, 2011), although this has been a controversial topic (Bull, 2001). Hallucinations or delusions associated with psychosis could cause the brain to produce experiences that may be perceived as demonic, such as malevolent voices, frightening visions, dark presences, or thoughts of persecution (Gearing et al., 2011). More commonly, neurotically focused problems—such as depression, anxiety, insecure attachment, or chronic mistrust of others—could also feed into a demonic worldview, but in a different way: By predisposing people to see themselves, others, or circumstances in a negative light, they bring more opportunities to feel opposed or victimized—and the adversaries they perceive could include supernatural ones.

Demonic Attributions for Specific Events

Now we shift from background factors to consider specific situations where people might make demonic attributions. Earlier, when we discussed meanings of demonic struggles, we sketched out a range of situations that might make people consider the possibility of demonic involvement. These situations all shared the theme of being opposed by a malevolent adversary, with some of the most common involving a sense of being tempted, lied to, tormented, or attacked. For now, let's assume that some situation has occurred that falls into one of those categories. What predicts whether the person will make a demonic attribution? Our work on supernatural attributions (Exline, Stauner, et al., 2020) suggests that people should be more likely to make demonic attributions if such attributions are accessible, plausible, meaningful, and motivating. Let's consider each of these in turn.

Demonic Ideas Are Accessible. Of course, people can only attribute events to the devil if the devil comes to mind. Certain situational cues could make people think of the devil: watching a movie about demons or poltergeists, for instance, or listening to a sermon about the devil. And, not surprisingly, negative events direct people's thoughts to the devil more than positive events do (Lupfer, Tolliver, & Jackson, 1996; Ray et al., 2015). But the many worldview factors that we just discussed could play a huge role here as well: People who see the world as a demonically influenced place may make a mental habit of attributing certain types of events to the devil or other evil entities, to the point where such a process might become almost automatic—thus, demonic explanations would be highly accessible for them. But people who do not believe in supernatural evil, or who see it as irrelevant to their daily lives, might require a truly extraordinary experience in order to consider demonic explanations. In such experiences, questions about plausibility often loom large.

Demonic Explanations Seem Plausible. People are more likely to make attributions, including demonic ones, if they seem logical and reasonable—if they seem to fit well with the situation at hand. This brings us back to the idea of supernatural operating rules (Exline, Wilt, et al., in press): People will be more likely to attribute events to the devil if the event fits with their beliefs about the devil's abilities and modes of operation. Can the devil affect human thoughts? If so, then a demonic attribution for a temptation will seem more credible. Can the devil work through people? If so, then it might make sense to see someone as an agent or messenger of Satan. (See Ray et al., 2015, for a study focusing on these ideas.) Does the devil have the intention and power to pull people away from God? If so, then it might make sense to worry about demonic threats to personal salvation.

Demonic Explanations Are Meaningful. People should also be more likely to embrace demonic attributions if such attributions help to satisfy desires to make meaning (cf. Park, 2013). At a cognitive level, does adding the devil to the equation add explanatory power, making the story of the event more believable, logically consistent, interesting, or memorable? Or, at a more intuitive level, does adding the devil to the story deepen the sense of personal meaning or resonance associated with it? If so, then people should be more likely to reach for demonic explanations (Routledge, Abeyta, & Roylance, 2016). Consider all of the different story lines that might accompany demonic struggles: narratives of being attacked, tempted to do wrong, or diverted from important goals could all resonate with people, echoing themes from more familiar, interpersonal experiences of opposition while imbuing them with a sense of cosmic significance. The language of supernatural evil might also give people a way to label experiences so horrible that other explanations or words simply seem inadequate to capture them. Given the cognitive or emotional appeal of certain story lines or concepts, people might actually *want* to make demonic attributions in some cases. We consider this possibility next.

Demonic Explanations Are Motivating. As shown in the literature on motivated reasoning (Kunda, 1990), people's beliefs are shaped not only by rational factors but also by emotional factors. At some level, we believe what we want to believe, and we push away ideas that we do not want to believe. And people may indeed find that demonic beliefs and attributions, though troubling in some ways, can also serve some useful functions.

Demonic attributions may help people to affirm their basic values, pinpointing certain things as clearly wrong (and subject to divine punishment) so that they will choose to steer away from them and stay on a good, safe moral path. Further, if they fail to meet their goals, blaming the devil could provide a ready excuse. Much as people sometimes defer control to God (Pargament et al., 1988) or blame God for negative events (Exline et al., 2011), they could also see the devil as a controlling force in their lives—and a convenient scapegoat when trouble arises. Blaming the devil might help them to stay on God's good side (Beck & Taylor, 2008), while divesting them of a sense of personal responsibility for their actions.

Demonic attributions could also energize people by framing their actions in terms of an epic, cosmic battle: People can fight against demons rather than blaming God or themselves. On the darker side, people could turn to demonic attributions as a moral justification for hostile attitudes or behaviors toward outgroups, ranging from prejudice to genocide. A potent and terrible example comes from the historical demonization of Jews, who have been framed as devils, satanic, and ritual murderers (Goldhagen, 2013). Even given these potentially serious problems, the sense of being on the heroic side of a battle could provide a major boost of self-esteem and energy, making people feel powerful, purposeful, and safe, secure in the rightness of their beliefs and opinions. Examples such as these highlight that demonic attributions do not always lead to demonic struggle. On the contrary, such attributions could actually be quite rewarding in some cases, especially if people see themselves heroically conquering their supernatural adversaries.

Threat Appraisals

In order to cross the line from demonic attribution to demonic struggle, we propose that something else is required: a sense of threat. Demonic struggle should be greatest in high-stakes situations: those that carry the potential for serious negative consequences. The idea of demonic operating rules comes back into play here: Do people see the devil as an extremely powerful, skilled, well-equipped adversary that is out to harm or destroy them? If so, they might fear physical or psychological pain, loss of resources, or damaged relationships resulting from demonic attack. Worse, they might fear the consequences of following the devil instead of God—a choice that might lead them toward divine disapproval, punishment, rejection, or even annihilation. On the other hand, if people see the devil as less powerful than God, they may feel secure in God's protection—assuming they believe they are still on God's side and haven't gone over to the enemy's side. People who are having divine struggles might have extreme difficulties here, being terrified of evil forces but also afraid to approach God for help.

Stress arises when people not only perceive a threat but see themselves as having insufficient resources to cope with the threat (Lazarus & Folkman, 1984). Our own model of spiritual struggles suggests that if people see themselves as weak or compromised, or if they see themselves as unable to access effective resources to stop the adversary's attacks, their sense of struggle should increase. In cases of demonic struggle, as we have seen with other forms of spiritual struggle, physical or psychological exhaustion, combined with negative emotions or difficulty discerning the best course of action, should intensify distress. A lack of (actual or perceived) social support could also make things worse: People could believe that they are all alone or that other would-be helpers are weak, unreliable, or disloyal. A sense of threat could also come from a sense of personal weakness or badness that could be amplified by low self-esteem, strong predispositions toward guilt, or depressive symptoms.

Summary

This section introduced many potential predictors of demonic struggle. Some focused on basic worldviews: Does supernatural evil exist, and what role might it play in everyday life? We then turned to demonic attributions in specific situations—attributions that could reflect not only worldviews but a host of other cognitive, emotional, and social factors. One take-home point from this multilayered, admittedly complex analysis is that demonic struggles cannot be explained by any one factor: They do not stem simply from psychology, from cultural beliefs, or from dramatic violations of natural laws. Having explored these many factors that might set the stage for demonic struggles, we now turn to their potential consequences.

Consequences of Demonic Struggles

There is little research on the direct consequences of demonic struggles. And unfortunately, there is potential for studies to provide misleading results as well, largely because demonic struggles usually show moderate positive correlations with religiousness (Exline, Pargament, Grubbs, & Yali, 2014). Thus, associations that are actually due to religiousness might be credited to demonic struggles if religiousness is not controlled. For example, in a study in which all RSS subscales are competing with one another in a regression model, demonic struggle could end up predicting spiritual growth or closeness to God—but only because of its connection with religiousness (which might have been left out of the model). For such analyses to yield accurate results, we reiterate the importance of controlling for religiousness (or another, belief-related variable, such as orthodoxy, fundamentalism, or belief in the devil). With this important caveat in mind, what ideas can we offer about possible consequences of demonic struggles?

Demonic Struggles and Decline

Many studies show that demonic struggles, like other spiritual struggles, are linked with greater psychological distress. For example, demonic struggles correlated positively with depression and anxiety in a national sample of U.S. adults (Abu-Raiya, Pargament, Krause, et al., 2015), a group of Christians going through training in spiritual warfare (Tanksley, 2010), a large U.S. undergraduate sample (Exline, Pargament, Grubbs, & Yali, 2014), and undergraduate samples of Israeli Jews (Abu-Raiya, Pargament, Weissberger, et al., 2016) and Israeli Palestinian Muslims (Abu-Raiya, Pargament, Exline, et al., 2015). Perhaps the most compelling finding is that in a sample of medically ill older adults, demonic appraisals predicted higher mortality rates over a 2-year period (Pargament, Koenig, et al., 2001). Given that so little longitudinal research exists on demonic struggles, it is difficult to fully assess the implications of demonic struggles for mental health or to determine whether demonic struggles are causes or effects of psychological problems.

In this section, we move beyond these correlations with psychological distress to consider some possible underlying mechanisms: Why would demonic attributions lead to distress or other problems? The ideas introduced here, though speculative, are ones that we are beginning to examine in our research program.

Some of these ideas were foreshadowed in earlier sections, especially the preceding one on threat appraisals.

Threat of Being on the "Bad Side." In the context of moral struggles, people may worry about committing a sin—but here it goes a step further. Rather than being seen as errors or poor choices, people may fear that sins imply a switch of coalitions: Rather than following God or fighting for the cause of good, they have now switched sides, following the devil or aligning themselves with forces of evil. Seeing themselves as having sold out to evil forces could foster a sense of weakness, low self-esteem, or—worse, self-hatred or a complete abandonment of moral principles and spiritual connections. A hopeless sense of having given oneself over to destructive forces might even open the door to tragic outcomes, such as suicide or homicide.

Inner Conflict. Struggling to make good moral choices or to follow their principles, people may feel torn within themselves. Like the familiar image of a person with a devil on one shoulder and an angel on the other, people may see one part of themselves as evil and another part as good, leading to a paralyzing sense of inner conflict. A sense of personal wholeness may be elusive here, as this dualistic view of the self might make integration of desires and emotions more difficult. Some of the greatest challenges here may be faced by people with conditions such as dissociative identity disorder, who by definition have difficulty integrating different parts of themselves into a coherent whole, and people suffering from psychosis, who may have to struggle against voices commanding them to harm others or themselves.

Difficulty in Moral Decision Making. Worries about demonic influence could strip people of confidence in moral decision making. People often associate the devil with trickery and lies, all aimed at luring people down a destructive path. Thus, when people try to look inward and follow their moral instincts, they may question whether their logic and intuitions can be trusted: Has their moral compass been compromised by sin—perhaps even hijacked by the devil? Such problems may be especially salient when people go against religious authority or engage in behaviors that suggest a "slippery slope" in moral terms.

Scrupulosity. Some people facing demonic struggles may fear that if evil overtakes them, they will face eternal damnation or eternal punishment from God. Especially among people with obsessive–compulsive tendencies, the terrifying prospect of divine punishment or rejection could feed tendencies toward scrupulosity, as people try desperately to maintain a sense of control and stay in God's good graces. People might also focus their anxiety about damnation or punishment on other people, leading to aggressive, relationship-straining attempts to persuade other people to turn away from behaviors or beliefs seen as wicked.

Sense of Victimhood. If people see themselves as being attacked by powerful, malevolent forces, they may feel weak and powerless. Even if not worried about being pulled over to the dark side, they might live in constant fear of ongoing attacks. Feeling oppressed or worn down by evil forces, they may find it difficult to seek out resources or sources of positive energy. Some may also take on the passive role of a victim, with its attendant disavowal of responsibility, rather than engaging in more active problem-solving strategies.

Antisocial Attitudes and Behaviors. Although not always directly traceable to demonic struggles per se, some of the most serious negative consequences of demonic attributions arise when people demonize other individuals or groups. A major risk of using evil as a pejorative category and a way of marking religious boundaries is that it can lead people to demonize others, essentially labeling them as evil or assuming that they are under the devil's control. And from here, it is a frighteningly small step to be able to justify hostility and aggression toward these groups by framing one's actions as part of a valiant struggle to combat evil. For instance, in a community sample of divorced women (Krumrei et al., 2011), demonization of one's ex-spouse was tied to higher levels of state aggression. And another study showed that if Christian students saw Jews as demonically influenced by having killed Jesus, they reported more anti-Semitic attitudes (Pargament, Trevino, Mahoney, & Silberman, 2007). At even greater extremes, excluding people from one's moral circle could easily justify prejudice, discrimination, and expulsion from communities. Along these lines, O'Donnell's (2020) discourse analysis explores how the spiritual warfare framing used by some religious (in this case, Christian) nationalists could feed into hostility toward immigrants; liberals; lesbian, gay, bisexual, and transgender (LGBT) individuals; and others seen as outsiders. And the possibilities become even more horrifying if people start trying to annihilate these evil forces by burning accused witches, torturing apostates, or murdering people they see as infidels, devil followers, or simply evil at their core.

Demonic Struggles and Growth

On initial reflection, it may seem counterintuitive to think that demonic struggles (or the associated attributions) could possibly lead to growth. But, as we foreshadowed in the section on motivation above, we believe that such struggles could prompt certain types of personal or spiritual growth, depending on how people choose to respond to the struggles. We suggest a few possibilities here. Once again, we need to note that these ideas are speculative, due to the lack of focused research in this area.

Sense of Empowerment. Belief in supernatural adversaries could offer some psychological benefits by providing people with an enemy, someone (or something) that they can fight. Anger is an approach-oriented emotion, one that can mobilize action. If this action can be focused in a prosocial direction (e.g., "I'm not going to let the devil destroy my marriage or my health!"), the associated energy and metaphors of battle could motivate certain people to stay strong, alert, active, and "on their game." In a related vein, if people see themselves as clearly on the side of good, even the perception of a demonic attack might feel like an affirmation of sorts: "If the devil is attacking me, I must be doing well!" The idea of being a personal threat to the powers of darkness—sufficiently important to target with an attack—could lead to a boost in self-esteem and confidence. Of course, this perception of being a threat to the powers of evil could take some very dark turns, particularly for people with narcissistic or sociopathic tendencies, or in cases in which people are demonizing other people or groups. But, psychologically, such a perception should still be affirming and empowering.

Clarification of Personal Values and Moral Boundaries. Working through demonic struggles, especially those involving tough discernment challenges, could help people to clarify their values and to mark moral boundaries, giving them a greater sense of confidence in their ability to discern right from wrong. Along the way, people might be able to advance to higher levels of moral or spiritual development and toward greater wholeness, perhaps by moving from narrow punishment or rule-focused concerns to a more universal ethic of care for others and the world. As part of this process, some people who previously followed external sources of authority in an unquestioning or passive way might be able to develop a set of values that are more internally guided, even if they still include influences from external sources.

Self-Control and Value-Driven Behavior. One way to combat a spiritual adversary would be to live a life of integrity and purpose, cultivating self-control and living in ways consistent with one's deepest values. As we describe in the second part of this chapter, certain religiously framed techniques can encourage people to choose the "good side" and to behave in virtuous ways. Successes in these areas, in turn, may help people to feel more confident, secure, and whole, with strengthened connections to other people and God.

ADDRESSING DEMONIC STRUGGLES IN CLINICAL PRACTICE

How can we help people to work through demonic struggles in positive ways? Given the lack of systematic intervention research focused on demonic struggles, we have drawn from existing theory, basic research, clinically oriented writing, and personal experience to offer some ideas about intervention. This is admittedly a challenging domain, and we certainly do not claim to offer definitive answers or foolproof solutions. Yet, even though our suggestions should be taken as tentative, we hope they may help to lay some groundwork for a nuanced, tailored approach to addressing demonic struggles. Given our emphasis on psychotherapy in this book, we focus mainly on the psychological lens. In a separate article (Exline, Pargament, Wilt, & Harriott, 2021), we offer a closer look at how people might use the mental illness, psychological, and supernatural lenses to frame reports of demonic activity.

In helping clients deal with spiritual struggles, one of our primary goals is to help them regain a sense of wholeness and integration. We want them to feel personally empowered, living a life rooted in meaningful values but also open to change and growth. And we want them to feel connected to their authentic selves, to other people, to the earth in which we live, and, for believers—to the divine. So let's begin to consider some ways that these struggles can be addressed respectfully and thoughtfully, with these key goals of wholeness and integration in mind. We start with a clinically focused example to help frame our discussion.

The Case of Michael

Michael, a 35-year-old Caucasian man from the Midwestern United States, married Karen, a college classmate, in his early 20s, and they now have two children in elementary school. His marriage to Karen, while pleasant enough, has always felt a bit bland, but he cares deeply about her and about his children. Michael has served as a deacon in a Pentecostal church for the last 5 years, and he actively strives to follow and serve God in his daily life. If asked, he would state his firm belief that God is all-loving. But he also has a strong sense of respect for God's laws, and he does fear that God will punish him if he commits a willful sin.

In his adolescent years, Michael began to experiment with alcohol and recreational drugs. He quickly found that alcohol offered a ready escape and found himself drinking regularly—and, at times, heavily—as a way to self-medicate. Having used marijuana many times with no ill effects, he once tried LSD in his college dorm room. But instead of the transcendent, mystical experience he had hoped for, Michael had a terrifying vision. At first, he was thrilled when he saw a beautiful Being of colorful light, who approached and extended a hand toward him. But once Michael tried to grasp the hand, everything changed. The Being immediately transformed into a monstrous, demonic figure, gripping his hand with sharp claws and dragging him through the dark toward a flaming pit. Plaintive wails and screams emanated from the pit, which was acrid with the smell of sulfur. Feeling horrified and completely helpless, Michael cried out for help from God and immediately found himself back in his dorm room, trembling and drenched with sweat. Not only was this a "scared-straight" experience for Michael in terms of hallucinogens, throughout his life he continued to think of this vision as a profound, very real encounter with the demonic realm. He also saw it as a warning from God to stay on the straight and narrow path. He stopped using all illegal drugs at that time, although he did continue drinking—sometimes in secret.

Over the course of his lifetime, and especially over the past few years, Michael has had many occasions when he fantasized about romantic and sexual encounters with women, and he has sometimes been plagued by repetitive thoughts along these lines, which he refers to as voices. The voices might seem to whisper ("You've gotta have her . . . ") or yell ("F___ it all, just DO IT!"), accompanied by intrusive sexual images that he can't get out of his mind. He has sometimes been tempted, especially when traveling for work, to have sexual encounters with other women, but so far he has managed to resist.

A few months ago, Michael confessed his sexual desires and thoughts to a close friend from his church. His friend expressed shock and deep concern. Although he praised Michael for resisting the ongoing temptations, he strongly suggested that Michael seek out deliverance ministry to rid himself of the spirit causing this temptation. His friend prayed with him, pleading with God to free Michael from the sinful desires, but Michael's desires did not change.

Now, the presenting problem: Michael is forming a close bond with a new coworker, Amelia. They have gone on several business trips together, often drinking and talking for hours on end. Amelia, who is single, and also Christian (but from a liberal Protestant denomination), is starting to feel like a true soul mate. Michael hasn't told anyone (including Amelia) about his strong attraction, but it continues to grow. Although deeply troubled by the prospect of harming his wife and children, he feels like he is falling in love. He has started drinking more heavily, and he is concerned because of some family history of alcohol abuse. Confused, frightened, and wracked with guilt, Michael is now reaching out to seek therapy for the first time in his life.

Michael's case contains many elements of demonic struggle. He believes firmly that supernatural evil is real and that the devil actively causes harm in people's lives. His beliefs come from several sources: biblical and church teaching, as well as his hallucinogenic experience, which he saw as a real supernatural encounter. The overlap with moral struggles is evident here, as Michael sees the devil as tempting him to take actions that could open himself and others to many risks: promiscuous (and perhaps unprotected) sexual encounters, an extramarital affair, breaking his marriage vows, and perhaps even wandering away from God and thus inviting divine punishment. Michael is also tormented by repetitive, intrusive thoughts and images that he attributes to demonic attack.

At the same time, though, much of Michael's distress centers on a problem of moral discernment: Are his desires for other women part of a dark temptation from the devil? Are they part of a scheming, targeted, intentional attack on his marriage—and even on his mortal soul? Or might they be part of a life-giving impulse and a reflection of his true identity—one that he's felt forced to suppress or deny? If framed in these latter terms, evil might be seen not as a temptation to a risky action but instead as a deadening, stifling force that could keep Michael from moving forward into a new season or domain of life.

Michael is also concerned about his heavy use of alcohol, which he frames straightforwardly as a self-destructive temptation from the devil. He knows that, given his past drinking habits and his family history of alcohol problems, this is an area that he needs to watch closely, although he does hope that he can continue to drink in moderation.

Assess and Explore Beliefs about Evil

When working with a client such as Michael, a first step would be to respectfully seek more information about his beliefs about supernatural evil. For example, how strongly does Michael believe in the devil and in hell, and what are these beliefs based on? Does he find that attributing events to the devil serves some valuable functions for him—helping him to stay on the straight and narrow path, for example—or do these beliefs simply oppress and frighten him? How does he think the devil operates? For instance, does the devil have the power to reach in and plant certain thoughts in Michael's mind? Finally, and very important in psychological terms, could temptations or tricks from the devil be powerful enough to cause Michael to go totally off course, ending up in hell? Or is he basically safe in God's care, with the devil's tricks being more akin to harassment, distractions, or illusions that do not ultimately jeopardize Michael's salvation or his relationship with God? Once you have this level of information, there are a number of directions you could take clinically, depending on how you frame the issues. We spend most of the chapter on those ideas, but first, let's consider another important piece of the assessment process: an honest self-assessment.

Reflect on Your Own Beliefs . . . and Potential Biases

A second layer of assessment focuses on your own beliefs, with the aim of making your likely approach to treatment more clear and explicit (see the "lenses" we discuss below), and pointing out possible blind spots or biases. This assessment could also help to clarify how large the gap is between your own worldview and that of the client. This is an important factor to consider in evaluating whether you can work effectively together or whether a referral to another professional within the client's tradition might be more appropriate.

Your Own Beliefs about the Supernatural, Including Evil

You might benefit from asking yourself questions similar to those you asked your client: What do you actually believe about the existence of a supernatural world, including the possibility of evil forces or entities? What do you want to believe? How do you tend to feel when these types of topics come up, and—honestly—how do you feel about people who believe (or do not believe) in supernatural evil?

It is important to ask these questions of yourself, because a lack of introspection and reflection could lead to ineffective treatment—perhaps even to harm. If you do not believe in supernatural evil, and especially if you do not *want* to believe in it, you could have a bias toward dismissing (or otherwise defending against) such beliefs when they are mentioned. You might find yourself trying to challenge clients in hopes that you can talk them out of their beliefs, or you might simply ignore references that the client makes to supernatural evil, instead staying in your more comfortable psychological territory. On the other hand, if you believe strongly in supernatural evil, you might go to the opposite extreme, assuming the attacks are real and perhaps jumping readily into supernaturally focused tactics. (See Exline, Pargament, Wilt, & Harriott, 2021, for more detail and cautions about this approach.)

Your Setting, Training, and Typical Treatment Modalities

The next question is more contextual: Are you working in a setting that would encourage you to frame these beliefs in a certain way? For example, if you work on an inpatient psychiatry unit, you may be predisposed to frame demonic struggles in terms of mental or medical illness. If you work in a secular psychotherapy practice, you might focus on sources of demonic beliefs and whether such beliefs serve a useful function in a person's life. But if you are part of a pastoral team, especially in a faith tradition that focuses on the reality of supernatural evil, you may be quick to think in terms of actual demonic activity. In hybrid settings, such as a treatment center that includes psychotherapy along with spiritual healing, or a Christian counselor's office where prayer with clients is common, you might be trained to focus on multiple levels of explanation—but in these cases, boundary issues could raise problems. Our focus here is mainly on the psychological lens, but first, let's consider the possible role of serious mental or physical health conditions.

The Mental Illness Lens: Focus on Serious Mental or Medical Conditions

Some demonic struggles could be secondary in nature—that is, they could stem from—or be exacerbated by—an underlying medical or mental health problem. Granted, some clinicians, not knowing the high base rates for belief in supernatural evil, might be too quick to assume that such beliefs indicate psychopathology, but there are indeed many clinical explanations to consider, and missing these could do a real disservice to the client. When unusual symptoms are encountered, an in-depth, standard psychological and/or medical assessment will hopefully help to clarify the diagnostic picture.

How might this type of assessment be important in Michael's case? It is clear that he had a vivid and intense hallucinatory experience many years ago after taking LSD. But what about his more recent intrusive and obsessive thoughts? Might they reflect an underlying anxiety disorder? He keeps using the term *voices*, which might simply be a metaphor for him, but they also raise the possibility of psychotic symptoms. Does his experience of demonic torment include any thoughts of suicide, homicide, or other harm to self or others? To what extent might alcohol abuse be amplifying his struggles?

Let's say that a clinical interview did suggest an underlying psychological or medical disorder. Clearly that diagnosis warrants clinical attention in its own right. But once these potential causes are uncovered, it is important to guard against another problem: It could be easy to brush demonic struggles to the side, simply framing them as a symptom of a psychological or medical condition (i.e., secondary struggles), even though they might be a key part of a person's psychological experience. Returning to Michael's case, perhaps a clinical interview would reveal an anxiety disorder, a substance use problem, or even some psychotic symptoms. But even if such issues were identified, it is important to keep in mind that Michael is framing his demonic struggles as real supernatural events, even though he holds natural explanations at the same time; in other words, he believes supernatural activity can be indirect, working through natural forces. We propose that in this case, demonic struggles deserve separate attention as part of Michael's complex struggle profile, even if other psychological conditions become the main focus of treatment. If Michael's demonic struggles are overlooked, we could be missing a vital opportunity to foster insight, healing, and growth.

William James (1902) wrote extensively about this possibility over 100 years ago in *The Varieties of Religious Experience*, reminding readers that diagnoses of psychological or medical illness do not rule out the possibility of profound, deeply meaningful spiritual experiences (whether positive or negative). In fact, James related how, throughout history, people who reported powerful mystical experiences and supernatural encounters—some of whom were later honored as saints—often suffered from serious mental or physical illness as well; the melancholy natures or unusual perceptions of these "sick souls" (as James labeled them) may have even opened the door to deeper, more profound spiritual experiences.

In short, there is a balance to strike here, and several extremes to avoid. One extreme response would be to automatically pathologize any and all perceptions of demonic activity even among people who otherwise appear psychologically and physically healthy. But at the other extreme, a clinician could too readily accept reports of demonic activity at face value and risk overlooking a serious medical or mental health condition. When such conditions are uncovered, especially if they are serious, they will likely become high priorities for treatment.

In some cases, demonic struggles might subside if these underlying conditions can be treated successfully. But in other cases, the struggles are still sufficiently central in a person's presenting problems to warrant individual attention.

The Psychological Lens: Focus on Thoughts, Emotions, and Behaviors

Broadly speaking, our therapeutic aim would be to help Michael find a greater sense of wholeness and experience growth. We want him to feel connected with his own deepest values, bringing him a sense of integrity, meaning, and strength. We want him to be "truly himself," living his life in an authentic way that brings joy and energy. And we want him to continue to deepen his loving bonds with other people and with God. On all of these fronts, we believe that standard psychotherapy techniques can offer a lot of help. Let's explore some of these next, keeping most of our focus on Michael's case.

Assessment of Basic Beliefs about Supernatural Evil

When using a psychological lens, a major aim would be to closely examine relevant beliefs and attributions, along with any function such thoughts might be serving, and to encourage clients to reflect on potential sources and consequences of such beliefs. Earlier in this section we discussed the value of a careful assessment of Michael's beliefs about the devil: what he believes about how the devil operates, the sources of such beliefs, his level of commitment to those beliefs, and any functions such beliefs might serve for him. Questions like these could provide a foundation for a therapy approach encouraging closer reflection on his beliefs, along with the emotions and behaviors that tend to accompany them.

Before going too deeply into assessment, it is important to keep in mind that demonic attributions do not always lead to demonic struggle—in fact, some people may see them as serving valuable psychological functions. As described in the first part of this chapter, belief in supernatural evil can help to reaffirm people's moral boundaries around actions that they see as being wrong. Some people may find it comforting to see the devil as a cause of problems in the world, because it protects them from blaming God for suffering and evil (Beck & Taylor, 2008). Others may find that demonic attributions give them an external explanation for difficulties they might otherwise blame on themselves or others, such as temptations to wrongdoing. If demonic attributions are not causing distress for the client, and if they are not encouraging harm to others (e.g., demonization of enemies or outgroup members), such beliefs might be worth briefly exploring in therapy without warranting direct intervention.

But what if demonic attributions do cause distress? Michael, for example, has come to therapy partly because of intrusive sexual thoughts and images—and he wonders whether the devil might be playing a role, trying to pull him off the path of righteousness and away from God. Michael is also feeling tormented by struggles around moral discernment, identity, and competing desires: to pursue a life-giving relationship and to preserve his loving commitments to his family. His questions about whether the devil might be feeding these ideas—not to mention his fear of being deceived and wandering away from God—are obviously causing a lot of strain. If he blames himself for his thoughts of sexual encounters, perhaps berating himself for indulging his fantasies or for allowing himself to become close to Amelia, he may worry that he has already chosen to follow the devil's path, whether intentionally or not.

A Closer Look at Personal Demonic Attribution and Struggle

Having considered his basic beliefs about the devil, Michael might now take a closer look at the demonic attributions that he has made (or considered) in reference to his own personal situation. Where does he see the devil at work, and why? Are there important messages that he can take from these ideas? And if these attributions are feeding directly into his sense of struggle, how can he respond?

Attributions Involving a Clear Sense of Harm to Self or Others. To start examining these attributions, it might be wise to begin with a demonic attribution that seems clear—one that seems straightforward in moral terms, where it is easy to imagine the devil being involved. In Michael's case, his drinking may be a good place to start. For him, it is easy to see impulses to drink heavily, secretly, or with the goal of self-medicating as being temptations from the devil. The risks to his own health and safety, as well as those of others, are very apparent. If asked to think about the function that a demonic attribution might serve, Michael could quickly see it as a benefit, in that it helps to keep heavy and secret drinking in the "bad, dangerous" category, and also gives him an external adversary to blame.

If Michael does see himself as being in a battle against evil—whether he himself is seeing this battle through a psychological or a supernatural lens—there could be value in exploring whether his religious tradition might offer him some strategies or resources that might help him to "fight back" against these impulses that have clear potential for harm. For example, in the Christian practice of *spiritual warfare* (Evans, 2018; Thigpen, 2014), people seek to protect themselves from the devil by putting on the "armor of God," which includes elements such as the breastplate of righteousness, the belt of truth, and the shield of faith. Similarly, within Islam (and especially within the Sufi tradition), the concept of *spiritual jihad* (Saritoprak et al., 2018) uses a battle metaphor to frame an internal struggle between the higher self (aligned with God) and the lower self (influenced by the devil and/or our own selfish desires). As noted in the preceding chapter, in response to a specific moral struggle, endorsement of a spiritual jihad mindset was linked with reports of more positive religious coping and more spiritual and posttraumatic growth, along with lower levels of anxiety and depression. Seeking religious support from God and members of one's religious community could also strengthen people in such cases, helping people to see themselves as part of a powerful, effective coalition against a common spiritual enemy (cf. Kirkpatrick, 2005; Pargament et al., 2000).

Still, there are cautions to consider. One issue is that the heavy focus on battle and conflict, whether seen literally or metaphorically, promotes a dualistic, good-versus-evil view of the world. Although such a worldview might empower some, others could find it distasteful, scary, or depressing. And even for people who favor dualistic worldviews, framing the world as a supernatural battleground could make it challenging to foster some therapeutic goals of connectedness, wholeness, and integration. It may be all too easy for people to demonize their enemies, or at least to find inner peace elusive, if they see their lives in terms of an epic battle.

Attributions Emphasizing Personal Responsibility. Michael might also see that, while blaming the devil for the temptation might protect him in some ways, it could also cut the attributional process short—perhaps absolving him of too much personal responsibility and also reducing his sense of efficacy about being able to find solutions. To fill out the attributional picture, Michael might be guided to consider other causes of his temptation to drink: the rewarding effects of alcohol itself; his family history of alcohol abuse; and triggering events, such as sexual temptation and anger at the church. Michael might still see the devil as operating through these natural mechanisms, but he might gain a greater sense of insight and control by considering these other reasons. Michael may also decide that he wants more social support to help keep his drinking in moderation, perhaps by addressing the alcohol issues in therapy or by joining a support group. He may also turn to religious coping for help, perhaps by praying for divine help and protection, listening to online sermons about alcohol use, or reading Scripture verses that emphasize self-control.

Another broad therapeutic aim here could be to help Michael to accept and integrate his dark thoughts and impulses as part of his shadow self (cf. Jung, 1954/1985), recognizing that all human beings carry the potential for both good and evil (May, 1969; Peck, 1983). Along these lines, consider the first stanzas from a poem by Thich Nhat Hanh (2001) entitled "Please Call Me by My True Names":

> I am a mayfly metamorphosing
> on the surface of the river.
> And I am the bird
> that swoops down to swallow the mayfly.

I am a frog swimming happily
in the clear water of a pond.
And I am the grass-snake
that silently feeds itself on the frog.

I am the child in Uganda, all skin and bones,
my legs as thin as bamboo sticks.
And I am the arms merchant,
selling deadly weapons to Uganda. (pp. 72–73)

Michael could then go through a similar process focused on his sexual thoughts, though here the process will likely be more challenging and complex. Here, too, it is probably easiest to start with demonic attributions that might seem straightforward to him: those tempting him toward promiscuous, unprotected sexual encounters or a secret extramarital affair, for example. As with the alcohol use, Michael could identify both potential triggers of such temptations and strategies to help him remain steadfast and safe. Because Michael sees the devil not only as a source of temptation but also as a source of torment, it might be easy for him to see the repetitive, intrusive thoughts and images of sexual encounters as being demonically influenced as well. But even if he sees the devil as causing these torments, he can still identify situational cues that tend to prompt such ruminations (e.g., too much time alone, boredom, questions about his marriage). He can also consider some of his long-standing predispositions that might feed his ruminations, such as his tendencies toward anxiety.

Attributions about One's Own Moral Compass. This brings us to some of the most difficult issues: Michael's deep desires for an intimate, passionate, sexually satisfying relationship and his questions about his marriage. Here, some key struggles would center on moral decision making or discernment (Gallagher, 2005; Liebert, 2008). Michael may need to decide whether it would be morally wrong for him to seek a divorce—or perhaps a more sexually open marital arrangement. Here, demonic struggle could center on Michael's uncertainty about whether he can trust his moral decisions. He may worry that the devil, through lies and deception, could have essentially hijacked his moral compass, with the aim of taking him away from God and toward destruction. As such, he fears that going against his church's understanding of biblical teaching could lead him straight into the devil's trap.

How could a therapist help Michael to take steps to restore his confidence in his moral compass, so that fears of demonic influence will not paralyze him? One priority would be to help reconnect Michael with his most deeply held values and sources of significance. Clearly he wants to please God, to stay close to God, and to steer clear of evil (and, along with it, the threat of hell). He also wants to show love and care for his wife and children, and he wants to keep his commitments to them. But he also wants to have a satisfying intimate relationship that will help him to thrive as a person. And, along these lines, he wants to give voice to the possibility that he may prefer another relationship. A therapist might ask, "Does Michael have a clear sense of priorities about these goals?" Also, "Does he see these goals as fundamentally conflicting, or might there be creative strategies that could help him to meet all of these goals?"

Reexamining Core Beliefs

As Michael explores his ideas and options, he may need to revisit his beliefs about the devil and about God. Even though beliefs in the devil and demons are non-negotiable within his tradition, he does have some questions. He's in a mode of exploration now, which is part of his reason for seeking therapy. Why wasn't the devil mentioned more prominently in the Hebrew Bible, for example? He might also ponder the mysteries of the biblical book of Job, in which God and the devil seem to be playing a game, after which God gave Satan permission to torment Job. He may wonder, Are God and the devil mortal enemies, or collaborators of a sort? Michael might benefit from exploring some books from a historical perspective, to better understand how views about the devil and hell have evolved over time (Poole, 2009; Russell, 1975; Turner, 1993). Even if he feels certain that the devil and demons exist, he might question some of his ideas about how they operate and communicate. For example, does the devil have the power to influence thoughts—or to pull a person completely off of God's path, especially when that person is trying to stay close to God?

Other questions might focus on Michael's beliefs about God, marriage, and the authority of religious texts. Does God speak only through the Bible? Is God likely to condemn someone to hell for breaking marriage vows? As a therapist, it is outside of your bounds to try to answer these questions, but you can provide encouragement and a safe space to explore the questions. Depending on your own knowledge base in the client's faith tradition, you might be able to recommend specific resources—or to at least guide the client in brainstorming about resources. In Michael's case, for example, he might benefit from reading about perspectives on sexuality and divorce from both conservative and liberal perspectives.

You could also support clients, such as Michael, in the transition from reflection to action. For example, Michael might decide that he wants to spend more time with his family and to reduce his alcohol use. He might want to strengthen his emotional and sexual bond with Karen, but he might also want to learn more about diverse religious views on divorce. He also needs to decide what actions to take with Amelia: pulling away, drawing closer, or putting the relationship on hold for a time. In each case, Michael may benefit from help considering the potential pros and cons of certain choices, assessing his readiness to take action, developing strategies, and reflecting on consequences after he does take action. With demonic struggles, there may be a lot of fear around making bad decisions—but also the potential for a real sense of triumph when a person takes steps in directions that feel strong and right.

CONCLUSIONS

The topic of supernatural evil is a controversial one, and the ideas presented here may be the most provocative of all the material covered in this book. People think about evil in a staggering variety of ways. For some, the language of evil and the demonic become compelling in response to life's most horrific events: abuse, betrayal, rape, genocide, pandemics, and war. Others might become convinced that supernatural evil exists by witnessing something that seems to violate natural laws, such as a possible demonic possession or haunting. And some see the world through a supernatural lens, one including evil beings who are active and powerful in the world. For them, demonic attributions and struggles could be a normal part of daily life.

When demonic struggles find their way into the therapy office, therapists face thorny questions about how to approach the demonic in a treatment context. There is, as yet, little systematic research to guide us through this thicket, although we hope that the material covered here triggers more thought and progress in this often overlooked domain.

We have tried to offer some admittedly tentative guidelines to help people address demonic struggles in therapy. But as with other spiritual struggles, we believe therapists can do a great deal of good simply by serving as respectful, reliable, caring companions for people who see themselves as engaged in a battle against formidable adversaries. They are wrestling to make good choices, and they may have tremendous fear of making bad ones. When people are facing intense demonic struggles, simply having a supportive companion alongside may be a big part of the battle. And whether this companion sees these dark forces and places as real or metaphorical, much of the remedy is essentially the same: Keep pursuing wholeness and growth. Keep turning toward the light, toward life, toward love.

CHAPTER 13

Interpersonal Struggles

> It's another exhausting part of everything—the struggle—and . . . just
> wanting to be safe. . . . You're constantly on guard . . . I've come to
> associate religion so much with the people that have hated me so much.
> So when I'm walking down the street or something, and I really hone in
> on a religious shirt or cross or something . . . I should stay away from
> them just in case.
>
> —CHRISTIAN LESBIAN COLLEGE STUDENT;
> ROCKENBACH ET AL. (2012, p. 65)

At their best, religion and spirituality are forces for more than simply tolerance of others, but also compassion, connectedness, and wholeness. After all, one of the main functions of religion is to join people into a social, moral, and spiritual community. "The idea of society is the soul of religion" is the way sociologist Émile Durkheim (1915, p. 433) put it. And a considerable body of research has shown that people who involve themselves more in religious and spiritual communities experience a number of mental health and physical health benefits, including greater longevity (see Koenig et al., 2012; Oman, 2018). Relationships, from a spiritual perspective, can also be imbued with deeper meaning and value because people are said to carry within them something of the sacred (Mahoney, 2013). When relationships are sanctified, research indicates, they are more likely to be treated with special care and generate special rewards (Mahoney et al., 2013, 2021).

Spirituality and religion are not always at their best, however, as we hear in the opening words from the student above. Religion may offer compassion and support to those who fall within the boundaries of a community, but those who do not share the beliefs, practices, values, or identity of the group may be treated quite differently. Further, because relationships are so often instilled with sacred meaning, conflicts in the interpersonal sphere can have special power.

Juergensmeyer (2000) explains how spirituality can magnify the effects of interpersonal conflict, leading at times to extreme results:

> When a struggle becomes sacralized, incidents that might previously have been considered minor skirmishes or slight differences of understanding are elevated to monumental proportions. The use of violence becomes legitimized, and the slightest provocation or insult can lead to terrorist assaults. What had become simply opponents become cosmic foes. (p. 163)

No book on spiritual struggles could possibly ignore the tensions, strains, and conflicts about sacred matters that arise in the relational realm. In this chapter, we turn our attention to interpersonal religious and spiritual struggles (interpersonal struggles for short).

UNDERSTANDING INTERPERSONAL STRUGGLES

We begin by considering how best to understand these struggles, including their frequency, their consequences, and their roots. We then focus on how practitioners can address interpersonal struggles when they arise in treatment.

Prevalence and Types of Interpersonal Struggles

The world seems ripe for interpersonal struggles involving religion and spirituality. As people across the globe have become increasingly interconnected, they are more and more likely to encounter others who hold different religious and spiritual orientations. This may be particularly true in the United States, where "Hindu yogis teach next door to South American shamans, and Congregationalist churches share their space with Buddhist and Taoist communities. Jewish men and women become Zen masters and Catholic priests learn Japanese forms of healing and purification" (Anderson & Hopkins, 1991, p. 122). Even among those who share a religious affiliation, there are likely to be many variations among individual beliefs and practices. And, as we have noted, there has been a rise in the numbers of people who see themselves as "spiritual, not religious" and prefer to create their own individualized approaches to spirituality. As a result of these forces of religious pluralization and individualization, today people are likely to encounter a wide range of religious and spiritual expressions. Although this diversity could conceivably lead to a sharing of experiences and worldviews that enlighten, enliven, and enrich the quality of relationships, it may also set the stage for interpersonal religious and spiritual conflicts.

Clearly, struggles with other people about sacred issues are far from rare. Pick up any newspaper and it will not be hard to find disturbing accounts of religiously based violence, terrorism, and war. In 2018, Federal Bureau of Investigation (FBI) data indicated that over 20.0% of single-bias hate crimes—more than three per day—were religiously motivated (*https://ucr.fbi.gov/hate-crime/2018/topic-pages/incidents-and-offenses*). Though not all are so dramatic, conflicts over sacred matters are fairly commonplace within the general population. Our large survey of U.S. adults revealed that, over the past few weeks, 45.5% had experienced interpersonal struggles, such as conflicts with other people about religious or spiritual matters or anger at organized religion (Exline, Pargament, & Grubbs, 2014). Among military veterans in college, 22.0% indicated that they were encountering a high degree of interpersonal struggle; these struggles were more common than any other type of spiritual struggles (Currier, McDermott, McCormick, et al., 2018). Members of religious communities are not spared from conflicts in the relational arena, either. In one study of religious American families, 89.0% reported at least one relational struggle around religion (Dollahite, Marks, & Young, 2019).

A closer look reveals that interpersonal struggles come in many shapes and sizes. First, some of these struggles focus on tensions with the individual's immediate social network, including his or her own religious congregation, clergy, religious leaders, family, friends, or community. Here, for example, is one woman describing the reaction of a fellow church member to her unplanned pregnancy when she was 16: "'We don't want you standing in the church pregnant.' So I said, 'Okay, when I'm done with the baby you know pregnancy, can I come back?' And she didn't answer me. She didn't want pregnancy in that church at all so I just quit" (Fletcher et al., 2020).

Other interpersonal struggles around religion involve outsiders to one's own group, including other faiths, organized religion as a whole, or the larger culture. By way of illustration, one Congolese refugee woman who had survived sexual violence described her struggles not with her faith or God, but with the lack of support for her faith from the larger U.S. culture: "America is like job first and then God after. . . . If I go to work and tell my manager I need Sunday off, it's not going to happen" (Smigelsky, Gill, Foshager, Aten, & Im, 2017).

Second, interpersonal struggles vary in their content. Some of these struggles center around disagreements or disunities in spiritual beliefs, practices, and values. In one striking example, Thomas Aquinas, who was to become a central Catholic theologian and philosopher, experienced a powerful spiritual struggle with his father. To prevent him from becoming a priest, his father went to lengths that ranged from imprisoning the young Aquinas to trying to have him seduced (Martin, 2006). Today, religious and spiritual disagreements are also fairly common. For example, among college students in Israel, 26% of Muslims and 10% of Jews reported conflicts with other people about religious and spiritual matters at high levels over the past few months (Abu-Raiya, Pargament, Exline, et al., 2015;

Abu-Raiya, Pargament, Weissberger, et al., 2016). In our U.S. college student sample, 46% of the students reported some degree of these conflicts in the past few months (Exline et al., 2014b).

Other relational struggles have to do with feelings of hurt, anger, or disappointment when individuals are targeted for mistreatment because of their spiritual orientation. In this vein, 25% of college students reported that their friends ridiculed others because of their religious and spiritual beliefs (Kane, 2010). Like their religious counterparts, atheists can also experience interpersonal spiritual tensions and conflicts—in this case, because of their lack of belief in God (Sedlar et al., 2018). Studies indicate that atheists are among the least liked and most distrusted of all people, particularly in areas with religious majorities (e.g., Gervais, Shariff, & Norenzayan, 2011).

Still other relational struggles center around the negative feelings that accompany experiences of religious or spiritual hypocrisy, rejection, or abuse. One woman who had been abused by the pastor of her church described the struggle she experienced after the abuse became public: "When I walked into the church everyone stared. You know, everyone would whisper . . . or shake their head. And so, I think it's more that uncomfortable feeling that kept me out of church" (Flynn, 2008).

Third, interpersonal struggles vary in their intensity. On one end of the scale, they may take the form of relatively mild annoyances and tensions with other people over religious and spiritual issues that may be expressed or go unspoken. Struggles of this kind may focus on boring sermons, dislike for some of the rules of a congregation, dissatisfaction with the music or the structure of religious services, or feeling put off by some of the members. Relational struggles can also involve painful family conflicts, such as those that arise from differences in the religious orientations of family members. Here's a child who is caught up in this type of struggle in his family: "My mom wants me to go to church, and my dad, depending on the sport, would want me to go to the sport. . . . We'd be split and there'd be a brawl between them" (Dollahite et al., 2019, p. 15). On the more extreme end, interpersonal struggles can be marked by deep hurt, feelings of abandonment, and powerful anger often tied to social traumas, such as religiously based abuse, discrimination, hate crimes, and violence. One survivor of clergy sexual abuse voiced the intense and chronic pain that accompanied her interpersonal struggle:

> The pain I was experiencing was like cancer pain. It had no meaning. It was endless. There was nothing I could do about it that could bring it relief. . . . That is the truth until this very day. . . . It invades my life all the time. It is always there. (Flynn, 2008, p. 221)

In short, struggles with other people over spiritual matters are not at all unusual and take many forms.

Consequences of Interpersonal Struggles

Regardless of their particular shape, these relational tensions and conflicts can lead to decline on the one hand and, perhaps, growth on the other.

Interpersonal Struggles and Decline

Here is the way one woman described the impact of her struggle with her Mormon church, a struggle that ultimately resulted in her being stricken from the records of the institution:

> It was like they had stolen my identity right out from underneath me. It was this feeling of groundlessness, like I had nothing to stand on. I had no idea who I was or what I believed in. I wasn't prepared for that. I wasn't prepared for it to have an effect on me like it did. (Zuckerman, 2012, p. 65)

Religious and spiritual relationships are more than social relationships. They are often filled with a deeper spiritual significance. Because religious and spiritual relationships are so intertwined with our most basic beliefs about the world, so deeply tied to our identity, so connected to the ultimate purposes we seek in life, and so involved in how we understand and relate to the sacred, conflicts in this relational sphere are likely to be especially distressing and disorienting.

People who experience conflicts and tensions with other people around spiritual issues report higher levels of psychological distress and problems, according to several studies. A large-scale investigation in the United States revealed that interpersonal struggles were associated with higher levels of depression and anxiety, even after controlling for the effects of other types of spiritual struggles (Abu-Raiya, Pargament, Krause, et al., 2015). Similar effects have been shown among other groups, such as college students (Exline, Pargament, Grubbs, & Yali, 2014) and Palestinian Muslims (Abu-Raiya, Pargament, Exline, et al., 2015). In one of the few longitudinal studies on this topic, interpersonal struggles with clergy and congregation members were predictive of increases in depression over 2 years among medically ill older adult patients (Pargament et al., 2004).

Several studies have zeroed in on more specific interpersonal struggles and yielded similar results. Struggles with various types of religiously based discrimination have been associated with psychological distress; these include studies of religious individuals encountering religious microaggressions, such as religious stereotyping (Cheng, Pagano, & Shariff, 2017), people with same-sex attractions struggling with religious stigma (Lauricella, Phillips, & Dubow, 2017), and atheists facing personal and group discrimination (Doane & Elliott, 2015). Conflicts within one's own religious and spiritual community have also been tied to greater psychological distress and problems. For example, in a study of lesbian, gay, and bisexual adults, higher levels of spiritual struggles and internalized homophobia mediated the relationship between the effects of religiously based stigma from participants' religious communities on greater psychological distress and lower well-being (Szymanski & Carrettta, 2020). Similarly, negative interactions with members of one's own religious community were linked to greater depressive symptoms in samples of older Mexican Americans (Krause & Hayward, 2012b) and Polish Catholics (Zarzycka, 2019). These findings may apply to clergy as well as lay members. In a national study of Presbyterian clergy, higher levels of interpersonal struggles with fellow church members (along with divine struggles and religious doubts) were associated with greater psychological distress (Ellison, Roalson, Guillory, Flannelly, & Marcum, 2010). Moreover, conflicts between clergy and church members exacerbated the effects of life stressors on distress.

Perhaps unsurprisingly, interpersonal struggles around religion and spirituality appear to have negative implications for not just individual mental health but also social relationships. Consider the powerful social impact of one man's struggles with childhood clergy sexual abuse:

> There's virtually nothing I have done or experienced since he (the priest) raped me that hasn't been affected. From my choice of marital partner . . . school experiences . . . career . . . parenting skills . . . relationships with everybody. . . . It's all connected. It changes who you are, how you feel . . . how you interact with people. (Fater & Mullaney, 2000, p. 281)

Some individuals choose to keep their religious struggles with others a secret for fear of stigma and condemnation. In a qualitative study of bisexual black church members, Jeffries, Dodge, and Sandfort (2008) offered the example of a bisexual Muslim man who noted that "It feels dangerous, sometimes, because I've got to be careful who I run into, who I mess with, you know? I've got to be careful" (p. 468).

Empirical research also shows how interpersonal struggles in the religious realm can affect relationships. For example, in a large-scale national study of parenting practices and their effects on children, Bartkowski, Xu, and Levin (2008) found that parents who argued more frequently about religious issues were more likely to have children who showed poorer self-control, poorer social skills, and more sadness and loneliness according to the ratings of their parents. Differences between spousal religious beliefs, practices, and affiliations have also been consistently associated with more marital conflict (e.g., Curtis & Ellison, 2002) and a greater likelihood of divorce (Vaaler, Ellison, & Powers, 2009). And spiritual struggles of an adult child with a parental divorce have been tied to more painful feelings about the divorce, intrusive thoughts, and depression (Warner et al., 2009).

Clearly, interpersonal struggles can be accompanied by distress and decline, both psychologically and socially. Even so, questions remain about whether these struggles are primary (the cause of distress), secondary (the effect of distress), or complex (both cause and effect of distress). It is also important to consider whether these findings represent the full story. Can struggles with relationships around sacred matters foster growth?

Interpersonal Struggles and Growth

Only a few studies have examined whether people who struggle interpersonally experience growth through the process. They have yielded some mixed results. Among young adults with same-sex attraction, those who struggled more with religious stigma over their sexuality reported significantly less spiritual growth, but these struggles were unrelated to stress-related growth more generally (Lauricella et al., 2017). Older adults who were medically ill and struggled to a greater extent with clergy and congregation members described less spiritual and stress-related growth (Pargament et al., 2004).

On the other hand, in a study of college students coping with physical and verbal aggression in a dating relationship, those who were more discontented with their religious communities were more motivated to end their hostile romantic relationship; perhaps interpersonal struggles in this instance helped to motivate a desirable but difficult life change (Mahoney, Abadi, & Pargament, 2015). Forgiveness of others within a religious community may also facilitate growth through relational struggles. In a study of Polish Catholics struggling with church tensions, higher levels of forgiveness were associated with more life satisfaction, better general health, and lower levels of anxiety and depression (Zarzycka, 2019). Remember, however, that forgiveness is a very sensitive and complex topic, and must be handled gingerly in therapy, especially in dealing with interpersonal struggles that involve physical and sexual abuse (Pargament et al., 2008).

Interpersonal struggles can also result in important changes in the person's orientation to religious institutions and relationships. Experiences of gay, lesbian, and bisexual individuals offer a case in point. Schuck and Liddle (2001) conducted a survey of these sexual minorities who felt conflict between their religion and their sexual orientation, and found that 53% reported a shift from being religious to being spiritual, 33% indicated that they had changed their religious affiliations, 33% had left their previous religion and no longer identify with any religion, and 16% tried to create change within their institution and faith. Many of these strugglers experienced their religious and spiritual changes as helpful and transformational. Some described growth while remaining in the community of faith that had been a source of conflict. One said, "I accepted being gay during Mass. I just realized that God loved me as I am" (Schuck & Liddle, 2001, p. 74). Others described positive life changes when they found more affirming congregations within their denomination, new denominations, or supportive groups associated with a particular faith, such as Dignity for Catholics and Integrity for Episcopalians (Schuck & Liddle, 2001). Still other interpersonal strugglers talked about their efforts to bring change to their religious institutions, such as programs to train and inform religious institutions about LGBT issues (Schuck & Liddle, 2001). It is important to add, any of these shifts in religious orientation could be associated with both pain and growth.

Overall, the jury is out on whether interpersonal struggles are associated with growth, as we have found with some other types of specific struggles. The lack of longitudinal studies on this topic may contribute to this lack of clarity. As we noted earlier, it may take some time for people to realize greater wholeness and growth following these relational struggles. It is clear though that struggles with religious and spiritual issues are tied to a variety of signs of personal and social stress and decline, and deserve attention in clinical practice. As a prelude to this practical conversation, let's examine some of the roots of interpersonal struggles.

Roots of Interpersonal Struggles

Like other spiritual struggles, interpersonal struggles are nested in an interrelated set of situational, social, personal, and spiritual factors. Below we highlight three of these roots.

Stressful Life Events

We have seen how major life stressors can disrupt and disorient the individual's core beliefs, practices, and significant purposes in life. These stressors also have the potential to ripple out and destabilize connections with other people, including spiritual connections. Stauner, Exline, Pargament, et al. (2019) demonstrate this point in their large-scale study of four samples from private, public, and Christian universities, and an online sample of adults. All of the participants indicated whether they had experienced each of 17 major life events, such as parental divorce, the death of a loved one, and sexual abuse or assault. In each of the four samples, those who had encountered more life stressors also reported significantly higher levels of interpersonal struggle.

Tensions, strains, and conflicts surrounding religion and spirituality may come even more to the fore when people experience religiously related stressors. Some of these struggles are triggered by encounters with outsiders to the individual's religious tradition. Consider the struggle of a Muslim woman on wearing a hijab in public: "Because I wear *hijab* . . . [when I am out] in the community. . . . I have to be different. I cannot be friends with everybody because their reaction to my *hijab* is different. I can only communicate with friends that I have from childhood" (Marks, Dollahite, & Young, 2019, p. 250, emphasis in original).

Other interpersonal struggles are generated by stressors that come from the individual's own religious tradition. Not surprisingly, major assaults perpetrated by religious individuals are likely to trigger interpersonal struggles. For example, according to a national survey of survivors of clergy sexual abuse, 71% "wondered whether my church had abandoned me" (Murray-Swank, 2010). However, struggles in the relational area can also follow less intense religiously related stressors. Several forms of religiously based mistreatment experienced by LGBT individuals often elicit interpersonal struggles (Wood & Conley, 2014). These range from spiritual bullying by religious leaders or peers to using God to legitimize denunciations of particular groups to more subtle, though still impactful, microassaults and invalidations.

Because of their sacred mission, religious institutions, clergy, and leaders are generally held to a higher standard. And when they fall short, many people struggle with disappointment, anger, and resentment about religious hypocrisy. This is the kind of struggle an older church member encountered with other members of her congregation: "They get off in a corner and talk about you and you're the one that's there on Saturday working with their children and washing the dishes on Sunday afternoon. They don't have the Christian spirit" (Krause, Chatters, Meltzer, & Morgan, 2000, p. 519). Similarly, violations and harm that are rooted in religious contexts often come as a greater surprise and disappointment and, as a result, are especially disturbing. One young woman described the double trauma she experienced: the first, a rape by an older member of her church; and the second, intense pressure to forgive him by church members. "Where is the justice in that?" she asked. "I got wronged in church and I'm supposed to be the one forgiving? . . . I've gotten more support from some of my non-religious friends" (Teng et al., 2015). When interpersonal events such as these are appraised as violations of the sacred, their painful effects may be magnified (Davis et al., 2014; Warner et al., 2009). To this point, a study of young adults whose parents had divorced showed that those who appraised the marital breakup as a desecration and sacred loss reported significantly higher levels of spiritual struggle with the divorce (Warner et al., 2009).

Marginal Religious Status

Religion, as we have noted, can draw people together or pull them apart. Individuals whose religious orientations and lifestyles lie outside of those acceptable to the larger religious context are especially likely to encounter tensions with others around religious and spiritual issues. Interpersonal struggles can grow out of individual marginalization from the dominant cultural and religious context. In this vein, Marks et al. (2019) studied the spiritual struggles of religious minority families (Jewish, Muslim, minority Christian faiths) and found that 61% reported conflicts with people outside of the family. For instance, an orthodox Jewish professional musician said, "Playing with the symphony, we have rehearsal schedules and . . . they would never ever dream of scheduling a rehearsal on a Sunday morning, ever . . . but they do not think twice about when we [Jewish persons] have our services" (p. 251).

Interpersonal struggles can also result from marginalization within the individual's own institution. Groups marginalized by many religious institutions—people identifying as atheist, agnostic, homosexual, and bisexual—show higher levels of interpersonal struggles (Exline, Pargament, Grubbs, & Yali, 2014), and interpersonal struggles were the most endorsed type of struggle in a sample of individuals who identified as transgender or gender nonconforming (Exline, Przeworski, et al., in press). When the sense of marginalization is internalized—as in the case of sexual minority individuals who take to heart the message that they are spiritually flawed—these struggles may become even stronger (Brewster, Velez, Foster, Esposito, & Robinson, 2016). The fit of the individual with his or her religious institution can also shape the likelihood of interpersonal struggles. A study by Stauner, Exline, Pargament, et al. (2019) illustrated this point. Among students at a Christian college where religious involvement is the norm, higher levels of religious commitment were associated with lower levels of interpersonal struggles. In contrast, at a secular university where religious involvement is less normative, higher levels of religious commitment were tied to higher levels of interpersonal struggles.

How do we explain these findings? Intolerance of differences, especially in the religious realm, may play a key role here.

Intolerance of Differences

"Tolerance is not a Sapiens trademark," Yuval Harari (2014, p. 18) observed in his book *Sapiens: A Brief History of Humankind*. On the face of it, there is no necessary reason why this should be the case. After all, as we mentioned earlier, differences between people could be an opportunity for mutual enrichment and growth rather than conflict. Yet, the reality is that differences of all kinds—national, ethnic, religious, lifestyle, cultural customs, beliefs, and practices—*are* often tied to interpersonal conflicts. Theorists and researchers have considered many reasons for intolerance. To name a few:

- A limitation in the capacity to empathize with others by understanding and sensing their emotions (Baron-Cohen, 2011).
- An authoritarian worldview that considers the social world to be a dangerous place that requires social domination if it is to be kept under control (Duckitt & Sibley, 2009).
- A lack of communication skills that makes it hard to share, understand, manage, and reconcile different points of view (Markman, Renick, Floyd, Stanley, & Clements, 1993).

- Cultural ethnocentrism that judges others from the standards of one's own culture, and assumes the superiority of one's own worldview (Kinder & Kam, 2009).
- Perceptions that outgroups represent a threat to one's personal and social identity (Tajfel & Turner, 2001).

When we add religion to the mix of intolerance, tension, and conflict, the result can be especially inflammatory. Consider the added power that threats from outsiders take on when they are perceived to be directed toward sacred values, beliefs, and practices. Anti-Semitism provides one case in point. Historically, Jews have been perceived as a threat to the sacred values of non-Jews. In the words of Prager and Telushkin (1983), "Literally hundreds of millions of people have believed that Jews drink the blood of non-Jews, that they cause plagues and poison wells, that they murdered G-d himself" (p. 17). Do these beliefs play any part in the record of horrific acts perpetrated against Jews over the centuries or the levels of anti-Semitism that continue today? Pargament et al. (2007) tested whether Christians who perceive Jews to be a threat to Christianity would be more likely to hold anti-Semitic attitudes and report greater conflicts with Jews. Perceptions of Jews as desecrators of Christianity were measured by items such as "The Jews represent a threat to the ultimate mission of Christ." It is important to note that only 10% of the participants agreed with these items. Those who did, however, were more likely to report anti-Semitic attitudes and conflicts with Jews. None of the other measures often used to study the roots of antireligious prejudice (e.g., fundamentalism, right-wing authoritarianism) predicted anti-Semitism after the effects of desecration were controlled. These findings have been largely replicated in studies of prejudice toward Muslims (Abu-Raiya, Pargament, Mahoney, & Trevino, 2008) and lesbian and gay individuals (Trevino, Desai, Lauricella, Pargament, & Mahoney, 2012). This research suggests that perceptions that an outgroup poses a threat to the sacred values of one's own religious group may be of special importance in efforts to understand religious prejudice.

The potential for intolerance and interpersonal struggle can also be magnified by religiously based forms of ethnocentrism—that is, the presumed superiority of one's own religious culture based on the perception that it is imbued with an exclusive sacred status. Of course, this sense of being a part of a religious institution that has special spiritual significance can also provide members with many benefits, including a clear and convincing sense of truth, identity, community, purpose, and orientation to life. However, these within-group benefits may not apply to people from other religious traditions when they are seen as false and inferior forms of faith. Outsiders, in this case, may be viewed as less deserving of love and compassion.

Relevant here is a large national phone survey of people from eight European countries conducted by Küpper and Zick (2010). The researchers reported that superior/exclusivist views of one's own religion were strongly linked with enmity to a variety of outgroups. Specifically, people who more strongly agreed that "My religion is the one true religion in the world" were more likely to report prejudice toward immigrants, women, Jews, Muslims, and other races.

Finally, intolerance and interpersonal struggles can come sharply to the foreground when religious and spiritual issues enter conversations. Consider how sensitive each of the following religiously loaded questions can become: Should we get married in a religious setting and, if so, which one? Should we raise our children in a particular religious tradition and, if so, which one? Should a loved one who has died have a religious funeral?

Annette Mahoney (2005), a pioneer in the study of relational spirituality, points out that spirituality can be weaponized in communication, as when people engage in spiritual one-upmanship by arguing that God is disappointed with the other or the other is taking positions that are inconsistent with religious principles. She and other researchers have found that spiritual one-upmanship is associated with more verbal aggression between mothers and college-age children (Brelsford & Mahoney, 2009) and between fathers and college-age students (Brelsford, 2011). Spiritual one-upmanship has also been tied to poorer marital communication around conflicts (Mahoney, Pargament, & DeMaris, 2019).

In short, intolerance of differences, particularly when rooted in religion, can be a major source of interpersonal struggle. That is not the full story, however. We will see shortly that there are counterbalancing, universalistic elements within religion that can foster greater interconnectedness rather than tension between religious groups. As Allport (1954) famously pointed out, religion can both make and unmake prejudice. A study by Preston and Ritter (2013) highlights this double-sided character of religion. When participants in their study were primed to think about the religious leaders of their institutions, they engaged in more prosocial behavior with members of their religious ingroup than with outgroup members. In striking contrast, when primed to think about what God would want them to do, the participants were more likely to engage in prosocial behavior with outsiders than insiders. Whether religion is a force for connection or disconnection, this and other studies suggest, very much depends on the kind of religion we are talking about. Having examined some roots of interpersonal struggles, we turn our attention now to ways therapists can address these struggles in treatment to reduce distress and encourage greater wholeness and growth, not only within people but among people as well.

ADDRESSING INTERPERSONAL STRUGGLES IN CLINICAL PRACTICE

Spiritual struggles, as we have seen, can be interwoven into many of the problems that clients bring to therapy. The point is no less true for interpersonal struggles. Relational conflicts around sacred issues can be a part of depression, anxiety, PTSD and stress-related disorders, addiction, marital and family conflicts, and social alienation. In the process of resolving any of these problems, clients may find themselves facing several key relational questions: How do I come to terms with religiously based mistreatment? How can I talk to members of my family about sensitive religious issues without things going ballistic? How do I decide what kind of relationship I want (if any) with my religious community? Is there a way for me to be true to both my own personal identity and my identity as a member of my faith? How do I accept the religious and spiritual views of others that I find objectionable? How can I find or create a religious home for myself?

These are difficult questions for both clients and therapists, and easy answers will not do. The therapeutic task is to help clients reduce the potentially harmful effects of interpersonal struggles and move toward greater wholeness and growth. This may call for new or deepened skills and resources for clients, including greater self-understanding, spiritual intimacy, communication skills, empathy, compassion, humility, empowerment, and openness to religious diversity. Therapists themselves may need to develop a deeper understanding of the relational side of religious life, one that includes not only an appreciation of the religious diversity of clients but also the religious diversity of their faith traditions, institutions, and cultures (Vieten & Scammell, 2015). Complicating matters further is the reality that work with interpersonal strugglers may require a shift at times in focus from individual therapy to therapy with couples, families, and clergy. Even so, as challenging as work with interpersonal struggles may be, it offers an opportunity for transformational changes involving not only individual clients but also their most important social relationships.

We turn our attention next to some of the practical issues that therapists should address in working with interpersonal struggles.

Assessing Whether Interpersonal Struggles Are Primary or Secondary to Psychological Problems

Leandra, a 24-year-old African American married woman and member of a Christian nondenominational fellowship, came to therapy complaining of occasional panic attacks when she left the safety of her apartment and found herself in places that she feared would leave her trapped. On more than one occasion, she had experienced symptoms of a racing heartbeat, pressure in her chest, dizziness, and trouble breathing that convinced her she was having a heart attack and she had ended up in the emergency room. However, the medical staff found no physical basis to her problems and encouraged her to seek counseling. Following her initial assessment, Leandra's therapist, a 50-year-old Christian psychologist, diagnosed Leandra with agoraphobia and began exposure therapy to help desensitive her to her fears. The therapy was only modestly helpful.

Leandra had become more able to go shopping by herself and pick up her daughter at kindergarten, but being in large open spaces still triggered panic in her. Antianxiety medications also provided only slight relief. To explore the roots of her panic further, Leandra's therapist asked her whether particular places outside of the home were especially likely to trigger her anxiety. This led to the following exchange:

LEANDRA: Last week you asked me whether some places really pushed my panic buttons and I said no. But I thought about it some more and realized that's not really true . . . I get nervous when I start to think about my church.

THERAPIST: When you think about your church, you begin to feel anxious.

LEANDRA: [looking uncomfortable] Yeah.

THERAPIST: How are you feeling now as you talk about your church here?

LEANDRA: Well, actually I'm getting very nervous.

THERAPIST: Okay, I appreciate your telling me that. Let's take it slow. Just focus on your breathing now and let me know when you start to feel better. [Long pause]

LEANDRA: It's funny. I never put two and two together and connected my problem with panic to anything about the church. I thought I was high-strung and just a little crazy.

THERAPIST: But your thinking has shifted?

LEANDRA: Yeah, your question made me start to wonder whether my panic might be tied to some bad things that happened to me in my church when I was an adolescent.

THERAPIST: Is that something you can talk about now?

LEANDRA: Maybe I need some time to prepare myself for that first.

THERAPIST: That's fine. I just want you to know how much I appreciate your honesty and courage in bringing up something that sounds really sensitive.

In the following session, Leandra's therapist learned that Leandra had been sexually molested by her Sunday school teacher in seventh and eighth grade. She had never spoken of this abuse to anyone, but since that time, she had kept her distance from her church. Her admission was a turning point in therapy and treatment shifted from an exclusive focus on agoraphobia to Leandra's struggle with a religiously based trauma.

The relationship between interpersonal struggles and psychological problems can be difficult to unravel. As illustrated by Leandra, what may seem to be a straightforward psychological disorder, with further assessment, may emerge as a case of interpersonal struggles, one in which the religious conflict plays a primary role in the development of the psychological problem. On the other hand, interpersonal struggles may mask more basic problems in relationships. The religious struggles in this instance are secondary to the other psychological problems.

Rotz, Russell, and Wright (1993) present the case of a married couple that illustrates this point. The couple came to therapy focusing on their conflicts around spirituality and church attendance. They argued about the husband's unwillingness to go to church and the state of his soul. The couple, it seemed, was looking for the therapist to adjudicate this contest about the spiritual superiority of the partners. The therapist instead shifted the focus of the therapy. After watching the couple enact their religious argument several times, the therapist wondered whether they might be too concerned about their individual relationships with God and not enough with their connection to each other. Is God, he wondered, truly interested in being an exclusive partner to either the husband or the wife? The therapist's comment prompted an admission from the husband that he felt jealous of his wife's relationship with her church and pastor. The wife, in turn, voiced her worries about her husband's level of commitment to the marriage. In this case, the couples' interpersonal struggle over God had masked their deeper questions of love and commitment to each other, and by focusing on these more basic concerns, the couple was able to reestablish intimacy in their marriage.

It is important to assess whether interpersonal struggles are a primary source of psychological problems, a secondary expression of these problems, or reciprocally related in a more complex way because that determination can affect the direction of treatment—in particular, the degree to which interpersonal struggles become a key focus of therapy.

Creating a Safe Space

> THERAPIST: Last session, you said that you hadn't spoken before about being molested by your Sunday school teacher in your church. I wondered why you kept that a secret?
>
> LEANDRA: I felt I didn't have much choice. The church meant everything to my grandmother. She had single-handedly raised five children and eight grandchildren, including me, and she always said that she couldn't have done it without the strength of her church. . . . And the Sunday school teacher was someone she admired. If she had known what he was doing, it would have killed her.
>
> THERAPIST: It sounds like you loved your grandmother a lot.
>
> LEANDRA: I did, and I never wanted to hurt her. That was one of the hardest things—after the troubles with the church started, I kind of went away somewhere in my head. I couldn't talk to anyone. And most of all, I missed being able to talk to my grandmother.

THERAPIST: That must have been such a terribly lonely time for you. Do you have anyone you talk to now about what happened to you?

LEANDRA: Well, now it's even more complicated. My husband, Dominic, is best friends with our pastor.

THERAPIST: So, as with your grandmother, you're fearful of hurting Dominic?

LEANDRA: That's right. And I'm not sure he'd understand how I feel.

THERAPIST: You've been keeping a lot of feelings to yourself. Where do all of those feelings go, Leandra? What do you do with them?

LEANDRA: I don't know. I don't even know what I've been feeling. I've tried not to pay any attention to all that feeling stuff and just get by. That's been hard enough.

THERAPIST: I hear that you've been carrying a heavy burden around for a long time. Maybe now you have a chance to unpack and explore some of that burden.

LEANDRA: I'm not sure it will really matter. Nothing's really changed. The church is still the center for my husband and family, and I still can't talk about it.

THERAPIST: Well, maybe we're getting a little ahead of ourselves here. It seems like you're thinking a lot about how your husband will react to your feelings. But before we talk about that, why don't we put your husband and family aside for the moment and focus first on exploring just what it is you're feeling?

LEANDRA: [*pauses*] This is just between you and me, right? I mean, I know you're a Christian and all that.

THERAPIST: I am a Christian, but my commitment is to helping you learn more about how you feel and how you can live a more fulfilling life, whatever you may decide and wherever that may take you. And please know that everything we talk about stays in this room, unless there's someone's safety at risk.

LEANDRA: You think what happened to me has something to do with my panic attacks?

THERAPIST: I do, and even more, I think talking about your feelings and experience will be really helpful to you.

LEANDRA: I hope you're right.

One of the most important jobs of the therapist is to create a space in the therapy room where clients can explore their concerns in safety and security. Clients must be reassured that they can talk about their struggles without fear of negative repercussions. Leandra, for example, needed to know that the conversation with her therapist would not be shared with anyone else. As importantly, she needed reassurance that her therapist's own Christian identification would not stand in the way of helping Leandra deal with such religiously sensitive issues. Finally, Leandra had been so preoccupied with how her family might react to her sexual abuse in the church that she had put aside the chance to process her own feelings. By shifting the initial treatment focus from her relationship with her family to her own feelings, Leandra's therapist was offering Leandra much needed breathing space in which she could begin to make sense of her traumatic experience.

To be able to explore their struggles, clients need a safe space not only inside the therapy room but outside of it as well. Therapists should help clients assess whether important relationships in their lives are safe or toxic. Griffith (2010), for example, raises some relevant questions to help clients determine whether their religious settings in particular are life enriching or life limiting: Is the client physically safe in the setting? Does the setting evoke fear and aggression, or reflection and creativity? Can individuals be heard, understood, and respected in the setting regardless of their role or status? How are people with different points of view and lifestyles treated? How are people outside of the religious group regarded? Clearly, when clients' physical safety is at risk, therapists must help them to extricate themselves from dangerous situations and locate a safe place. When the risk is less dire, however, therapists can work with clients to evaluate various options to find a safer community: trying to create a more supportive niche in the current congregation, looking for an entirely new religious home, or taking a break from involvement in a congregation. Leandra had been able to sidestep these questions. Constricting as it was, her agoraphobia had the benefit of providing a temporary sense of protection by preventing her from going anywhere near the church that had caused havoc in her life.

Foster, Bowland, and Vosler (2015) present the stories of many gay and lesbian Christians who struggled with their religious communities and succeeded in their search for safer religious settings. One man described his experience in a new congregation:

> I came to the Sunday school class and they were talking about homosexuality. They weren't, oh hush, we gotta be careful. . . . They were talking about acceptance and I'm going like, I spent 30 years trying to get to this point and now I'm just a baby in self-acceptance. This church is accepting and they're talking about it in Sunday school class, about diversity and so forth. So I began to start coming here and I've been coming here ever since. (p. 197)

Processing Interpersonal Struggles

With safety and security established, clients who are struggling interpersonally can start to process their feelings and make sense of their struggles. Often, clients need help to identify their own thoughts, emotions, and desires, and differentiate them from those of others (Sandage, Rupert, Stavros, & Devor, 2020). After all, until clients know themselves better, they are not in a position to work through tensions with other people. However, ongoing spiritual conflicts can sidetrack people from sorting out their own feelings about key issues.

Over the course of several months, Leandra began to explore the feelings that surrounded her experience of sexual abuse in the church. She described a confusing array of emotions: initial flattery that her Sunday school teacher had invited her to private Bible study lessons; happiness with the special attention she was receiving; confusion when he began to sit close to her and stroke her; fear when he made her sit on his lap as he read Bible stories to her; terror and paralysis when he began to fondle her and rub up against her sexually; and panic every time she had to go to church. These sessions led to the following important exchange:

THERAPIST: You've done some very difficult and important work describing the feelings you experienced in Sunday school. You've been able to talk about a host of feelings and every single one of them is totally understandable. But I noticed one set of feelings that you haven't talked about yet.

LEANDRA: What's that?

THERAPIST: Anger. Where did anger fit into your feelings?

LEANDRA: [*long pause*] Anger doesn't really describe what I felt. . . . I hated it and I hated him. I mean, I really despised him. I went to bed wishing he were dead. The funny thing was that he did die when I was in high school, and all I felt was relief that this horrible man was gone from the world. Isn't that terrible?

THERAPIST: I think that's another totally understandable feeling. I should tell you, too, that as you've described your experiences, I've also felt a lot of anger toward this man.

LEANDRA: Really?

THERAPIST: Yes, what kind of man would take advantage of a young student?

LEANDRA: I think I felt that, too, but I never let myself get into those feelings.

THERAPIST: Why not?

LEANDRA: They just seemed so strong. I think I felt if I lost my temper, I would go crazy and never be able to stop screaming.

THERAPIST: You're talking about it now and don't seem to be going crazy.

LEANDRA: Yeah, but I'm just getting started.

THERAPIST: Your anger toward the Sunday school teacher is very much alive.

LEANDRA: There's not a day that goes by that I don't think about that awful man. I used to love going to Sunday school. I used to love hearing the stories about Jesus and the children. He took something beautiful and smeared it with filth. He took an innocent child and touched her with his dirty fingers, all the while reading stories from the Bible! And this happened in a place that was supposed to be God's house. For me, he turned it into the house of the devil. [*Now yelling*] I hate him! I hate him! I hate him! And I never want to step foot in that church again!

THERAPIST: [*long pause*]. This has been very painful for you. It's taken a lot of guts for you to talk about these feelings. And I want you to know that, painful as all this is, to me you're sounding less confused and more sure of yourself. I hear you speaking from your heart with a lot of strength and power.

LEANDRA: I didn't know I had all of these feelings inside of me.

THERAPIST: Well, I wonder whether in some ways your agoraphobia protected you from those feelings. Those panic attacks kept you away from the church.

LEANDRA: Maybe so, but those panic attacks were awful.

THERAPIST: So what would it be like if that anxiety faded into the background?

LEANDRA: That would be great . . . but I guess I'd have to face all of those other feelings about my abuse and my church . . . and maybe I'd need to be more honest with my husband, too.

THERAPIST: What do you think about that?

With a deeper understanding of themselves and their feelings, clients like Leandra are better equipped to address and resolve the real tensions and conflicts in their lives, including those that center around religious and spiritual relationships.

Reconnecting with Other People

Perhaps because interpersonal struggles around religious and spiritual issues can be such sensitive, emotionally loaded topics, many people prefer to avoid them. In the process, however, they may distance themselves from potentially rewarding relationships, as we saw with Leandra. Avoiding interpersonal struggles, painful as they may be, is not likely to be an effective strategy for reducing conflicts or creating closeness. On the contrary, several studies have shown that interaction between groups that are in conflict is a better way to ameliorate these tensions (Putnam, 2000; Schmid, Hewstone, Küpper, Zick, & Tausch, 2014). For instance, simply knowing someone from another religion can reduce interreligious prejudice.

More direct conversations about interpersonal struggles, however, are not risk-free. Because interpersonal struggles in the religious and spiritual realm often center around fundamental questions about the trustworthiness of others, social identity, and personal safety, they are frequently accompanied by strong feelings of anger, disappointment, and fear of rejection or a ruptured relationship. Dialogue about these conflicts and emotions can easily descend into destructive arguments, including pitched battles between what are perceived to be the warring sides of good versus evil, right versus wrong, and moral versus immoral, with each partner claiming the higher spiritual ground. Consider, for example, how Leandra's first attempt to talk with her husband about her experience of sexual abuse quickly became combative in therapy:

DOMINIC: All of this talk about being molested came as a real shock to me. But I was glad to know why you've been so weird about the church. Now maybe we can start to go as a family.

LEANDRA: [*shaking her head violently*] No, I can't go back to that place. That's no church. The devil lived there. And every time I even go near, I feel like I'm choking.

DOMINIC: I know the abuse was bad and all that, but it happened over 10 years ago. And that teacher died. It's time to move on, Lea.

LEANDRA: You don't know what the hell you're talking about.

DOMINIC: Whoa! You're talking crazy.

LEANDRA: I'll tell you what's crazy, you care more about the pastor and your damned meetings at church than you do about me!

DOMINIC: That man saved my life, so don't you ever disrespect him!

LEANDRA: What about you disrespecting me?

In working with interpersonal struggles, therapists face the task of helping clients find an alternative to the avoidance of painful struggles on the one hand, and heated, unproductive arguments on the other. Mahoney and colleagues have coined a useful concept in this regard: They emphasize the importance of fostering spiritual intimacy among family members struggling to communicate effectively around core differences. Spiritual intimacy is defined as "engaging in spiritual disclosure and providing support when a partner offers spiritual disclosures" (Kusner, Mahoney, Pargament, & DeMaris, 2014, p. 605). Spiritual intimacy does not sidestep or minimize important spiritual tensions—instead, it focuses on the creation of an atmosphere in which partners can safely risk speaking from the heart and listening to each other with compassion and empathy. In two observational longitudinal studies of pregnant married couples in the transition to parenthood, higher levels of spiritual intimacy were predictive of stronger observed emotional intimacy as the couples communicated about their conflicts (Kusner et al., 2014) and vulnerabilities (Padgett, Mahoney, Pargament, & DeMaris, 2019). This research leads to an important practical question: How can therapists help clients move from divisive interpersonal struggles to greater spiritual intimacy?

Finding Common Ground

Studies have shown that people who can identify points of commonality with others are less likely to engage in conflict and discrimination (e.g., Kunst, Kimel, Shani, Alayan, & Thomsen, 2019). Chaplain Sue Jelinek (personal communication, January 17, 2019) applied this lesson in her counseling with religious families with a child who identifies as transgender or gender nonconforming (TGNC). One father of a transgender teen, Ben, wondered how he could talk to his biblically conservative parents who, he feared, would judge their grandson to be sinful. Jelinek offered this suggestion:

> "[Tell them] that they all love Ben and want him to be happy, safe, reach his God-given potential and be able to share the gifts and talents he has been blessed with. [Tell them] that the person Ben is now is still the same person he was prior to his transitioning—his personality, thoughtfulness, sense of humor are all still a part of who he is."

Baron-Cohen (2011) provided another powerful example of finding common ground. This came from efforts to encourage dialogue between Israeli and Palestinian parents who had lost children through violence in Israel. At a community forum on a Sabbath, two of the parents introduced themselves this way:

> I am Ahmed, and I am a Palestinian. My son died in the Intifada, killed by an Israeli bullet. I come to wish you all Shabbat Shalom. Then the other man spoke: "I am Moishe, and I am an Israeli. My son also died in the Intifada, killed by a home-made petrol bomb thrown by a Palestinian teenager. I come to wish you all Salaam Aleikem." (p. 193)

Seeing the Sacred Spark

Possibilities for reconnection also emerge when we are able to view people more deeply, looking beneath surface labels to see beings who carry something of a common sacred spark within them. This is the way Griffith (2010) explained the Hutu Protestant pastor who protected a Tutsi woman during the Rwandan genocide by hiding her in his home: "Her category—Tutsi—was an aspect of who she was as a person; her person was not an aspect of her category" (Griffith, 2010, p. 159). In studies of married couples communicating about their conflicts and emotional vulnerabilities, the capacity to see the sacred in others, including those who may be a source of tension and conflict, was associated with greater connectedness and intimacy (Kusner et al., 2014; Padgett et al., 2019).

Similarly, other studies have shown that Christians who remind themselves more frequently that God loves all of his children, including those who belong to different religions and manifest different lifestyles, are less likely to be prejudiced toward Jews, Muslims, and gays and lesbians (Abu-Raiya, Pargament, Mahoney, & Trevino, 2008; Pargament et al., 2007; Trevino, Desai, et al., 2012).

Some evidence suggests that it may be possible to foster the ability to view others in more of their humanness. Bassett et al. (2005) developed a brief intervention to help Christian college students develop more positive views of gay and lesbian individuals. The students watched four scenes of a movie that depicted the life of a gay man grappling with common human experiences, such as tensions with families and friends. The students then read three passages from scriptures that emphasized living a life of love, living a life of acceptance, and living peaceably. Although the findings were somewhat complex, the intervention generally improved the attitudes of students toward gays and lesbians, particularly students who had been the most uniformly rejecting of these groups.

Accepting Differences and Beyond

Reconnection does not mean denying or minimizing differences in values, beliefs, and practices between people. Rather it rests on an acceptance of these differences. One Jewish woman described her process of reaching acceptance in an article aptly titled "My Jewish Sons Have a Christmas Tree and I Need to Deal" (Ingber, 2019). Growing up, she had viewed "not decorating our front lawn in lights as much a part of my Jewish identity as celebrating Passover and going to Hebrew school on Thursdays." In contrast, her husband, a Hindu, had had positive memories of putting up a Christmas tree in his family as a child. The couple never settled their difference before their marriage and eventually they divorced in part because of their unresolved religious conflict. Nevertheless, the woman remained concerned about her adult sons having a Christmas tree in their homes. She said, "It has shaken me to my core to know my boys may not end up being Jewish the way I am." Over time, however, she was able to find greater acceptance. "I have to move on," she realized:

> Frankly, I need to get over the damn tree. My boys are different from me, and that has a special beauty to it. They are "both" [Jewish and Indian]. And while I will do everything I can to instill in them the same love for Judaism that I have, who they are and what "both" looks like will ultimately be up to them.

When strugglers go beyond accepting differences to seeing positive value in differences, the process of reconnection may be facilitated even further. In a study of German adolescents, Streib and Klein (2014) found that those who were more able to appreciate and find wisdom in the religions of others reported less anti-Semitic and anti-Islamic prejudice.

Disentangling Tensions and Conflicts

Helping clients come to terms with complicated tensions and conflicts about religious and spiritual issues is often challenging. This point is even more true when these struggles manifest themselves in relationships. One person's struggles may trigger the struggles of another and, as was the case with Leandra and Dominic, the conversation can quickly heat up and boil over. Helping couples, families, and other relationships move from spiritual struggles to spiritual intimacy requires active efforts by the therapist to lower the emotional temperature in the room and disentangle the complex feelings that can arise. Consider how Leandra's therapist approached this task with the couple:

THERAPIST: Things got pretty hot between the two of you the last time we met. I know that was uncomfortable, but I think the two of you were trying to share some important feelings with each other. These are feelings that do need to come out and do need to be heard. I'd like to help the two of you do that by suggesting a way of talking that slows things down, lowers the temperature in the room, and makes sure you both will be able to say important things and feel heard. How does that sound?

LEANDRA AND DOMINIC: [*Both nod.*]

THERAPIST: Great! Here's what I have in mind. I want each of you to have a chance to be a "speaker" and each of you to have a chance to be a "listener." When you are a speaker, you will have the floor and your job will be to try to share an important message with your partner in a sensitive way. When you are a listener, your job will be to try to hear and understand what your partner is saying. You may feel the urge to make some points of your own, but you'll need to put that urge aside for the time being while your partner has the floor. Your job will be simply to listen. We'll then reverse the roles of speaker and listener. Is that clear?

LEANDRA AND DOMINIC: Yes [*in unison*].

THERAPIST: Leandra, I wonder if you might go first and share something about your experience in the church with the teacher. Do you feel ready to do that? Dominic, do you feel ready to listen?

LEANDRA AND DOMINIC: [*Both nod.*]

LEANDRA: Well, this won't be easy. I haven't really talked much about what really happened with you, Dominic. [*Deep breath*] Okay, well, I guess it's time. I was only 12 when that teacher had me come into his office after Sunday school and sit on his lap while he read Bible stories to me. At first it seemed okay. I mean, I had never had an adult give me that kind of special attention. But then he started to rub my back, and then his hands started to wander to the front of my blouse, and he would rub my chest.

DOMINIC: Sweet Jesus.

LEANDRA: I wish Jesus were there, but it was just the teacher and me, and he didn't stop there. He started stroking my legs and began to fondle me under my panties. [*Crying*] I wanted to run, but I felt paralyzed. He would tell me to sit still and "just be a good girl." And then he would be rubbing himself against my bottom. I didn't know what he was doing at first, but then I knew he was, you know, doing himself. [*Crying harder now.*]

DOMINIC: [*crying too*] I'm so sorry, baby. He had no right to do that.

LEANDRA: I didn't know what to do. My grandmother was so proud of me, and she loved the church so much. I couldn't let myself hurt her, so I didn't feel I could say or do anything. Every week I worried about Sundays. I knew what was coming, and I would get so nervous sometimes that I'd throw up. I just tried to turn all my feelings off.

DOMINIC: I didn't know. I didn't know.

LEANDRA: One week, he tried to get me to take my panties off and he unzipped himself. I ran out of the room, and I never went back. He never said anything, and I never did, either.

DOMINIC: [*holding Leandra's hand*] I wish I could have killed that man.

LEANDRA: Me too.

THERAPIST: [*long pause*] The two of you shared a very sensitive and very powerful conversation together. Leandra, you did a wonderful job talking. And, Dominic, you did a wonderful job listening. It took you both a lot of strength and courage. Next session, I'd like to give you a chance to be the speaker, Dominic, and you'll have a chance to be the listener, Leandra.

Just as communication in conjoint therapy can quickly cycle down to arguments and fighting, communication can also quickly cycle upward to greater intimacy and closeness when self-disclosure is met with empathy and compassion. That occurred in the following session in which Dominic had his chance to be the speaker and described how the pastor of their church had helped guide him away from criminal activity and drug use as an adolescent to sobriety, continued education, and a good job. In tears, he talked about how he couldn't turn his back on the pastor—the man, he felt, had saved his life. Leandra was able to hear Dominic and offer him support and affirmation.

When people are able to establish spiritual intimacy, their spiritual conflicts often become easier to resolve and even fade in importance. As they grew closer, Leandra and Dominic were able to talk more freely about ways to deal with their very different feelings about the church. Dominic voiced his willingness to explore other churches they would both feel comfortable attending while he continued counseling with the pastor and attending his church-based 12-step program. Leandra said she would be open to meeting with the pastor to talk about her abuse and what the church could do to become a safer place for its members, particularly children and adolescents. The couple ended their therapy having taken significant steps from interpersonal spiritual struggle to spiritual intimacy and a stronger marriage.

CONCLUSIONS

Spiritual struggles involve not only individuals but relationships as well. Signs of struggle about religious and spiritual issues are all too familiar in the world today. These struggles can be found at every level of human interaction: cultural, national, institutional, familial, and dyadic. In this chapter, we focused on how practitioners can understand and address interpersonal struggles in the clinical context. The therapy process does become more complex when spiritual struggles manifest themselves in relationships. Adding to the challenge is the relative lack of attention interpersonal struggles have received in clinical research and practice. This is, in short, a new topic for practitioners. Even so, we believe it is a vital topic. We have seen that interpersonal struggles around religion are not at all uncommon. Moreover, they can be significant sources of psychological and social distress and decline. These struggles can also be embedded in the problems that clients bring to treatment. By broadening the scope of clinical work to include interpersonal struggles around religion, practitioners have the opportunity to help clients move from fragmentation to greater wholeness within themselves and, as importantly, in relationship to significant others in their lives.

CHAPTER 14

Concluding Thoughts

Spiritual struggles can be found wherever people encounter life's most fundamental tensions and challenges. Struggles are "in-between" phenomena, located in between belief and unbelief, meaningfulness and meaninglessness, connection and disconnection, morality and impulsivity, security and insecurity, and good and evil. Because they often lay concealed in the cracks and crevices of basic human experience, spiritual struggles have been easy to overlook. Fortunately, this picture has begun to change. In this book, we introduced readers to a rapidly growing body of theory, research, and clinical practice to shine some light directly on spiritual struggles. We would like to leave our readers with a few concluding points.

Spiritual struggles are a natural part of life, an outgrowth of the situations we face, our orientation to life, and our efforts to realize significance. Stories of struggle are age-old. They are embedded in the epic accounts of the origins of virtually every major religious tradition. Indeed, it may be no exaggeration to say that stories of struggle and their resolution lie at the very heart of religion. Struggles are by no means a thing of the past, however. Today, people from every walk of life, and every religious and spiritual orientation, from the most devout to the most disengaged, report spiritual struggles. And, we strongly suspect, spiritual struggles will continue to figure large in the lifelong journeys of future generations. Following her interviews with one of the fastest growing groups in the United States—the "nones": people who do not affiliate with any religion, including agnostics, atheists, and the "spiritual but not religious," Linda Mercadante (2020) reached this conclusion:

> Struggles with the existential issues that all humans face will continue. Nones may experience them differently, define them as primarily psychological or biological, or dismiss them as a residue of the past. But many may instead recognize them for

the spiritual struggles they genuinely are and seek appropriate resources that will lead toward resolution and growth. Increasingly, those in the helping professions will encounter spiritual struggles in their clients.

Spiritual struggles carry important implications for the trajectory of our lives. An impressive body of study demonstrates how spiritual struggles have the capacity to shake us to our core, leaving us dizzied, disoriented, and distressed. If not addressed, they can lead to serious decline. Struggles can be intertwined with virtually every kind of psychological problem, including anxiety, depression, impulse control, addictions, personality disorders, bipolar illness, schizophrenia, and marital/family problems. The picture that emerges from this literature is one that should caution us against any tendency to shrug off, make light of, or sentimentalize spiritual struggles.

This is not to diminish the possibility of a brighter side to spiritual struggles. Developmental theorists have stressed that without conflict, strain, and struggle, we would remain frozen, unable to respond to change, vulnerable to being shattered by any force that throws us off balance. Inherent in spiritual struggles is the possibility of meaningful change. We struggle not only reactively *with* life challenges, but proactively *to* find significance in life. And when mastered, struggles can push people into higher levels of cognitive, moral, and faith maturity. Stories of dramatic transformation through spiritual struggles—from the narratives of the founders of religious traditions to contemporary accounts—illustrate just this point. If spiritual struggles can lead to problems, these stories suggest, they can also lead to growth. And perhaps they may be accompanied by both pain and gain. Elizabeth Kübler-Ross (1975) put it elegantly:

> The most beautiful people we have known are those who have known defeat, known suffering, known struggle, known loss, and have found their way out of the depths. These persons have an appreciation, a sensitivity, and an understanding of life that fills them with compassion, gentleness, and a deep loving concern. Beautiful people do not just happen. (p. 96)

While theory and personal testimonies highlight the potential of spiritual struggles for growth, the empirical research presents a more sobering picture: Growth through struggles, these studies show, may be possible but it is certainly not inevitable. Why should that be the case? Perhaps it takes more time for growth to occur in the aftermath of spiritual struggles than has been allowed in current research. Perhaps growth itself needs to be assessed through more nuanced indicators, such as the ability to experience the melancholy of both sadness and happiness, greater compassion for the suffering of others, a deeper sense of humor, and virtues, including the courage to raise hard questions and the humility to admit we don't have all the answers. Further research is needed to test these possibilities.

In this book, we have suggested a third explanation for the tenuous links between spiritual struggles and growth: the possibility that spiritual struggles are in fact pivotal times in life, forks in the road that can lead to growth, decline, or both. The trajectory of spiritual struggles, we have asserted, depends on the degree of wholeness of the individual. In support of this idea, research has begun to show that markers of wholeness—a broad and deep perspective, a life-affirming orientation, the ability to put the bits and pieces of life together into a cohesive pattern—may be important precursors of growth through spiritual struggles (e.g., Hart et al., 2020).

In short, scientific research makes it clear that spiritual struggles are too important a part of peoples' lives to ignore. More than that, however, the state of the science leads naturally to a vital practical question: How do we help spiritual strugglers at this critical juncture? More specifically, how can we help individuals come to terms with their spiritual struggles before they result in serious problems? And, to consider a brighter side, how can we use times of spiritual struggle as springboards for life-transforming changes and greater wholeness that foster growth? These are questions of direct concern to mental health professionals.

Therapists are well positioned to assist clients during these pivotal times. After all, therapy is designed to help people come to terms with all kinds of sensitive, painful, and challenging tensions and conflicts. Nevertheless, some therapists may draw the line at spiritual struggles for several reasons. Let's briefly review each of their concerns and our response.

- *Talking about spiritual struggles in therapy will be off-putting to clients.* As we have noted, surveys indicate that a majority of clients would welcome the chance to talk about deeper spiritual issues in therapy, including spiritual struggles (Exline et al., 2000; Rosmarin, 2018). Fearing pressure or critical responses from others, clients may particularly appreciate the more objective perspective of therapists and their commitment to helping clients find their own answers to spiritual questions and conflicts.

- *Spiritual struggles fall outside the boundary of psychotherapy.* Certainly, practitioners are not theologians or clergy, and it is not the role of therapists to offer religious rituals or expert opinions on the truth or falsity of religious claims, including God's existence or nonexistence. We have tried to show, however, that therapists can approach spiritual struggles with the same caring, compassion, perspective, and skills as they would any other sensitive topic. And when religious expertise and legitimacy are needed, consultation and collaboration with clergy, as with other helping professionals, can be appropriate as well.

- *Will talking about spiritual struggles in therapy really make a difference to my clients?* By overlooking or avoiding spiritual struggles in therapy, therapists miss an opportunity for meaningful discussion and significant change.

After all, as the empirical research has indicated, many clients manifest spiritual struggles that are interwoven with the psychological problems they bring to therapy. Not only that, spiritual struggles have been linked to a greater risk of distress, disorientation, and decline. Clinical case studies, including our own experiences, have shown that the process of therapy is enriched when spiritual struggles are included in the therapeutic conversation. Promising evaluative studies also suggest that the therapist's willingness to talk about spiritual struggles can help clients move toward greater wholeness and growth rather than brokenness and decline.

- *To deal with spiritual struggles in therapy requires a great deal of specialized knowledge and skill.* We have emphasized that work with struggles does not require a whole new model of treatment but rather a broadening and deepening of therapy to encompass spirituality as both a potential resource and a source of struggle and problems. There is no need for expert answers on the part of the therapist to the profound existential and spiritual dilemmas the client may be facing—only guiding wisdom (cf. Jones, 2019).

- *I just don't know how to deal with spiritual struggles in therapy.* In this book we have tried to provide practitioners with a basic foundation of knowledge and skills that will help them assess and address spiritual struggles with greater confidence in psychotherapy. This base of knowledge and skill is part of an emerging definition of spiritual competency in mental health care (Vieten & Scammell, 2015). Hopefully, it will also become more a regular part of clinical training in the mental health professions.

- *Spiritual struggles are a painful topic for me personally.* Mistreatment at the hands of religious institutions, heartfelt prayers that go unanswered, encounters with trauma so horrific that only the language of evil seems to explain it— the stuff of which spiritual struggles are made can raise troubling questions and conflicts not only for clients but therapists as well. And practitioners may prefer to avoid their own struggles that are raw, unresolved, or unrecognized. With a few exceptions (Strosky et al., 2018), little research has been conducted on the spiritual struggles of therapists. This research, however, suggests that, as with clients, spiritual struggles may be a source of distress for practitioners. But the solution, we believe, is not to avoid spiritual struggles in clinical work. Rather, with the support of others and perhaps some of the tools in this book, therapists can try to understand and address their own spiritual struggles. Doing so, we believe, may prove beneficial not only to clients but to practitioners themselves.

There is, in short, a strong rationale for bringing spiritual struggles into the therapeutic arena. To make that integration more of a reality, however, we have more work to do. We are just beginning to learn how to help clients facing spiritual struggles in psychotherapy, and there is plenty of room for innovation in this area. For example, our approach to spiritual struggles has been eclectic, drawing on resources from multiple therapeutic orientations. This work could be tailored to more specific therapeutic orientations as well, and some encouraging initial efforts have been made in this direction, involving ACT (Santiago & Gall, 2016) and CBT (Pearce & Koenig, 2016). We also need to learn more about the best ways to assist people grappling with specific forms of struggle: divine, doubt-related, moral, interpersonal, and demonic struggles, and struggles of ultimate meaning. And we need to better understand how to work with people from other religious worlds, particularly non-Western traditions (e.g., Hinduism, Islam, folk religions) who may experience and approach spiritual struggles differently from their Western counterparts. We look forward to creative new approaches to spiritual struggles in therapy.

Although this book has focused on bringing new knowledge about spiritual struggles to the attention of mental health practitioners, we cannot conclude without at least brief mention of the relevance of spiritual struggles to contexts outside of the psychotherapy room. Religious institutions represent one such context. We believe spiritual struggles should be a topic that is regularly considered on the pulpit and within religious education programs. These programs could be of value to any age group. However, because raising questions is a natural part of the development of adolescents, the "coming-of-age" period could be an especially appropriate time for discussions about spiritual struggles. Serious tensions and conflicts about spiritual matters could be anticipated, normalized, and discussed openly without criticism or stigma. Religious educators, leaders, and clergy could serve as valuable models in this regard by discussing their own experiences of spiritual struggles and how they have handled them in their own lives. Without these resources, adolescents may be more likely to withdraw entirely from religious and spiritual life when spiritual struggles arise.

Even though religious institutions represent a natural place to talk about spiritual struggles, we believe the subject should not simply be delegated to religious congregations. Spiritual struggles represent a relevant topic for families as well. Curiosity and questions about religious and spiritual issues are a normal outgrowth of the intellectual, social, moral, and spiritual development of children and adolescents (Mahoney, 2013). Parents could help children along in their development by encouraging rather than discouraging these questions, difficult though they may be, and by sharing their own thoughts and experiences about spiritual struggles. We don't think it too much of a stretch to imagine family conversations around the dinner table about religious and spiritual matters, including spiritual struggles. With greater education and involvement from religious institutions and families, young adults may be better equipped to anticipate, understand, and deal with the spiritual struggles that arise over the course of their lives.

Most, if not all of us, encounter periods when we are shaken to the core, when the beliefs, practices, connections, and values that we have relied on can no longer be counted on to orient and guide us in the pursuit of our aspirations. Make no mistake, being shaken in this fundamental way is a disturbing experience, made worse when there is no way to understand it and no one to provide the guidance and support that might help us move through it. Perhaps as a result, for some, being shaken to the core can be a shattering experience. That doesn't have to be the case. In this book, we have talked about ways that spiritual struggles can lead to wholeness and growth rather than brokenness and decline. We hope that this work contributes to our ability to understand and address this easy-to-overlook, but pivotal and very human experience.

References

Aarnio, K., & Lindeman, M. (2007). Religious people and paranormal believers: Alike or different? *Journal of Individual Differences, 28*(1), 1–9.

Abramowitz, J. S., Huppert, J. D., Cohen, A. B., Tolin, D. F., & Cahill, S. P. (2002). Religious obsessions and compulsions in a non-clinical sample: The Penn Inventory of Scrupulosity (PIOS). *Behavior Research and Therapy, 40*(7), 825–838.

Abu-Raiya, H., Pargament, K. I., Exline, J. J., & Agbaria, Q. (2015). Prevalence, predictors, and implications of religious/spiritual struggles among Muslims. *Journal for the Scientific Study of Religion, 54*(4), 631–648.

Abu-Raiya, H., Pargament, K. I., & Krause, N. (2016). Religion as problem, religion as solution: Religious buffers of the links between religious/spiritual struggles and well-being/mental health. *Quality of Life Research, 25*(5), 1265–1274.

Abu-Raiya, H., Pargament, K. I., Krause, N., & Ironson, G. (2015). Robust links between religious/spiritual struggles, psychological distress, and well-being in a national sample of American adults. *American Journal of Orthopsychiatry, 85*(6), 565–575.

Abu-Raiya, H., Pargament, K. I., Mahoney, A., & Stein, C. (2008). A psychological measure of Islamic religiousness: Development and evidence for reliability and validity. *International Journal for the Psychology of Religion, 18*(4), 291–315.

Abu-Raiya, H., Pargament, K. I., Mahoney, A., & Trevino, K. (2008). When Muslims are perceived as a religious threat: Examining the connection between desecration, religious coping, and anti-Muslim attitudes. *Basic and Applied Social Psychology, 30*(4), 311–325.

Abu-Raiya, H., Pargament, K. I., Weissberger, A., & Exline, J. (2016). An examination of religious/spiritual struggle among Israeli Jews. *International Journal for the Psychology of Religion, 26*(1), 61–79.

Abu-Raiya, H., Sasson, T., Palachy, S., Mozes, E., & Tourgeman, A. (2017). The relationships between religious coping and mental and physical health among female survivors of intimate partner violence in Israel. *Psychology of Religion and Spirituality, 9*(Suppl. 1), S70–S78.

Abu-Raiya, H., & Sulleiman, R. (2020, October). Direct and indirect links between religious coping and posttraumatic growth among Muslims who lost their children due to traffic accidents. *Journal of Happiness Studies.* Advance online publication.

Adom-Fynn, D., Asamoah, D., Quainoo, E. A., Tetteh, S. Q., & Acquah, D. (2019/2020). Religious coping and self-esteem of women living with cervical cancer in Ghana. *International Journal of Healthcare Sciences, 7*(2), 162–179.

Affleck, G., Tennen, H., Croog, S., & Levine, S. (1987). Causal attribution, perceived benefits, and morbidity after a heart attack: An 8-year study. *Journal of Consulting and Clinical Psychology, 55*(1), 29–35.

Ahles, J. J., Mezulis, A. H., & Hudson, M. R. (2016). Religious coping as a moderator of the relationship between stress and depressive symptoms. *Psychology of Religion and Spirituality, 8*(3), 228–234.

Ahrens, C. E., Abeling, S., Ahmad, S., & Hinman, J. (2010). Spirituality and well-being: The relationship between religious coping and recovery from sexual assault. *Journal of Interpersonal Violence, 25*(7), 1242–1263.

Ai, A. L., Seymour, E. M., Tice, T. N., Kronfol, Z., & Bolling, S. F. (2009). Spiritual struggle related to plasma interleukin-6 prior to cardiac surgery. *Psychology of Religion and Spirituality, 1*(2), 112–128.

Ai, A. L., Tice, T. N., Huang, B., & Ishisaka, A. (2005). Wartime faith-based reactions among traumatized Kosovar and Bosnian refugees in the United States. *Mental Health, Religion and Culture, 8*(4), 291–308.

Ai, A. L., Tice, T. N., Lemieux, C. M., & Huang, B. (2011). Modeling the post-9/11 meaning-laden paradox: From deep connection and deep struggle to posttraumatic stress and growth. *Archive for the Psychology of Religion, 33*(2), 173–204.

Ake, G. S., III, & Horen, S. G. (2003). The influence of religious orientation and coping on the psychological distress of Christian domestic violence victims. *Journal of Religion and Abuse, 5*(2), 5–28.

Allen, J. G. (2013). *Restoring mentalizing in attachment relationships: Treating trauma with plain old therapy.* New York: American Psychiatric Publishing.

Alimujiang, A., Wiensch, A., Boss, J., Fleischer, N. L., Mondul, A. M., McLean, K., et al. (2019). Association between life purpose and mortality among US adults older than 50 years. *JAMA Network Open, 2*(5), e194270.

Allport, G. W. (1950a). *The individual and his religion.* New York: Macmillan.

Allport, G. W. (1950b). A psychological approach to the study of love and hate. In P. A. Sorokin (Ed.), *Explorations in altruistic love and behavior* (pp. 145–164). Boston: Beacon Press.

Allport, G. W. (1954). *The nature of prejudice.* Cambridge, MA: Perseus Books.

Allport, G. W., & Ross, J. M. (1967). Personal religious orientation and prejudice. *Journal of Personality and Social Psychology, 5*(4), 432–443.

Altemeyer, B., & Hunsberger, B. (1997). *Amazing conversions: Why some turn to faith and others abandon religion.* Amherst, MA: Prometheus Books.

American Psychological Association. (2017). *Ethical principles of psychologists and code of conduct.* Washington, DC: Author.

Anderson, S. R., & Hopkins, P. (1991). *The feminine face of God: The unfolding of the sacred in women.* New York: Bantam Books.

Anderson-Mooney, A. J., Webb, W., Mvududu, N., & Charbonneau, A. M. (2015). Dispositional forgiveness and meaning-making: The relative contributions of forgiveness and adult attachment style to struggling or enduring with God. *Journal of Spirituality in Mental Health, 17*(2), 91–109.

Ano, G. G., & Pargament, K. I. (2013). Predictors of spiritual struggles: An exploratory study. *Mental Health, Religion and Culture, 16*(4), 419–434.

Ano, G. G., Pargament, K. I., Wong, S., & Pomerleau, J. (2017). From Vice to Virtue: Evaluating a manualized intervention for moral spiritual struggles. *Spirituality in Clinical Practice, 4*(2), 129–144.

Ano, G. G., & Vasconcelles, E. G. (2005). Religious coping and psychological adjustment to stress: A meta-analysis. *Journal of Clinical Psychology, 61*(4), 461–480.

Appel, J. E., Park, C. L., Wortmann, J. H., & van Schie, H. T. (2020). Meaning violations, religious/spiritual struggles, and meaning in life in the face of stressful life events. *International Journal for the Psychology of Religion, 30*(1), 1–17.

Arendt, H. (1963). *Eichmann in Jerusalem.* New York: Viking Press.

Avants, S. K., Beitel, M., & Margolin, A. (2005). Making the shift from "addict self" to "spiritual self": Results from a stage I study of Spiritual Self-Schema (3-S) therapy for the treatment of addiction and HIV risk behavior. *Mental Health, Religion and Culture, 8*(3), 167–177.

Aveni, A. (2017). *In the shadow of the moon: The science, magic, and mystery of solar eclipses.* New Haven, CT: Yale University Press.

Bader, C. D., Mencken, F. C., & Baker, J. O. (2010). *Paranormal America: Ghost encounters, UFO sightings, Bigfoot hunts, and other curiosities in religion and culture.* New York: New York University Press.

Baider, L., & Sarell, M. (1983). Perceptions and causal attributions of Israeli women with breast cancer concerning their illness: The effects of ethnicity and religiosity. *Psychotherapy and Psychosomatics, 39*(3), 136–143.

Baird, J. (2014, September 15). Doubt as a sign of faith. Retrieved from *https://www.nytimes.com/2014/09/26/opinion/julia-baird-doubt-as-a-sign-of-faith.html.*

Baird, R. M. (1980). The creative role of doubt in religion. *Journal of Religion and Health, 19*(3), 172–179.

Bakan, D. (1966). *The duality of human existence: An essay on psychology and religion.* Chicago: Rand McNally.

Baker, J. (2008). Who believes in religious evil? An investigation of sociological patterns of belief in Satan, hell, and demons. *Review of Religious Research, 50*(2), 206–220.

Balboni, T. A., Balboni, M., Paulk, M. E., Phelps, A., Wright, A., Peteet, J., et al. (2011). Support of cancer patients' spiritual needs and associations with medical care costs at the end of life. *Cancer, 117*(23), 5383–5391.

Baltazar, T., & Coffen, R. D. (2011). The role of doubt in religious identity development and psychological maturity. *Journal of Research on Christian Education, 20*(2), 182–194.

Baltes, P. B., & Staudinger, U. M. (2000). Wisdom: A metaheuristic (pragmatic) to orchestrate mind and virtue toward excellence. *American Psychologist, 55*(1), 122–136.

Baron-Cohen, S. (2011). *The science of evil: On empathy and the origins of cruelty.* New York: Basic Books.

Barrett, J. L. (2011). *Cognitive science, religion, and theology: From human minds to divine minds.* West Conshohocken, PA: Templeton Press.

Barrett, J. L. (2012). *Born believers: The science of children's religious belief.* New York: Free Press.

Bartkowski, J. P., Xu, X., & Levin, M. L. (2008). Religion and child development: Evidence from the Early Childhood Longitudinal Study. *Social Science Research, 37*(1), 18–36.

Bassett, R. L., van Nikkelin-Kuyper, M., Johnson, D., Miller, A., Carter, A., & Grimm, J. P. (2005). Being a good neighbor: Can students come to value homosexual persons? *Journal of Psychology and Theology, 33*(1), 17–26.

Batson, C. D. (1975). Rational processing or rationalization? The effect of disconfirming information on a stated religious belief. *Journal of Personality and Social Psychology, 32*(1), 176–184.

Batson, C. D., Schoenrade, P., & Ventis, W. L. (1993). *Religion and the individual: A social–psychological perspective.* New York: Oxford University Press.

Baumeister, R. F. (1997). *Evil: Inside human violence and cruelty.* New York: W. H. Freeman.

Baumeister, R. F., & Bushman, B. J. (2008). *Social psychology and human nature.* Belmont, CA: Wadsworth/Thomson.

Baumeister, R. F., & Exline, J. J. (1999). Virtue, personality, and social relations: Self-control as the moral muscle. *Journal of Personality, 67*(6), 1165–1194.

Baumeister, R. F., Gailliot, M., DeWall, C. N., & Oaten, M. (2006). Self-regulation and personality: How interventions increase regulatory success, and how depletion moderates the effects of traits on behavior. *Journal of Personality, 74*(6), 1773–1801.

Baumeister, R. F., & Vonasch, A. J. (2015). Use of self-regulation to facilitate and restrain addictive behavior. *Addictive Behaviors, 44*(May), 3–8.

Beck, J. S. (2011). *Cognitive behavior therapy: Basics and beyond* (2nd ed.). New York: Guilford Press.

Beck, R. (2007). The winter experience of faith: Empirical, theological, and theoretical perspectives. *Journal of Psychology and Christianity, 26*(1), 68–78.

Beck, R., & Taylor, S. (2008). The emotional burden of monotheism: Satan, theodicy, and relationship with God. *Journal of Psychology and Theology, 36*(3), 151–160.

Becker, E. (1973). *The denial of death.* New York: Free Press.

Begelman, D. A. (1993). Possession: Interdisciplinary roots. *Dissociation, 6*(4), 201–212.

Belavich, T. G., & Pargament, K. I. (2002). The role of attachment in predicting spiritual coping with a loved one in surgery. *Journal of Adult Development, 9*(1), 13–29.

Benhabib, S. (2014, September 21). Who's on trial, Eichmann or Arendt? Retrieved from *https://opinionator.blogs.nytimes.com/2014/09/21/whos-on-trial-eichmann-or-anrendt.*

Benjet, C., Bromet, E., Karam, E. G., Kessler, R. C., McLaughlin, K. A., Ruscio, A. M., et al. (2016). The epidemiology of traumatic event exposure worldwide: Results from the World Mental Health Survey Consortium. *Psychological Medicine, 46*(2), 327–343.

Benore, E., Pargament, K. I., & Pendleton, S. (2008). An initial examination of religious coping in children with asthma. *International Journal for the Psychology of Religion, 18*(4), 267–290.

Benore, E. R., & Park, C. L. (2004). Death-specific religious beliefs and bereavement: Belief in an afterlife and continued attachment. *International Journal for the Psychology of Religion, 14*(1), 1–22.

Bentzen, J. (2020). In crisis, we pray: Religiosity and the COVID-19 pandemic. Retrieved from *https://www.dropbox.com/s/jc8vcx8qqdb84gn/Bentzen_religiosity_covid.pdf?dl=0.*

Berg, G. (2011). The relationship between spiritual distress, PTSD and depression in Vietnam combat veterans. *Journal of Pastoral Care and Counseling, 65*(5), 1–11.

Bergin, A. E. (1991). Values and religious issues in psychotherapy and mental health. *American Psychologist, 46*(4), 394–403.

Berkman, E. T. (2017). Self-regulation training. In K. D. Vohs & R. F. Baumeister (Eds.),

Handbook of self-regulation: Research, theory, and applications (3rd ed., pp. 440–457). New York: Guilford Press.

Berkovits, E. (1979). *With God in hell: Judaism in the ghettos and deathcamps.* New York: Sanhedrin Press.

Bermúdez, J. M., & Bermúdez, S. (2002). Altar-making with Latino families: A narrative therapy perspective. In T. D. Carlson & M. J. Erickson (Eds.), *Spirituality and family therapy* (pp. 329–347). New York: Haworth Press.

Berzengi, A., Berzenji, L., Kadim, A., Mustafa, F., & Jobson, L. (2017). Role of Islamic appraisals, trauma-related appraisals, and religious coping in the posttraumatic adjustment of Muslim trauma survivors. *Psychological Trauma: Theory, Research, Practice, and Policy, 9*(2), 189–197.

Bhikkhu, S. (1985). *The giving rise of the ten kinds of mind of the Bodhisattva/The discourse on the ten wholesome ways of action.* Kuala Lumpur, Malaysia: Syarikat Dharma.

Binau, B. A. (2007). "Holding on" and "letting go": The dynamics of forgiveness. *Word and World, 27*(1), 23–31.

Bjorck, J. P., & Thurman, J. W. (2007). Negative life events, patterns of positive and negative religious coping, and psychological functioning. *Journal for the Scientific Study of Religion, 4*(2), 159–167.

Bockrath, M. F., Pargament, K. I., Wong, S., Harriott, V. A., Pomerleau, J. M., Homolka, S. J., et al. (2021). Religious and spiritual struggles and their links with psychological adjustment: A meta-analysis of longitudinal studies. *Psychology of Religion and Spirituality.* Advance online publication.

Boisen, A. T. (1955). *Religion in crisis and custom: A sociological and psychological study.* Westport, CT: Greenwood Press.

Bojuwoye, O. (2013). Integrating principles underlying ancestral spirits belief in counseling and psychotherapy. *IFE Psychologia, 21*(1), 74–89.

Borowiecki, K. J. (2017). How are you, my dearest Mozart?: Well-being and creativity of three famous composers based on their letters. *The Review of Economics and Statistics, 99*(4), 591–605.

Boshan, Y. (2016). *Great doubt: Practicing Zen in the world* (J. Shore, Trans.). Somerville, MA: Wisdom.

Bourguignon, E. (1976). *Possession.* San Francisco: Chandler & Sharp.

Bowland, S., Biswas, B., Kyriakakis, S., & Edmond, T. (2011). Transcending the negative: Spiritual struggles and resilience in older female trauma survivors. *Journal of Religion, Spirituality and Aging, 23*(4), 318–337.

Bowland, S., Edmond, T., & Fallot, R. D. (2012). Evaluation of a spiritually focused intervention with older trauma survivors. *Social Work, 57*(1), 73–82.

Bradley, D. F., Exline, J. J., & Uzdavines, A. (2015). The god of nonbelievers: Characteristics of a hypothetical god. *Science, Religion and Culture, 2*(3), 120–130.

Bradley, D. F., Exline, J. J., & Uzdavines, A. (2017). Relational reasons for nonbelief in the existence of gods: An important adjunct to intellectual nonbelief. *Psychology of Religion and Spirituality, 9*(4), 319–327.

Bradley, R., Schwartz, A. C., & Kaslow, N. J. (2005). Posttraumatic stress disorder symptoms among low-income, African American women with a history of intimate partner violence and suicidal behaviors: Self-esteem, social support, and religious coping. *Journal of Traumatic Stress, 18*(6), 685–696.

Breines, J. G., & Chen, S. (2012). Self-compassion increases self-improvement motivation. *Personality and Social Psychology Bulletin, 38*(9), 1133–1143.

Brelsford, G. (2011). Divine alliances to handle family conflict: Theistic mediation and triangulation in father–child relationships. *Psychology of Religion and Spirituality, 3*(4), 285–297.

Brelsford, G. M., & Doheny, K. K. (2020). Parents' spiritual struggles and stress: Associations with mental health and cognitive well-being following a neonatal intensive care unit experience. *Psychology of Religion and Spirituality.* Advance online publication.

Brelsford, G. M., & Mahoney, A. (2009). Relying on God to resolve conflict: Theistic mediation and triangulation in relationships between college students and mothers. *Journal of Psychology and Christianity, 28*(4), 291–301.

Breuninger, M. M., Wilt, J. A., Bautista, C. L., Pargament, K. I., Exline, J. J., Fletcher, T. L., et al. (2019). The invisible battle: A descriptive study of religious/spiritual struggles in veterans. *Military Psychology, 31*(6), 433–449.

Brewster, M. E., Velez, B. L., Foster, A., Esposito, J., & Robinson, M. A. (2016). Minority stress and the moderating role of religious coping among religious and spiritual sexual minority individuals. *Journal of Counseling Psychology, 63*(1), 119–126.

Brocas, J. (2018). *Deadly departed: Do's, don'ts, and dangers of afterlife communication.* Stockbridge, MA: Soul Odyssey.

Brontë, A. (1920). The doubter's prayer. In C. Shorter (Ed.), *The complete poems of Anne Brontë* (pp. 38–40). London: Hadden and Stroughton.

Brooks, D. (2015). *The road to character.* New York: Random House.

Brooks, D. (2019, July 5). Will Gen-Z save the world? The revolt against boomer morality. Retrieved from *www.nytimes.com/2019/07/04/opinion/gen-z-boomers.html*.

Bryant, A. N. (2011). The impact of campus context, college encounters, and religious/spiritual struggle on ecumenical worldview development. *Research in Higher Education, 52*(5), 441–459.

Bryant, A. N., & Astin, H. S. (2008). The correlates of spiritual struggle during the college years. *Journal of Higher Education, 79*(1), 1–27.

Buber, M. (1950). *The way of man: According to Hasidic teaching.* New York: Kensington.

Bull, D. L. (2001). A phenomenological model of therapeutic exorcism for dissociative identity disorder. *Journal of Psychology and Theology, 29*(2), 131–139.

Burke, L. A., Neimeyer, R. A., Holland, J. M., Dennard, S., Oliver, L., & Shear, M. K. (2014). Inventory of Complicated Spiritual Grief: Development and validation of a new measure. *Death Studies, 38*(4), 239–250.

Burley, M. (2000). *Hatha yoga: Its context, theory, and practice.* Delhi, India: Motilal Banarsidass.

Büssing, A., Baumann, K., Jacobs, C., & Frick, E. (2017). Spiritual dryness in Catholic priests: Internal resources as possible buffers. *Psychology of Religion and Spirituality, 9*(1), 46–55.

Büssing, A., Michalsen, A., Khalsa, S. B. S., Telles, S., & Sherman, K. J. (2012). Effects of yoga on mental and physical health: A short summary of reviews. *Evidence-Based Complementary and Alternative Medicine, 2012.*

Calhoun, L. G., Cann, A., Tedeschi, R. G., & McMillan, J. (2000). A correlational test of the relationship between posttraumatic growth, religion, and cognitive processing. *Journal of Traumatic Stress, 13*(3), 521–527.

Calhoun, L. G., & Tedeschi, R. G. (2004). The foundations of posttraumatic growth: New considerations. *Psychological Inquiry, 15*(1), 93–102.

Campbell, J. (2008). *The hero with a thousand faces*. Novato, CA: New World Library.

Campbell, W. K., Brunell, A. B., & Foster, J. D. (2004). Sitting here in limbo: Ego shock and posttraumatic growth. *Psychological Inquiry, 15*(1), 26–25.

Camus, A. (1946). *The stranger* (S. Gilbert, Trans.). New York: Knopf.

Cashwell, C. S., Bentley, D. P., & Yarborough, P. (2007). The only way out is through: The peril of spiritual bypass. *Counseling and Values, 51*(2), 139–148.

Castaneda, C. (1971). *The teachings of Don Juan: A Yaqui way of knowledge*. New York: Washington Square Press.

Chan, C. S., & Rhodes, J. E. (2013). Religious coping, posttraumatic stress, psychological distress, and posttraumatic growth among female survivors four years after Hurricane Katrina. *Journal of Traumatic Stress, 26*(2), 257–265.

Chardon, M. L., Brammer, C., Madan-Swain, A., Kazak, A. E., & Pai, A. L. H. (2021). Caregiver religious coping and posttraumatic responses in pediatric hematopoietic stem cell transplant. *Journal of Pediatric Psychology, 46*(4), 465–473.

Chen, Y., Kim, E. S., Koh, H. K., Frazier, A. L., & VanderWeele, T. J. (2019). Sense of mission and subsequent health and well-being among young adults: An outcome-wide analysis. *American Journal of Epidemiology, 188*(4), 664–673.

Chen, Z. J., Bechara, A. O., Worthington, E. L., Jr., Davis, E. B., & Csikszentmihalyi, M. (2019). Trauma and well-being in Colombian disaster contexts: Effects of religious coping, forgiveness, and hope. *Journal of Positive Psychology, 16*(1), 82–93.

Cheng, Z. H., Pagano, L. A., Jr., & Shariff, A. F. (2017). The development, validation and clinical implications of the Microaggressions Against Religious Individuals Scale (MARIS). *Psychology of Religion and Spirituality, 11*(4), 327–338.

Childs, R. E. (1985). Maternal psychological conflicts associated with the birth of a retarded child. *Maternal–Child Nursing Journal, 14*(3), 175–182.

Chittister, J. D. (2003). *Scarred by struggle, transformed by hope*. Grand Rapids, MI: Eerdmans.

Chochinov, H. M. (2002). Dignity-conserving care—a new model for palliative care: Helping the patient feel valued. *Journal of the American Medical Association, 287*(17), 2253–2260.

Chouhoud, Y. (2018). *What causes Muslims to doubt Islam? A quantitative analysis*. Dallas, TX: Yaqeen Institute for Islamic Research. Available online at *https://yaqeen-institute.org/youssef-chouhoud/what-causes-muslims-to-doubt-islam-a-quantitative-analysis*.

Chow, E. O. W., & Nelson-Becker, H. (2010). Spiritual distress to spiritual transformation: Stroke survivor narratives from Hong Kong. *Journal of Aging Studies, 24*(4), 313–324.

Cloninger, C. R., Svrakic, D. M., & Przybeck, T. R. (1993). A psychobiological model of temperament and character. *Archives of General Psychiatry, 50*(12), 975–990.

Coe, G. A. (1916). *The psychology of religion*. Chicago: University of Chicago Press.

Cole, B., & Pargament, K. (1999). Re-creating your life: A spiritual/psychotherapeutic intervention for people diagnosed with cancer. *Psycho-Oncology, 8*(5), 395–407.

Cole, B. S., Hopkins, C. M., Tisak, J., Steel, J. L., & Carr, B. I. (2008). Assessing spiritual growth and spiritual decline following diagnosis of cancer: Reliability and validity of the Spiritual Transformation Scale. *Psycho-Oncology, 17*(2), 112–121.

Collins, D. J. (Ed.). (2015). *The Cambridge history of magic and witchcraft in the west: From antiquity to the present*. New York: Cambridge University Press.

Cooper, L. B., Bruce, A. J., Harman, M. J., & Boccaccini, M. T. (2009). Differentiated styles of attachment to God and varying religious coping efforts. *Journal of Psychology and Theology, 37*(2), 134–141.

Cotton, S., Pargament, K. I., Weekes, J. C., McGrady, M. E., Grossoehme, D., Luberto, C. M., et al. (2013). Spiritual struggles, health-related quality of life and mental health outcomes in urban adolescents with asthma. *Research in the Social Scientific Study of Religion, 24*, 259–280.

Cowden, R. G., Pargament, K. I., Chen, Z. J., Davis, E. B., Lemke, A. W., Glowiak, K. J., et al. (in press). Religious/spiritual struggles and psychological distress: A test of three models in a longitudinal study of adults with chronic health conditions. *Journal of Clinical Psychology.*

Currier, J. M., Fadoir, N., Carroll, T. D., Kuhlman, S., Marie, L., Taylor, S. E., et al. (2020). A cross-sectional investigation of divine struggles and suicide risk among men in early recovery from substance use disorders. *Psychology of Religion and Spirituality, 12*(3), 324–333.

Currier, J. M., Foster, J. D., & Isaak, S. L. (2019). Moral injury and spiritual struggles in military veterans: A latent profile analysis. *Journal of Traumatic Stress, 32*(3), 393–404.

Currier, J. M., Foster, J. D., Witvliet, C. V. O., Abernethy, A. D., Luna, L M. R., Schnitker, S. A., et al. (2019). Spiritual struggles and mental health outcomes in a spiritually integrated inpatient program. *Journal of Affective Disorders, 249*(15), 127–135.

Currier, J. M., Holland, J. M., & Drescher, K. D. (2015). Spirituality factors in the prediction of outcomes of PTSD treatment for U.S. military veterans. *Journal of Traumatic Stress, 28*(1), 57–64.

Currier, J. M., McDermott, R. C., Hawkins, D. E., Green, C. L., & Carpenter, R. (2018). Seeking help for religious and spiritual struggles: Exploring the role of mental health literacy. *Professional Psychology: Research and Practice, 49*(1), 90–97.

Currier, J. M., McDermott, R. C., McCormick, W. H., Churchwell, M. C., & Milkeris, L. (2018). Exploring cross-lagged associations between spiritual struggles and risk for suicidal behavior in a community sample of military veterans. *Journal of Affective Disorders, 230*(1), 93–100.

Currier, J. M., Smith, P. N., & Kuhlman, S. (2017). Assessing the unique role of religious coping in suicidal behavior among U.S. Iraq and Afghanistan veterans. *Psychology of Religion and Spirituality, 9*(1), 118–123.

Curtis, K. T., & Ellison, C. G. (2002). Religious heterogamy and marital conflict: Findings from the national survey of families and households. *Journal of Family Issues, 23*(4), 551–576.

Dabrowski, K. (1964). *Positive disintegration.* Boston: Little, Brown.

Damen, A., Exline, J., Pargament, K., Yao, Y., Chochinov, H., Emanuel, L., et al. (in press). Prevalence, predictors and correlates of religious and spiritual struggles in palliative cancer patients. *Journal of Pain and Symptom Management.*

Davis, C. G., Nolen-Hoeksema, S., & Larson, J. (1998). Making sense of loss and benefiting from experience: Two construals of meaning. *Journal of Personality and Social Psychology, 75*(2), 561–574.

Davis, D. E., Ho, M. Y., Griffin, B. J., Bell, C., Hook, J. N., Van Tongeren, D. R., et al. (2015). Forgiving the self and physical and mental health correlates: A meta-analytic review. *Journal of Counseling Psychology, 62*(2), 329–335.

Davis, D. E., Van Tongeren, D. R., Hook, J. N., Davis, E. B., Worthington, E. L., Jr., & Foxman, S. (2014). Relational spirituality and forgiveness: Appraisals that may hinder forgiveness. *Psychology of Religion and Spirituality, 6*(2), 102–112.

de Castella, R., & Simmonds, J. G. (2013). "There's a deeper meaning as to what suffering's all about": Experiences of religious and spiritual growth following trauma. *Mental Health, Religion and Culture, 16*(5), 536–556.

Decker, L. R. (1993). The role of trauma in spiritual development. *Journal of Humanistic Psychology, 33*(4), 33–46.

Dees, M. K., Vernooij-Dassen, M. J., Dekkers, W. J., Vissers, K. C., & van Weel, C. (2012). "Unbearable suffering": A qualitative study on the perspectives of patients who request assistance in dying. *Journal of Medical Ethics, 37*(12), 727–734.

Dein, S., & Illaiee, A. S. (2013). Jinn and mental health: Looking at jinn possession in modern psychiatric practice. *The Psychiatrist, 37*(9), 290–293.

Delaney, H. D., Miller, W. R., & Bisonó, A. M. (2013). Religion and spirituality among psychologists: A survey of clinician members of the American Psychological Association. *Spirituality in Clinical Practice, 1*(S), 95–106.

Desai, K. M., & Pargament, K. I. (2015). Predictors of growth and decline following spiritual struggles. *International Journal for the Psychology of Religion, 25*(1), 42–56.

DeSteno, D. (2018). *Emotional success: The power of gratitude, compassion, and pride.* New York: Houghton Mifflin Harcourt.

Dickens, C. (1902). *A tale of two cities.* London: Nisbet.

Dillard, A. (1974). *Pilgrim at Tinker Creek.* New York: HarperCollins.

Doane, M. J., & Elliott, M. (2015). Perceptions of discrimination among atheists: Consequences for atheist identification, psychological and physical well-being. *Psychology of Religion and Spirituality, 7*(2), 130–141.

Doehring, C. (1993). *Internal desecration: Traumatization and representations of God.* Lanham, MD: University Press of America.

Doehring, C. (2015). *The practice of pastoral care: A postmodern approach* (Rev. ed.). Louisville, KY: Westminster John Knox Press.

Doehring, C. (2019). Searching for wholeness amidst traumatic grief: The role of spiritual practices that reveal compassion in embodied, relational, and transcendent ways. *Pastoral Psychology, 68*(3), 241–259.

Doehring, C., & Clarke, A. (2002, August). *Perceiving sacredness in life: Personal, religious, social, and situational predictors.* Paper presented at the annual meeting of the American Psychological Association, Chicago, IL.

Dollahite, D. C., Marks, L. D., & Young, K. P. (2019). Relational struggles and experiential immediacy in religious American families. *Psychology of Religion and Spirituality, 11*(1), 9–21.

Done, D. (2019). *When faith fails: Finding God in the shadow of doubt.* Nashville, TN: Nelson Books.

Dostoevsky, F. (2017). *The Brothers Karamazov.* St. Petersburg, Russia: Palmyra.

Dransart, D. A. C. (2018). Spiritual and religious issues in the aftermath of suicide. *Religions, 9*(5), 153.

Drescher, K. D., Foy, D. W., Kelly, C., Leshner, A., Schutz, K., & Litz, B. (2011). An exploration of the viability and usefulness of the construct of moral injury in war veterans. *Traumatology, 17*(1), 8–13.

Drescher, K. D., Smith, M. W., & Foy, D. W. (2007). Spirituality and maladjustment following war-zone experiences. In C. R. Figley & W. P. Nash (Eds.), *Combat stress injury: Theory, research, and management* (pp. 295–310). New York: Routledge/ Taylor & Francis Group.

Driscoll, M. (2015). *Demons, deliverance, and discernment.* San Diego, CA: Catholic Answers.

Duckitt, J., & Sibley, C. G. (2009). A dual-process motivational model of ideology, politics, and prejudice. *Psychological Inquiry, 20*(2–3), 98–109.

Durà-Vilà, G., & Dein, S. (2009). The dark night of the soul: Spiritual distress and its psychiatric implications. *Mental Health, Religion and Culture, 12*(6), 543–559.

During, E. H., Elahi, F. M., Taieb, O., Moro, M.-R., & Baubet, T. (2011). A critical review of dissociative trance and possession disorders: Etiological, diagnostic, therapeutic, and nosological issues. *Canadian Journal of Psychiatry, 56*(4), 235–242.

Durkheim, E. (1915). *The elementary forms of religious life.* New York: Free Press.

Dworsky, C. K. O., Pargament, K. I., Gibbel, M. R., Krumrei, E. J., Faigin, C. A., Haugan, M. R. G., et al. (2013). Winding road: Preliminary support for a spiritually integrated intervention addressing college students' spiritual struggles. *Research in the Social Scientific Study of Religion, 24,* 309–339.

Dworsky, C. K. O., Pargament, K. I., Wong, S., & Exline, J. J. (2016). Suppressing spiritual struggles: The role of experiential avoidance in mental health. *Journal of Contextual Behavioral Science, 5*(4), 258–265.

Earl, T. R., Fortuna, L. R., Gao, S., Williams, D. R., Neighbors, H., Takeuchi, D., et al. (2015). An exploration of how psychotic-like symptoms are experienced, endorsed, and understood from the National Latino and Asian American Study and National Survey of American Life. *Ethnicity and Health, 20*(3), 273–292.

Ebadi, A., Ahmadi, F., Ghanei, M., & Kazemnejad, A. (2009). Spirituality: A key factor in coping among Iranians chronically affected by mustard gas in the disaster of war. *Nursing Health Science, 11*(4), 344–350.

Ecklund, E. H. (2010). *Science vs. religion: What scientists really think.* New York: Oxford University Press.

Edinger-Schons, L. M. (2020). Oneness beliefs and their effect on life satisfaction. *Psychology of Religion and Spirituality, 12*(4), 428–439.

Efrati, Y. (2019). God, I can't stop thinking about sex! The rebound effect in unsuccessful suppression of sexual thoughts among religious adolescents. *Journal of Sex Research, 56*(2), 146–155.

Einstein, A. (1956). *The world as I see it.* New York: Kensington.

Elkins, D. N. (1995). Psychotherapy and spirituality: Toward a theory of the soul. *Journal of Humanistic Psychology, 35*(2), 78–98.

Ellis, M. R., Thomlinson, P., Gemmill, C., & Harris, W. (2013). The spiritual needs and resources of hospitalized primary care patients. *Journal of Religion and Health, 52*(4), 1306–1318.

Ellison, C. G., Fang, Q., Flannelly, K. J., & Steckler, R. A. (2013). Spiritual struggles and mental health: Exploring the moderating effects of religious identity. *International Journal for the Psychology of Religion, 23*(3), 214–229.

Ellison, C. G., & Lee, J. (2010). Spiritual struggles and psychological distress: Is there a dark side of religion? *Social Indicators Research, 98*(3), 501–517.

Ellison, C. G., Roalson, L. A., Guillory, J. M., Flannelly, K. J., & Marcum, J. P. (2010). Religious resources, spiritual struggles, and mental health in a nationwide sample of PCUSA clergy. *Pastoral Psychology, 59*(3), 287–304.

Emmons, R. A. (1999). *The psychology of ultimate concerns: Motivation and spirituality in personality.* New York: Guilford Press.

Emmons, R. A., Cheung, C., & Tehrani, K. (1998). Assessing spirituality through personal goals: Implications for research on religion and subjective well-being. *Social Indicators Research, 45*(1–3), 391–422.

Emmons, R. A., & Crumpler, C. A. (2000). Gratitude as a human strength: Appraising the evidence. *Journal of Social and Clinical Psychology, 19*(1), 56–69.

Emmons, R. A., & Schnitker, S. A. (2013). Gods and goals: Religion and purposeful action. In R. F. Paloutzian & C. L. Park (Eds.), *Handbook of the psychology of religion and spirituality* (2nd ed., pp. 256–273). New York: Guilford Press.

Epictetus. (1888). The Enchiridion or manual, of Epictetus (G. Long, Trans.). Retrieved from *www.hermitary.com/solitude/epictetus_enchiridion.html*.

Erdrich, L. (2001). *The last report on the miracles at Little No Horse*. New York: Harper Collins.

Erikson, E. H. (1968). *Identity: Youth and crisis*. New York: Norton.

Erikson, E. H. (1998). *The life cycle completed*. New York: Norton.

Eskin, M., Baydar, N., El-Nayal, M., Asad, N., Noor, I. M., Razaeian, M., et al. (2020, November). Associations of religiosity, attitudes towards suicide and religious coping with suicidal ideation and suicide attempts in 11 Muslim countries. *Social Science and Medicine, 265*, 113390.

Evans, T. (2018). *Warfare: Winning the spiritual battle*. Chicago: Moody.

Evans, W. R., Stanley, M. A., Barrera, T. L., Exline, J. J., Pargament, K. I., & Teng, E. J. (2018). Morally injurious events and psychological distress among veterans: Examining the mediating role of religious and spiritual struggles. *Psychological Trauma: Theory, Research, Practice, and Policy, 10*(3), 360–367.

Exline, J. J. (2002a, August). *Rifts and reconciliation between humans and God: An overview*. Presentation at annual meeting of the American Psychological Association, Chicago, IL.

Exline, J. J. (2002b). Stumbling blocks on the religious road: Fractured relationships, nagging vices, and the inner struggle to believe. *Psychological Inquiry, 13*(3), 182–189.

Exline, J. J. (2013). Religious and spiritual struggles. In K. I. Pargament, J. J. Exline, & J. W. Jones (Eds.), *APA handbook of psychology, religion, and spirituality (Vol. 1): Context, theory, and research* (pp. 459–476). Washington, DC: American Psychological Association.

Exline, J. J. (2019). [Undergraduates report more positive attitudes about those who believe in God versus the devil.] Unpublished raw data.

Exline, J. J. (2020). Anger toward God and divine forgiveness. In E. L. Worthington & N. G. Wade (Eds.), *Handbook of forgiveness* (2nd ed., pp. 117–127). New York: Routledge.

Exline, J. J. (in press). Psychopathology, normal psychological processes, or supernatural encounters? Three ways to frame reports of after-death communication (ADC). *Spirituality in Clinical Practice*.

Exline, J. J., Deshea, L., & Holeman, V. T. (2007). Is apology worth the risk? Predictors, outcomes, and ways to avoid regret. *Journal of Social and Clinical Psychology, 26*(4), 479–504.

Exline, J. J., & Grubbs, J. B. (2011). "If I tell others about my anger toward God, how will they respond?" Predictors, associated behaviors, and outcomes in an adult sample. *Journal for Psychology and Theology, 39*(4), 304–315.

Exline, J. J., Grubbs, J. B., & Homolka, S. J. (2015). Seeing God as cruel or distant: Links with divine struggles involving anger, doubt, and fear of God's disapproval. *International Journal for the Psychology of Religion, 25*(1), 29–41.

Exline, J. J., Hall, T. W., Pargament, K. I., & Harriott, V. A. (2017). Predictors of growth from spiritual struggle among Christian undergraduates: Religious coping and perceptions of helpful action by God are both important. *Journal of Positive Psychology, 12*(5), 501–508.

Exline, J. J., Homolka, S. J., & Grubbs, J. B. (2013). Negative views of parents and struggles with God: An exploration of two mediators. *Journal of Psychology and Theology, 41*(3), 200–212.

Exline, J. J., Homolka, S. J., & Harriott, V. A. (2016). Divine struggles: Links with body image concerns, binging, and compensatory behaviours around eating. *Mental Health, Religion and Culture, 19*(1), 8–22.

Exline, J. J., Kamble, S., & Stauner, N. (2017). Anger toward God(s) among undergraduates in India. *Religions, 8*(9), 194.

Exline, J. J., Kaplan, K. J., & Grubbs, J. B. (2012). Anger, exit, and assertion: Do people see protest toward God as morally acceptable? *Psychology of Religion and Spirituality, 4*(4), 264–277.

Exline, J. J., Krause, S. J., & Broer, K. A. (2016). Spiritual struggle among patients seeking treatment for chronic headaches: Anger and protest behaviors toward god. *Journal of Religion and Health, 55*(5), 1729–1747.

Exline, J. J., Pargament, K. I., & Grubbs, J. B. (2014). [Longitudinal study of religious/spiritual struggles among U.S. adults using Qualtrics panels.] Unpublished raw data.

Exline, J. J., Pargament, K. I., Grubbs, J. B., & Yali, A. M. (2014). The Religious and Spiritual Struggles Scale: Development and initial validation. *Psychology of Religion and Spirituality, 6*(3), 208–222.

Exline, J. J., Pargament, K. I., & Hall, T. (2014a). [Frequency of reports of post-traumatic growth following religious and spiritual struggles.] Unpublished raw data.

Exline, J. J., Pargament, K. I., & Hall, T. W. (2014b). [Religious and spiritual issues in college life: Results from three universities.] Unpublished raw data.

Exline, J. J., Pargament, K. I., & Wilt, J. A. (2020). *Six-item and one-item screeners to assess religious and spiritual struggle.* Manuscript in preparation.

Exline, J. J., Pargament, K. I., Wilt, J. A., Grubbs, J. G., & Yali, A. M. (2021). *The RSS-14: Development and preliminary validation of a 14-item form of the Religious and Spiritual Struggles Scale.* Manuscript submitted for publication.

Exline, J. J., Pargament, K. I., Wilt, J. A., & Harriott, V. A. (2021). Mental illness, normal psychological processes, or attacks by the devil? Three lenses to frame demonic struggle in therapy. *Spirituality in Clinical Practice.* Advance online publication.

Exline, J. J., Park, C. L., Smyth, J. M., & Carey, M. P. (2011). Anger toward God: Social-cognitive predictors, prevalence, and links with adjustment to bereavement and cancer. *Journal of Personality and Social Psychology, 100*(1), 129–148.

Exline, J. J., Prince-Paul, M., Root, B. L., & Peereboom, K. S. (2013). The spiritual struggle of anger toward God: A study with family members of hospice patients. *Journal of Palliative Medicine, 16*(4), 369–375.

Exline, J. J., Przeworski, A., Peterson, E., Turnamian, M. R., Stauner, N., & Uzdavines, A. (in press). Religious and spiritual struggles among transgender and gender nonconforming (TGNC) adults. *Psychology of Religion and Spirituality.*

Exline, J. J., Stauner, N., Fincham, F., & May, R. (2017, April). Supernatural and natural attributions in the wake of Hurricane Hermine. In J. J. Exline & A. Uzdavines (Chairs), *Could it be supernatural? Perceptions of divine, demonic and impersonal supernatural involvement in daily life.* Symposium presented at the Mid-Year Conference on Psychology, Religion, and Spirituality, Chattanooga, TN.

Exline, J. J., Stauner, N., Fincham, F. D., May, R. W., Wilt, J. A., Pargament, K. I., et al. (2020). *Supernatural attributions.* Manuscript in preparation.

Exline, J. J., Uzdavines, A., & Bradley, D. F. (2015, March). *If given clear evidence for the existence of a god, how do atheists and agnostics think they would respond?* Presentation at the annual Midyear Research Conference on Religion and Spirituality, Provo, UT.

Exline, J. J., Van Tongeren, D. R., Bradley, D. F., Wilt, J. A., Stauner, N., Pargament, K. I., et al. (2020). Pulling away from religion: Religious/spiritual struggles and religious disengagement among college students. *Psychology of Religion and Spirituality.* Advance online publication.

Exline, J. J., Wilt, J. A., Stauner, N., Harriott, V. A., & Saritoprak, S. N. (2017). Self-forgiveness and religious/spiritual struggles. In L. Woodyatt, E. L. Worthington, Jr., M. Wenzel, & B. J. Griffin (Eds.), *Handbook of the psychology of self-forgiveness* (pp. 131–145). New York: Springer.

Exline, J. J., Wilt, J. A., Stauner, N., Schutt, W. A., Pargament, K. I., Fincham, F., et al. (in press). Supernatural operating rules: How people envision and experience God, the devil, ghosts/spirits, fate/destiny, karma, and luck. *Psychology of Religion and Spirituality.*

Exline, J. J., Yali, A. M., & Lobel, M. (1999). When God disappoints: Difficulty forgiving God and its role in negative emotion. *Journal of Health Psychology, 4*(3), 365–379.

Exline, J. J., Yali, A. M., & Sanderson, W. C. (2000). Guilt, discord, and alienation: The role of religious strain in depression and suicidality. *Journal of Clinical Psychology, 56*(12), 1481–1496.

Faigin, C. A., Pargament, K. I., & Abu-Raiya, H. (2014). Spiritual struggles as a possible risk factor for addictive behaviors: An initial empirical investigation. *International Journal for the Psychology of Religion, 24*(3), 201–214.

Falb, M. D., & Pargament, K. I. (2013). Buddhist coping predicts psychological outcomes among end-of-life caregivers. *Psychology of Religion and Spirituality, 5*(4), 252–262.

Fallot, R. D., & Heckman, J. P. (2005). Religious/spiritual coping among women trauma survivors with mental health and substance use disorders. *Journal of Behavioral Health Services and Research, 32*(2), 215–226.

Fater, K., & Mullaney, J. A. (2000). The lived experience of adult male survivors who allege childhood sexual abuse by clergy. *Issues in Mental Health Nursing, 21*(3), 281–295.

FBI Data. (2018). 2018 hate crime statistics. Retrieved from *https://ucr.fbi.gov/hate-crime/2018/topic-pages/incidents-and-offenses.*

Feldman, D. (2012). *Unorthodox: The scandalous rejection of my Hasidic roots.* New York: Simon & Schuster.

Festinger, L., Riecken, H. W., & Schachter, S. (1956). *When prophecy fails.* New York: Harper & Row.

Finocchiaro, M. A. (1989). *The Galileo affair.* Berkeley: University of California Press.

Fisher, A. R. (2017). A review and conceptual model of the research on doubt, disaffiliation, and related religious changes. *Psychology of Religion and Spirituality, 9*(4), 358–367.

Fisher, M. L., & Exline, J. J. (2006). Self-forgiveness versus excusing: The roles of remorse, effort, and accepting responsibility. *Self and Identity, 5*(2), 127–146.

Fisher, M. L., & Exline, J. J. (2010). Moving toward self-forgiveness: Removing barriers related to shame, guilt and regret. *Social and Personality Psychology Compass, 4*(8), 548–558.

Fitchett, G., Murphy, P. E., Kim, J., Gibbons, J. L., Cameron, J. R., Davis, J. A., et al. (2004). Religious struggle: Prevalence, correlates and mental health risks in diabetic, congestive heart failure, and oncology patients. *International Journal of Psychiatry in Medicine, 34*(2), 179–196.

Fitchett, G., Rybarczyk, B. D., DeMarco, G. A., & Nicholas, J. J. (1999). The role of religion in medical rehabilitation outcomes: A longitudinal study. *Rehabilitation Psychology, 44*(4), 333–353.

Fitchett, G., Winter-Pfändler, U., & Pargament, K. I. (2013). Struggle with the divine in Swiss patients visited by chaplains: Prevalence and correlates. *Journal of Health Psychology, 19*(8), 966–976.

Flaherty, S. M. (1992). *Woman, why do you weep? Spirituality for survivors of childhood sexual abuse*. New York: Paulist Press.

Flannelly, K. J. (2017). Religious doubt and mental health. In K. J. Flannelly (Ed.), *Religious beliefs, evolutionary psychiatry, and mental health in America* (pp. 233–242). New York: Springer.

Fleischhack, M., & Schenkel, E. (Eds.). (2016). *Ghosts—or the (nearly) invisible: Spectral phenomena in literature and the media*. Frankfurt am Main, Germany: Peter Lang.

Fletcher, T. L., Farmer, A., Lamkin, J. P., Stanley, M. A., Exline, J. J., Pargament, K. I., et al. (2020). Characterizing religious and spiritual struggles in U.S. veterans: A qualitative study. *Spirituality in Clinical Practice, 7*(3), 162–177.

Flynn, K. A. (2008). In their own voices: Women who were sexually abused by members of the clergy. *Journal of Child Sexual Abuse, 17*(3–4), 216–237.

Folkman, S. (Ed.). (2011). *Oxford handbook of stress, health, and coping*. New York: Oxford University Press.

Fontana, A., & Rosenheck, R. (2004). Trauma, change in strength of religious faith, and mental health service use among veterans treated for PTSD. *Journal of Nervous and Mental Disease, 192*(9), 579–584.

Ford, M. E., & Nichols, C. W. (1987). A taxonomy of human goals and some possible applications. In M. E. Ford, & D. H. Ford (Eds.), *Humans as self-constructing living systems: Putting the framework to work* (pp. 289–311). London: Routledge.

Foster, K. A., Bowland, S. E., & Vosler, A. N. (2015). All the pain along with all the joy: Spiritual resilience in lesbian and gay Christians. *American Journal of Community Psychology, 55*(1–2), 191–201.

Fowler, J. W. (1981). *Stages of faith: The psychology of human development and the quest for meaning*. San Francisco: Harper & Row.

Frankel, E. (2005). *Sacred therapy: Jewish spiritual teachings on emotional healing and inner wholeness*. Boston: Shambhala.

Frankel, E. (2017). *The wisdom of not knowing: Discovering a life of wonder by embracing uncertainty*. Boulder, CO: Shambhala.

Frankl, V. E. (1959). *Man's search for meaning*. New York: Washington Square Press.

Frankl, V. E. (1985). *The unheard cry for meaning: Psychotherapy and humanism*. New York: Washington Square Press.

Frankl, V. E. (2000). *Man's search for ultimate meaning*. Cambridge, MA: Perseus.

Fraser, G. A. (Ed.). (1997). *The dilemma of ritual abuse: Cautions and guides for therapists*. Washington, DC: American Psychiatric Press.

Frazier, P., Tennen, H., Gavian, M., Park, C., Tomich, P., & Tashiro, T. (2009). Does self-reported posttraumatic growth reflect genuine positive change? *Psychological Science, 20*(7), 912–919.

Fredrickson, B. L. (1998). What good are positive emotions? *Review of General Psychology, 2*(3), 300–319.

Fredrickson, B. L., Mancuso, R. A., Branigan, C., & Tugade, M. M. (2000). The undoing effect of positive emotions. *Motivation and Emotion, 24*(4), 237–258.

Freud, S. (1961). *The future of an illusion.* New York: Norton. (Original work published 1927)

Friedman, T. L. (2014, October 21). Putin and the pope. Retrieved from *www.nytimes. com/2014/10/22/opinion/thomas-friedman-putin-and-the-pope.html?auth=login-google.*

Fromm, E. (1950). *Psychoanalysis and religion.* New Haven, CT: Yale University Press.

Fromm, E. (1973). *The anatomy of human destructiveness.* New York: Holt.

Fundaminsky, S. (2000). Memorial prayer for our six million martyrs who perished during the Nazi regime. In A. Rosenfeld (Ed.), *Selichot for the whole year* (2nd ed., p. 349). New York: Judaica Press.

Galek, K., Flannelly, K. J., Ellison, C. G., Silton, N. R., & Jankowski, K. R. B. (2015). Religion, meaning and purpose, and mental health. *Psychology of Religion and Spirituality, 7*(1), 1–12.

Galek, K., Krause, N., Ellison, C. G., Kudler, T., & Flannelly, K. J. (2007). Religious doubt and mental health across the lifespan. *Journal of Adult Development, 14*(1–2), 16–25.

Galilei, G. (1988). Letter to Grand Duchess Christina, 1614. In J. Rohr (Ed.), *Science and religion: Opposing viewpoints* (pp. 17–22). St. Paul, MN: Greenhaven Press.

Gall, T. L., & Guirguis-Younger, M. (2013). Religious and spiritual coping: Current theory and research. In K. I. Pargament, J. J. Exline, & J. W. Jones (Eds.), *APA handbook of psychology, religion, and spirituality (Vol. 1): Context, theory, and research* (pp. 349–364). Washington, DC: American Psychological Association.

Gall, T. L. (2006). Spirituality and coping with life stress among adult survivors of childhood sexual abuse. *Child Abuse and Neglect, 30*(7), 829–844.

Gall, T. L., Charbonneau, C., & Florack, P. (2011). The relationship between religious/ spiritual factors and perceived growth following a diagnosis of breast cancer. *Psychology and Health, 26*(3), 287–305.

Gall, T. L., Kristjansson, E., Charbonneau, C., & Florack, P. (2009). A longitudinal study on the role of spirituality in response to the diagnosis and treatment of breast cancer. *Journal of Behavioral Medicine, 32*(2), 174–186.

Gallagher, T. M. (2005). *The discernment of spirits: An Ignatian guide for everyday living.* New York: Crossroad.

Gallup, G., Jr., & Lindsay, D. M. (1999). *Surveying the religious landscape: Trends in U.S. beliefs.* Harrisburg, PA: Morehouse.

Gandhi, M. (1968). *The selected works of Mahatma Gandhi: An autobiography (Vol. I).* Ahmedabad, India: Navajivan.

Gateway to Wholeness (Pargament, K. I., Brown, M., Gao, F., & Reinert, K.). (2020, November). You can overcome. Retrieved from *gatewaytowholeness.com.*

Gauthier, K. J., Christopher, A. N., Walter, M. I., Mourad, R., & Marek, P. (2006). Religiosity, religious doubt, and the need for cognition: Their interactive relationship with life satisfaction. *Journal of Happiness Studies, 7*(2), 139–154.

Gearing, R. E., Alonzo, D., Smolak, A., McHugh, K., Harmon, S., & Baldwin, S. (2011). Association of religion with delusions and hallucinations in the context of schizophrenia: Implications for engagement and adherence. *Schizophrenia Research, 126*(1–3), 150–163.

Geertz, C. (1966). Religion as a cultural system. In M. Banton (Ed.), *Anthropological approaches to the study of religion* (pp. 1–46). London: Tavistock.

Genia, V. (1990). Interreligious encounter group: A psychospiritual experience for faith development. *Counseling and Values, 35*(1), 39–51.

George, L. S., & Park, C. L. (2016). Meaning in life as comprehension, purpose, and mattering: Toward integration and new research questions. *Review of General Psychology, 20(*3), 205–220.

Gerber, M. M., Boals, A., & Schuettler, D. (2011). The unique contributions of positive and negative religious coping to posttraumatic growth and PTSD. *Psychology of Religion and Spirituality, 3*(4), 298–307.

Gervais, W. M., Shariff, A. F., & Norenzayan, A. (2011). Do you believe in atheists? Distrust is central to anti-atheist prejudice. *Journal of Personality and Social Psychology, 101*(6), 1189–1206.

Ghaempanah, Z., Rafieinia, P., Sabahi, P., Hosseini, S. M., & Memaryan, N. (2020). Spiritual problems of women with breast cancer in Iran: A qualitative study. *Health, Spirituality, and Medical Ethics, 7*(1), 9–15.

Gilbert, P. (2010). *Compassion focused therapy.* New York: Routledge.

Goldhagen, D. J. (2013). *The devil that never dies: The rise and threat of global antisemitism.* New York: Little, Brown.

Goodman, M., Rubinstein, R. L., Alexander, B. B., & Luborsky, M. (1991). Cultural differences among elderly women in coping with the death of an adult child. *Journal of Gerontology: Social Sciences, 46*(6), S321–S329.

Grand, S. (2000). *The reproduction of evil: A clinical and cultural perspective.* New York: Analytic Press.

Granqvist, P., & Kirkpatrick, L. A. (2013). Religion, spirituality, and attachment. In K. I. Pargament, J. J. Exline, & J. W. Jones (Eds.), *APA handbook of psychology, religion, and spirituality (Vol. 1): Context, theory, and research* (pp. 139–155). Washington, DC: American Psychological Association.

Green, L. L., Fullilove, M. T., & Fullilove, R. E. (1998). Stories of spiritual awakening: The nature of spirituality in recovery. *Journal of Substance Abuse Treatment, 15*(4), 325–331.

Greenberg, D., & Huppert, J. D. (2010). Scrupulosity: A unique subtype of obsessive–compulsive disorder. *Current Psychiatry Reports, 12*(4), 282–289.

Greenberg, D., & Witztum, E. (2001). S*anity and sanctity: Mental health work among the ultra-orthodox in Jerusalem.* New Haven, CT: Yale University Press.

Greene, B. (1983, December 1). Muhammed Ali is the most famous man in the world: Now begins the toughest fight of his career. *Esquire*, 134–136, 139–142.

Greene, J. M. (2007). *Here comes the sun: The spiritual and musical journey of George Harrison.* New York: Wiley.

Griffith, J. L. (2010). *Religion that heals, religion that harms: A guide for clinical practice.* New York: Guilford Press.

Griffith, J. L., & Griffith, M. E. (2002). *Encountering the sacred in psychotherapy: How to talk with people about their spiritual lives.* New York: Guilford Press.

Groopman, J. (2004). *The anatomy of hope: How people prevail in the face of illness.* New York: Random House.

Grubbs, J. B., & Exline, J. J. (2014). Why did God make me this way? Anger at God in the context of personal transgressions. *Journal of Psychology and Theology, 42*(4), 315–325.

Grubbs, J. B., Exline, J. J., Pargament, K. I., Volk, F., & Lindberg, M. J. (2017). Internet pornography use, perceived addiction, and religious/spiritual struggles. *Archives of Sexual Behavior, 46*(6), 1733–1745.

Grubbs, J. B., Perry S. L., Wilt, J. A., & Reid, R. C. (2019). Pornography problems due to moral incongruence: An integrative model with a systematic review and meta-analysis. *Archives of Sexual Behavior, 48*(2), 397–415.

Grubbs, J. B., Wilt, J. A., Stauner, N., Exline, J. J., & Pargament, K. I. (2016). Self, struggle, and soul: Linking personality, self-concept, and religious/spiritual struggle. *Personality and Individual Differences, 101*, 144–152.

Gutierrez, I. A., Chapman, H., Grubbs, J. B., & Grant, J. (2020). Religious and spiritual struggles among military veterans in a residential gambling treatment programme. *Mental Health, Religion and Culture, 23*(2), 187–203.

Gutierrez, I. A., Park, C. L., & Wright, B. R. E. (2017). When the divine defaults: Religious struggle mediates the impact of financial stressors on psychological distress. *Psychology of Religion and Spirituality, 9*(4), 387–398.

Haar, J. M., Russo, M., Suñe, A., & Ollier-Malaterre, A. (2014). Outcomes of work–life balance on job satisfaction, life satisfaction, and mental health: A study across seven cultures. *Journal of Vocational Behavior, 85*(3), 361–373.

Haggar, M. S., Wood, C., Stiff, C., & Chatzisarantis, N. L. (2010). Ego depletion and the strength model of self-control: A meta-analysis. *Psychological Bulletin, 136*(4), 495–525.

Haidt, J. (2003). Elevation and the positive psychology of morality. In C. L. M. Keyes & J. Haidt (Eds.), *Flourishing: Positive psychology and the life well lived* (pp. 275–289). Washington, DC: American Psychological Association.

Haines, S. J., Gleeson, J., Kuppens, P., Hollenstein, T., Ciarrochi, J., Labuschagne, I., et al. (2016). The wisdom to know the difference: Strategy–situation fit in emotion regulation in daily life is associated with well-being. *Psychological Science, 27*(12), 1651–1659.

Hale-Smith, A., Park, C. L., & Edmondson, D. (2012). Measuring beliefs about suffering: Development of the Views of Suffering Scale. *Psychological Assessment, 24*(4), 855–866.

Hall, D. L., Matz, D. C., & Wood, W. (2010). Why don't we practice what we preach? A meta-analytic review of religious racism. *Personality and Social Psychology Review, 14*(1), 126–139.

Hall, T. W., & Fujikawa, A. M. (2013). God image and the sacred. In K. I. Pargament, J. J. Exline, & J. W. Jones (Eds.), *APA handbook of psychology, religion, and spirituality (Vol. 1): Context, theory, and research* (pp. 277–292). Washington, DC: American Psychological Association.

Hanh, T. N. (2001). *Call me by my true names: The collected poems of Thich Nhat Hanh.* Berkeley, CA: Parallax Press.

Haque, A., & Keshavarzi, H. (2014). Integrating indigenous healing methods in therapy: Muslim beliefs and practices. *International Journal of Culture and Mental Health, 7*(3), 297–314.

Harari, Y. N. (2014). *Sapiens: A brief history of humankind.* New York: Vintage.

Hardy, A. (1979). *The spiritual nature of man: A study of contemporary religious experience.* Oxford, UK: Clarendon Press.

Harris Interactive (2008, December 10). More people believe in the devil, hell and angels than in Darwin's theory of evolution: Nearly 25% of Americans believe they were once another person. Retrieved from *https://theharrispoll.com/wp-content/uploads/2017/12/Harris-Interactive-Poll-Research-Religious-Beliefs-2008-12.pdf*.

Harris, J. I., Erbes, C. R., Engdahl, B. E., Ogden, H., Olson, R. H. A., Winskowski, A. M. M., et al. (2012). Religious distress and coping with stressful life events: A longitudinal study. *Journal of Clinical Psychology, 68*(12), 1276–1286.

Harris, J. I., Erbes, C. R., Engdahl, B. E., Thuras, P., Murray-Swank, N., Grace, D., et al. (2011). The effectiveness of a trauma-focused spiritually integrated intervention for veterans exposed to trauma. *Journal of Clinical Psychology, 67*(4), 425–438.

Harris, J. I., Erbes, C. R., Winskowski, A. M., Engdahl, B. E., & Nguyen, X. V. (2014). Social support as a mediator in the relationship between religious comforts and strains and trauma symptoms. *Psychology of Religion and Spirituality, 6*(3), 223–229.

Harris, J. I., Meis, L., Cheng, Z. H., Voecks, C., Usset, T., & Sherman, M. (2017). Spiritual distress and dyadic adjustment in veterans and partners managing PTSD. *Spirituality in Clinical Practice, 4*(4), 229–237.

Harris, J. I., Park, C. L., Currier, J. M., Usset, T. J., & Voecks, C. D. (2015). Moral injury and psycho-spiritual development: Considering the developmental context. *Spirituality in Clinical Practice, 2*(4), 256–266.

Harris, J. I., Usset, T., Krause, L., Schill, D., Reuer, B., Donahue, R., et al. (2018). Spiritual/religious distress is associated with pain catastrophizing and interference in veterans with chronic pain. *Pain Medicine, 19*(4), 757–763.

Hart, A. C., Pargament, K. I., Grubbs, J. B., Exline, J. J., & Wilt, J. A. (2020). Predictors of self-reported growth following religious and spiritual struggles: Exploring the role of wholeness. *Religions, 11*(9), 445.

Hartog, K., & Gow, K. M. (2005). Religious attributions pertaining to the causes and cures of mental illness. *Mental Health, Religion and Culture, 8*(4), 263–276.

Haugen, M. R. G. (2011). *Does trauma lead to religiousness? A longitudinal study of the effects of traumatic events on religion and spirituality during the first three years at university* (Unpublished doctoral dissertation). Bowling Green State University, Bowling Green, OH.

Haugk, K. C. (2004). *Don't sing songs to a heavy heart: How to relate to those who are suffering*. St. Louis, MO: Stephen Ministries.

Hawking, S. (1988). *A brief history of time: From big bang to black holes*. New York: Bantam Books.

Hayes, S. C., Strosahl, K. D., & Wilson, K. G. (2016). *Acceptance and commitment therapy: An experiential approach to behavior change* (2nd ed.). New York: Guilford Press.

Hecht, J. M. (2003). *Doubt: A history. The great doubters and their legacy of innovation from Socrates and Jesus to Thomas Jefferson and Emily Dickinson*. New York: HarperOne.

Held, P., Klassen, B. J., Hall, J. M., Friese, T. R., Bertsch-Gout, M. M., Zalta, A. K., et al. (2019). "I knew it was wrong the moment I got the order": A narrative thematic analysis of moral injury in combat veterans. *Psychological Trauma: Theory, Research, Practice, and Policy, 11*(4), 396–405.

Helgeson, V. S., Reynolds, K. A., & Tomich, P. L. (2006). A meta-analytic review of benefit finding and growth. *Journal of Consulting and Clinical Psychology, 74*(5), 797–816.

Henning, K. R., & Frueh, B. C. (1997). Combat guilt and its relationship to PTSD symptoms. *Journal of Clinical Psychology, 53*(8), 801–808.

Herman, J. L. (1992/1997). *Trauma and recovery: The aftermath of violence—from domestic abuse to political terror.* New York: Basic Books.

Hodge, D. R. (2001). Spiritual assessment: A review of major qualitative methods and a new framework for assessing spirituality. *Social Work, 46*(3), 203–214.

Hodge, D. R. (2004). Working with Hindu clients in a spiritually sensitive manner. *Social Work, 49*(1), 27–38.

Hofmann, W., Vohs, K. D., & Baumeister, R. F. (2012). What people desire, feel conflicted about, and try to resist in everyday life. *Psychological Science, 23*(6), 582–588.

Holley, D. M. (2011). How can a believer doubt that God exists? *Philosophical Quarterly, 61*(245), 746–761.

Hood, R. W., Jr. (2003). The relationship between religion and spirituality. In A. L. Greil & D. G. Bromley (Eds.), *Defining religion: Investigating the boundaries between the sacred and secular* (Vol. 10, pp. 241–264). Bingley, UK: Emerald Group.

Hornbacher, M. (1999). *Wasted: A memoir of anorexia and bulimia.* New York: Harper Collins.

Horvath, A. O., Del Re, A. C., Flückiger, C., & Symonds, D. (2011). Alliance in individual psychotherapy. *Psychotherapy, 48*(1), 9–16.

Hunsberger, B., McKenzie, B., Pratt, M., & Pancer, S. M. (1993). Religious doubt: A social psychological analysis. *Research in the Social Scientific Study of Religion, 5*, 27–51.

Hunsberger, B., Pratt, M., & Pancer, S. M. (2001). Adolescent identity formation: Religious exploration and commitment. *Identity: An International Journal of Theory and Research, 1*(4), 365–386.

Hunsberger, B., Pratt, M., & Pancer, S. M. (2002). A longitudinal study of religious doubts in high school and beyond: Relationships, stability, and searching for answers. *Journal for the Scientific Study of Religion, 41*(2), 255–266.

Huppert, J. D., & Siev, J. (2010). Treating scrupulosity in religious individuals using cognitive-behavioral therapy. *Cognitive and Behavioral Practice, 17*(4), 382–392.

Idliby, R., Oliver, S., & Warner, P. (2007). *The faith club: A Muslim, a Christian, a Jew—three women search for understanding.* New York: Free Press.

Ingber, H. (2019, December 24). "My Jewish sons have a Christmas tree, and I need to deal." *New York Times.* Retrieved from *www.nytimes.com/2019/12/24/opinion/ christmas-hanukkah-divorce.html?searchResultPosition=1.*

Ironson, G., Kremer, H., & Lucette, A. (2016). Relationship between spiritual coping and survival in patients with HIV. *Journal of General Internal Medicine, 31*(9), 1068–1076.

Ironson, G., Stuetzle, R., Fletcher, M. A., & Ironson, D. (2006). View of God is associated with disease progression in HIV. *Annals of Behavior Medicine, 3*(Suppl.), S074.

Ironson, G., Stuetzle, R., Ironson, D., Balbin, E., Kremer, H., George, A., et al. (2011). View of God as benevolent and forgiving or punishing and judgmental predicts HIV disease progression. *Journal of Behavioral Medicine, 34*(6), 414–425.

James, F. A., III. (2010). In the shadow of Mount Hood: Meeting God in the mystery of grief. *Christianity Today, 54*(9), 57–60.

James, W. (1902). *The varieties of religious experience: A study in human nature.* New York: Modern Library.

Janoff-Bulman, R. (1992). *Shattered assumptions: Towards a new psychology of trauma.* New York: Free Press.

Janoff-Bulman, R., & Frantz, C. M. (1997). The impact of trauma on meaning: From meaningless world to meaningful life. In M. J. Power & C. R. Brewin (Eds.), *The transformation of meaning in psychological therapies: Integrating theory and practice* (pp. 91–106). Chichester, UK: Wiley.

Janů, A., Malinakova, K., Kosarkova, A., & Tavel, P. (2020). Associations of childhood trauma experiences with religious and spiritual struggles. *Journal of Health Psychology.* Advance online publication.

Jayawickreme, E., & Blackie, L. E. R. (2014). Post-traumatic growth as positive personality change: Evidence, controversies, and future directions. *European Journal of Personality, 28*(4), 312–331.

Jeffries, W. L., IV, Dodge, B., & Sandfort, T. G. M. (2008). Religion and spirituality among bisexual black men in the USA. *Culture, Health, and Sexuality, 10*(5), 463–477.

Jensen, L. A. (2009). Conceptions of God and the Devil across the lifespan: A cultural-developmental study of religious liberals and conservatives. *Journal for the Scientific Study of Religion, 48*(1), 121–145.

Johnson, C. V., & Hayes, J. A. (2003). Troubled spirits: Prevalence and predictors of religious and spiritual concerns among university students and counseling center clients. *Journal of Counseling Psychology, 50*(4), 409–419.

Johnson, S. K., & Armour, M. P. (2016). Finding strength, comfort, and purpose in spirituality after homicide. *Psychology of Religion and Spirituality, 8*(4), 277–288.

Johnson, T. H. (Ed.). (1960). *The complete poems of Emily Dickinson.* New York: Little, Brown.

Jones, J. W. (1991). *Contemporary psychoanalysis and religion: Transference and transcendence.* New Haven, CT: Yale University Press.

Jones, J. W. (2002). *Terror and transformation: The ambiguity of religion in psychoanalytic perspective.* London: Routledge.

Jones, R. S. (2019). *Spirit in session: Working with your client's spirituality (and your own) in psychotherapy.* West Conshohocken, PA: Templeton Press.

Jones, S. L. (1994). A constructive relationship for religion with the science and profession of psychology: Perhaps the boldest model yet. *American Psychologist, 49*(3), 184–199.

Jouriles, E. N., Rancher, C., Mahoney, A., Kurth, C., Cook, K., & McDonald, R. (2020). Divine spiritual struggles and psychological adjustment among adolescents who have been sexually abused. *Psychology of Violence, 10*(3), 334–343.

Juergensmeyer, M. (2000). *Terror in the mind of God: The global rise of religious violence.* Los Angeles: University of California Press.

Jung, C. G. (1985). *The practice of psychotherapy* (G. Adler & R. F. C. Hull, Trans.). Princeton, NJ: Princeton University Press. (Original work published 1954)

Jung, J. H. (2020). Does religious bonding moderate the association between divine struggles and depressive symptoms among married adults? *Psychology of Religion and Spirituality, 12*(3), 376–386.

Kane, M. N. (2010). Perceptions about the ridicule of religious and spiritual beliefs. *Journal of Contemporary Religion, 25*(3), 453–462.

Kao, L. E., Shah, S. B., Pargament, K. I., Griffith, J. L., & Peteet, J. R. (2019). "Gambling with God": A self-inflicted gunshot wound with religious motivation in the context of a mixed-mood episode. *Harvard Review of Psychiatry, 27*(1), 65–72.

Kaplan, A. (1964). *The conduct of inquiry: Methodology for behavioral science.* San Francisco: Chandler.

Karff, S. E. (1979). *Agada: The language of Jewish faith.* Cincinnati, OH: Hebrew Union College Press.

Karff, S. E. (2015). *For this you were created: Memoir of an American rabbi.* Houston, TX: Bright Sky Press.

Kashdan, T. B., & Rottenberg, J. (2010). Psychological flexibility as a fundamental aspect of health. *Clinical Psychology Review, 30*(7), 865–878.

Kass, J. D. (2017). *A person-centered approach to psychospiritual maturation: Mentoring psychological resilience and inclusive community in higher education.* New York: Palgrave Macmillan.

Keng, S.-L., Smoski, M. J., & Robins, C. J. (2011). Effects of mindfulness on psychological health: A review of empirical studies. *Clinical Psychology Review, 31*(6), 1041–1056.

Kesebir, P., & Kesebir, S. (2012). The cultural salience of moral character and virtue declined in twentieth century America. *Journal of Positive Psychology, 7*(6), 471–480.

Kézdy, A., Martos, T., Boland, V., & Horváth-Szabó, K. (2011). Religious doubts and mental health in adolescence and young adulthood: The association with religious attitudes. *Journal of Adolescence, 34*(1), 39–47.

Khan, Z. H., Sultana, S., & Watson, P. J. (2009). Pakistani Muslims dealing with cancer: Relationships with religious coping, religious orientation, and psychological distress. *Research in the Social Scientific Study of Religion, 20,* 217–237.

Kidd, S. M. (2016). *When the heart waits: Spiritual direction for life's sacred questions.* New York: HarperOne.

Kinder, D. R., & Kam, C. D. (2009). *Us against them: Ethnocentric foundations of American opinion.* Chicago: University of Chicago Press.

King, L. A., Heintzelman, S. J., & Ward, S. J. (2016). Beyond the search for meaning: A contemporary science of the experience of meaning in life. *Current Directions in Psychological Science, 25*(4), 211–216.

King, L. A., Scollon, C. K., Ramsey, C., & Williams, T. (2000). Stories of life transition: Subjective well-being and ego development in parents of children with Down syndrome. *Journal of Research in Personality, 34*(4), 509–536.

King, S. D. W., Fitchett, G., & Berry, D. L. (2013). Screening for religious/spiritual struggle in blood and marrow transplant patients. *Journal of Supportive Care in Cancer, 21*(4), 993–1001.

King, S. D. W., Fitchett, G., Murphy, P. E., Pargament, K. I., Harrison, D. A., & Loggers, E. T. (2017). Determining best methods to screen for religious/spiritual distress. *Journal of Supportive Care for Cancer, 25*(2), 471–479.

King, S. D. W., Fitchett, G., Murphy, P. E., Pargament, K. I., Martin, P. J., Johnson, R. H., et al. (2017). Spiritual or religious struggle in hematopoietic cell transplant survivors. *Psycho-Oncology, 26*(2), 270–277.

King, S. D., Fitchett, G., Murphy, P. E., Rajaee, G., Pargament, K. I., Loggers, E. T., et al. (2018). Religious/spiritual struggle in young adult hematopoietic cell transplant survivors. *Journal of Adolescent and Young Adult Oncology, 7*(2), 210–216.

Kirkpatrick, L. A. (2005). *Attachment, evolution, and the psychology of religion.* New York: Guilford Press.

Kirvan, J. (1999). *God hunger: Discovering the mystic in all of us.* Notre Dame, IN: Sorin Books.

Kitchens, M. B. (2015). Thinking about God causes internal reflection in believers and unbelievers. *Self and Identity, 14*(6), 724–747.

Klass, D. (1988). *Parental grief: Solace and resolution*. New York: Springer.

Koenig, H. G. (2018a). *Religion and mental health: Research and clinical applications*. New York: Elsevier.

Koenig, H. G. (2018b). Measuring symptoms of moral injury in veterans and active duty military with PTSD. *Religions, 9*(3), 86.

Koenig, H. G., King, D. E., & Carson, V. B. (2012). *Handbook of religion and health* (2nd ed.). New York: Oxford University Press.

Kojetin, B. A., McIntosh, D. N., Bridges, R. A., & Spilka, B. (1987). Quest: Constructive search or religious conflict? *Journal for the Scientific Study of Religion, 26*(1), 111–115.

Kooistra, W. P. (1990). *An empirical examination of religious doubt among Christian adolescents* (Unpublished doctoral dissertation). Bowling Green State University, Bowling Green, OH.

Kooistra, W. P., & Pargament, K. I. (1999). Religious doubting in parochial school adolescents. *Journal of Psychology and Theology, 27*(1), 33–42.

Kopacz, M. S., & Connery, A. L. (2015). The veteran spiritual struggle. *Spirituality in Clinical Practice, 2*(1), 61–67.

Korbman, M. D., Pirutinsky, S., Feindler, E. L., & Rosmarin, D. H. (2021). Childhood sexual abuse, spirituality/religion, anxiety and depression in a Jewish community sample: The mediating role of religious coping. *Journal of Interpersonal Violence*. Advanced online publication.

Kornfield, J. (1993). *A path with heart: A guide through the perils and promises of spiritual life*. New York: Bantam Books.

Krause, N. (2006). Religious doubt and psychological well-being: A longitudinal investigation. *Review of Religious Research, 47*(3), 287–302.

Krause, N., Chatters, L. M., Meltzer, T., & Morgan, D. L. (2000). Negative interaction in the church: Insights from focus groups with older adults. *Review of Religious Research, 41*(4), 510–533.

Krause, N., & Ellison. C. G. (2009). The doubting process: A longitudinal study of the precipitants and consequences of religious doubt in older adults. *Journal for the Scientific Study of Religion, 48*(2), 293–312.

Krause, N., & Hayward, R. D. (2012a). Humility, lifetime trauma, and change in religious doubt among older adults. *Journal of Religion and Health, 51*(4), 1002–1016.

Krause, N., & Hayward, R. D. (2012b). Negative interaction with fellow church members and depressive symptoms among older Mexican Americans. *Archive for the Psychology of Religion, 34*(2), 149–171.

Krause, N., & Hayward, R. D. (2012c). Religion, meaning in life, and change in physical functioning during late adulthood. *Journal of Adult Development, 19*(3), 158–169.

Krause, N., Pargament, K. I., Hill, P. C., Wong, S., & Ironson. G. (2017). Exploring the relationships among age, spiritual struggles, and health. *Journal of Religion, Spirituality and Aging, 29*(4), 266–285.

Krause, N., Pargament, K. I., Hill, P. C., & Ironson, G. (2020). Exploring religious and/or spiritual identities: Part 1. Assessing relationships with health. *Mental Health, Religion and Culture, 22*(9), 877–891.

Krause, N., Pargament, K. I., & Ironson, G. (2017). Spiritual struggles and health: Assessing the influence of socioeconomic status. *Journal for the Scientific Study of Religion, 56*(3), 620–636.

Krause, N., Pargament, K. I., Hill, P. C., & Ironson, G. (2018). Spiritual struggles and problem drinking: Are younger adults at greater risk than older adults? *Substance Use and Misuse, 53*(5), 808–815.

Krause, N., Pargament, K. I., Ironson, G., & Hill, P. C. (2017). Religious involvement, financial strain, and poly-drug use: Exploring the moderating role of meaning in life. *Substance Use and Misuse, 52*(3), 286–293.

Krause, N., & Wulff, K. M. (2004). Religious doubt and health: Exploring the potential dark side of religion. *Sociology of Religion, 65*(1), 35–56.

Krok, D., Brudek, P., & Steuden, S. (2019). When meaning matters: Coping mediates the relationship of religiosity and illness appraisals with well-being in older cancer patients. *International Journal for the Psychology of Religion, 29*(1), 46–60.

Krumrei, E. J., Mahoney, A., & Pargament, K. I. (2011). Spiritual stress and coping model of divorce: A longitudinal study. *Journal of Family Psychology, 25*(6), 973–985.

Kübler-Ross, E. (1975). *Death: The final stage of growth.* New York: Simon & Schuster.

Kunda, Z. (1990). The case for motivated reasoning. *Psychological Bulletin, 108*(3), 480–498.

Kunst, J. R., Kimel, S. Y., Shani, M., Alayan, R., & Thomsen, L. (2019). Can Abraham bring peace? The relationship between acknowledging shared religious roots and intergroup conflict. *Psychology of Religion and Spirituality, 11*(4), 417–432.

Küpper, B., & Zick, A. (2010). *Religion and prejudice in Europe: New empirical findings.* London: Alliance Publishing Trust.

Kurtz, E. (2007). *Shame and guilt.* New York: iUniverse.

Kurtz, E., & Ketcham, K. (1992). *The spirituality of imperfection: Storytelling and the search for meaning.* New York: Bantam Books.

Kushner, H. S. (1981). *When bad things happen to good people.* New York: Schocken Books.

Kushner, H. S. (1989). *Who needs God.* New York: Fireside.

Kusner, K. G., Mahoney, A., Pargament, K. I., & DeMaris, A. (2014). Sanctification of marriage and spiritual intimacy predicting observed marital interactions across the transition to parenthood. *Journal of Family Psychology, 28*(5), 604–614.

Kvande, M. N., Klöckner, C. A., Moksnes, U. K., & Espnes, G. A. (2015). Do optimism and pessimism mediate the relationship between religious coping and existential well-being? Examining mechanisms in a Norwegian population sample. *International Journal for the Psychology of Religion, 25*(2), 130–151.

LaMothe, R. (1998). Sacred objects as vital objects: Transitional objects reconsidered. *Journal of Psychology and Theology, 26*(2), 159–167.

LaMothe, R. (2009). The clash of Gods: Changes in a patient's use of God representations. *Journal of the American Academy of Psychoanalysis and Dynamic Psychiatry, 37*(1), 73–84.

Lane, C. (2011). *The age of doubt: Tracing the roots of our religious uncertainty.* New Haven, CT: Yale University Press.

Latzer, Y., Weinberger-Litman, S. L., Gerson, B., Rosch, A., Mischel, R., Hinden, T., et al. (2015). Negative religious coping predicts disordered eating pathology among Orthodox Jewish adolescent girls. *Journal of Religion and Health, 54*(5), 1760–1771.

Lauricella, S. K., Phillips, R. E., III, & Dubow, E. F. (2017). Religious coping with sexual stigma in young adults with same-sex attractions. *Journal of Religion and Health, 56*(4), 1436–1449.

Laycock, J. P. (Ed.). (2015). *Spirit possession around the world: Possession, communion, and demon expulsion across cultures.* Santa Barbara, CA: ABC-CLIO.

Lazarus, R. S., & Folkman, S. (1984). *Stress, appraisal, and coping.* New York: Springer.

Leaman, S. C., & Gee, C. B. (2012). Religious coping and risk factors for psychological distress among African torture survivors. *Psychological Trauma: Theory, Research, Practice, and Policy, 4*(5), 457–465.

Leavey, G. (2010). The appreciation of the spiritual in mental illness: A qualitative study of beliefs among clergy in the U.K. *Transcultural Psychiatry, 47*(4), 571–590.

Lee, M., Nezu, A. M., & Nezu, C. M. (2014). Positive and negative religious coping, depressive symptoms, and quality of life in people with HIV. *Journal of Behavioral Medicine, 37*(5), 921–930.

Lee, S. A., Roberts, L. B., & Gibbons, J. A. (2013). When religion makes grief worse: Negative religious coping as associated with maladaptive emotional responding patterns. *Mental Health, Religion and Culture, 16*(3), 291–305.

Lehman, D. R., Wortman, C. B., & Williams, A. F. (1987). Long-term effects of losing a spouse or child in a motor vehicle crash. *Journal of Personality and Social Psychology, 52*(1), 218–231.

Lerner, M. (1994). *Jewish renewal: A path to healing and transformation.* New York: Grosset/Putnam.

Lewis, C. S. (1955). *Surprised by joy: The shape of my early life.* New York: Harcourt Brace.

Lewis, C. S. (1961). *A grief observed.* London: Faber and Faber.

Lewis, C. S. (1982). *The Screwtape letters.* Bantam. (Original work published 1942)

Liebert, E. (2008). *The way of discernment: Spiritual practices for decision making.* Louisville, KY: Westminster John Knox.

Lim, A., Hoek, H. W., & Blom, J. D. (2015). The attribution of psychotic symptoms to jinn in Islamic patients. *Transcultural Psychiatry, 52*(1), 18–32.

Lin, C. Y., Saffari, M., Koenig, H. G., & Pakpour, A. H. (2018). Effects of religiosity and religious coping on medication adherence and quality of life among people with epilepsy. *Epilepsy and Behavior, 78*, 45–51.

Lindsay, E. K., Young, S., Smyth, J. M., Brown, K. W., & Creswell, J. D. (2018). Acceptance lowers stress reactivity: Dismantling mindfulness training in a randomized controlled trial. *Psychoneuroendocrinology, 87*, 63–73.

Linley, P. A., & Joseph, S. (2004). Positive change following trauma and adversity: A review. *Journal of Traumatic Stress, 17*(1), 11–21.

Lipsyte, R. (2016). The greatest. *Time, 187*(23), 20–44.

Litz, B. T., Stein, N., Delaney, E., Lebowitz, L., Nash, W. P., Silva, C., et al. (2009). Moral injury and moral repair in war veterans: A preliminary model and intervention strategy. *Clinical Psychology Review, 29*(8), 695–706.

Loevinger, J. (1976). *Ego development: Conceptions and theories.* San Francisco: Jossey-Bass.

Loewenthal, K. M. (2019). EMDR—eye movement desensitization and reprocessing therapy and religious faith among orthodox Jewish (Haredi) women. *Israeli Journal of Psychiatry, 56*(2), 20–27.

Lomax, J. W., & Pargament, K. I. (2011). Seeking "sacred moments" in psychotherapy and in life. *Psyche and Geloof, 22*(2), 79–90.

Lord, B. D., & Gramling, S. E. (2014). Patterns of religious coping among bereaved college students. *Journal of Religion and Health, 53*(1), 157–177.

Lupfer, M. B., Tolliver, D., & Jackson, M. (1996). Explaining life-altering occurrences: A test of the "God-of-the-gaps" hypothesis. *Journal for the Scientific Study of Religion, 35*(4), 379–391.

Luzzatto, M. C. (1997). *The way of God: Derech hashem* (A. Kaplan, Trans.). Nanuet, NY: Feldheim.

Lynberg, M. (2001). *Make each day your masterpiece: Practical wisdom for living an exceptional life.* Kansas City, MO: Andrews McMeel.

Lynch, T. R. (2018). *Radically open dialectical behavior therapy: Theory and practice for treating disorders of overcontrol.* New York: Context Press.

Lyons, M. E., Garvie, P. A., Kao, E., Briggs, L., He, J., Malow, R., et al. (2011). Spirituality in HIV-infected adolescents and their families: FAmily CEntered (FACE) Advance Care Planning and medication adherence. *Journal of Adolescent Health, 48*(6), 633–636.

Ma, Y-Y. (2016, March 3). Music happens between the notes. *On being.* Retrieved from *https://onbeing.org/programs/yo-yo-ma-music-happens-between-the-notes.*

Maercker, A., & Zoellner, T. (2004). The Janus face of self-perceived growth: Toward a two-component model of posttraumatic growth. *Psychological Inquiry, 15*(1), 41–48.

Magyar-Russell, G., Brown, I. T., Edara, I. R., Smith, M. T., Marine, J. E., & Ziegelstein, R. C. (2014). In search of serenity: Religious struggle among patients hospitalized for suspected acute coronary syndrome. *Journal of Religion and Health, 53*(2), 562–578.

Magyar-Russell, G., Pargament, K. I., Grubbs, J. B., Wilt, J. A., & Exline, J. J. (2020). The experience of sacred moments and mental health benefits over time. *Psychology of Religion and Spirituality.* Advance online publication.

Magyar-Russell, G., Pargament, K. I., Trevino, K. M., & Sherman, J. E. (2013). Religious and spiritual appraisals and coping strategies among patients in medical rehabilitation. *Research in the Social Scientific Study of Religion, 24*, 93–135.

Mahoney, A. (2005). Religion and conflict in marital and parent–child relationships. *Journal of Social Issues, 61*(4), 689–706.

Mahoney, A. (2013). The spirituality of us: Relational spirituality in the context of family relationships. In K. I. Pargament, J. J. Exline, & J. W. Jones (Eds.), *APA handbook of psychology, religion, and spirituality (Vol. 1): Context, theory, and research* (pp. 365–389). Washington, DC: American Psychological Association.

Mahoney, A., Abadi, L., & Pargament, K. I. (2015). Exploring women's spiritual struggles and resources to cope with intimate partner aggression. In A. J. Johnson (Ed.), *Religion and men's violence against women* (pp. 45–59). New York: Springer Science.

Mahoney, A., Pargament, K. I., Cole, B., Jewell, T., Magyar, G., Tarakeshwar, N., et al. (2005). A higher purpose: The sanctification of strivings in a community sample. *International Journal for the Psychology of Religion, 15*(3), 239–262.

Mahoney, A., Pargament, K. I., & DeMaris, A. (2019, November). *Couples' spiritual intimacy and one-upmanship predicting marital conflict across the transition to parenthood.* Paper presented at the meeting of the Association for Behavioral and Cognitive Therapies, Atlanta, GA.

Mahoney, A., Pargament, K. I., & Hernandez, K. M. (2013). Heaven on earth: Beneficial effects of sanctification for individual and interpersonal well-being. In S. A. David, I. Boniwell, & A. C. Ayers (Eds.), *Oxford book of happiness* (pp. 397–410). Oxford, UK: Oxford University Press.

Mahoney, A., Wong, S., Pomerleau, J. M., & Pargament, K. I. (2021). Sanctification of diverse aspects of life and psychosocial functioning: A meta-analysis of studies from 1999 to 2019. *Psychology of Religion and Spirituality.* Advance online publication.

Maltby, J., Lewis, C. A., Freeman, A., Day, L., Cruise, S. M., & Breslin, M. J. (2010). Religion and health: The application of a cognitive-behavioural framework. *Mental Health, Religion and Culture, 13*(7), 749–759.

Maltby, L. E., & Hall, T. W. (2012). Trauma, attachment and spirituality: A case study. *Journal of Psychology and Theology, 40*(4), 302–312.

Mandela, N. (1994). *Long walk to freedom: The autobiography of Nelson Mandela.* New York: Little, Brown.

Marcia, J. E. (1966). Development and validation of ego-identity status. *Journal of Personality and Social Psychology, 3*(5), 551–558.

Markman, H. J., Renick, M. J., Floyd, F. J., Stanley, S. M., & Clements, M. (1993). Preventing marital distress through communication and conflict management training: A 4- and 5-year follow-up. *Journal of Consulting and Clinical Psychology, 61*(1), 70–77.

Marks, L. D., Dollahite, D. C., & Young, K. P. (2019). Struggles experienced by religious minority families in the United States. *Psychology of Religion and Spirituality, 11*(3), 247–256.

Martela, F., & Steger, M. F. (2016). The three meanings of meaning in life: Distinguishing coherence, purpose, and significance. *Journal of Positive Psychology, 11*(5), 531–545.

Martin, J. (2006). *My life with the saints.* Chicago: Loyola Press.

Martínez-Taboas, A. (2018). The case of the shaking legs: Somatoform dissociation and spiritual struggles. *Frontiers in the Psychotherapy of Trauma and Dissociation, 1*(2), 124–134.

Marty, M. E. (1983). *A cry of absence: Reflections for the winter of the heart.* Grand Rapids, MI: Eerdmans.

Maslow, A. H. (1970). *Motivation and personality* (2nd ed.). New York: Harper & Row.

Maunu, A., & Stein, C. H. (2010). Coping with the personal loss of having a parent with mental illness: Young adults' narrative accounts of spiritual struggle and strength. *Journal of Community Psychology, 38*(5), 645–655.

May, R. (1969). *Love and will.* New York: Norton.

McAdams, D. P. (2013). *The redemptive self: Stories Americans live by.* Oxford, UK: Oxford University Press.

McCabe, G. (2008). Mind, body, emotions and spirit: Reaching to the ancestors for healing. *Counselling Psychology Quarterly, 21*(2), 143–152.

McCleary-Gaddy, A. T., & Miller, C. T. (2019). Negative religious coping as a mediator between perceived prejudice and psychological distress among African Americans: A structural equation modeling approach. *Psychology of Religion and Spirituality, 11*(3), 257–265.

McConnell, K. M., Pargament, K. I., Ellison, C. G., & Flannelly, K. J. (2006). Examining the links between spiritual struggles and symptoms of psychopathology in a national sample. *Journal of Clinical Psychology, 62*(12), 1469–1484.

McCormick, W. H., Carroll, T. D., Sims, B. M., & Currier, J. (2017). Adverse childhood experiences, religious/spiritual struggles, and mental health symptoms: Examination of mediation models. *Mental Health, Religion and Culture, 20*(10), 1042–1054.

McCullough, M. E., & Carter, E. C. (2013). Religion, self-control, and self-regulation: How and why are they related? In K. I. Pargament, J. J. Exline, & J. W. Jones (Eds.), *APA handbook of psychology, religion, and spirituality (Vol. 1): Context, theory and research* (pp. 123–138). Washington, DC: American Psychological Association Press.

McFarland, C., & Alvaro, C. (2000). The impact of motivation on temporal comparisons: Coping with traumatic events by perceiving personal growth. *Journal of Personality and Social Psychology, 79*(3), 327–343.

McGee, J. S., Myers, D. R., Carlson, H., Funai, A. P., & Barclay, P. A. (2013). Spirituality, faith, and mild Alzheimer's disease. *Research in the Social Scientific Study of Religion, 24*, 221–257.

McGee, J. S., Zhao, H. C., Myers, D. R., & Eaton, H. S. (2018). Spiritual diversity and living with early-stage dementia. *Clinical Gerontologist, 41*(3), 261–267.

McIntosh, D. N. (1995). Religion-as-schema, with implications for the relation between religion and coping. *International Journal for the Psychology of Religion, 5*(1), 1–16.

McIntosh, D. N., Inglehart, M. R., & Pacini, R. (1990). *Flexible and central religious belief systems and adjustment to college.* Paper presented at the meeting of the Midwestern Psychological Association, Chicago, IL.

McKay, R., Herold, J., & Whitehouse, H. (2013). Catholic guilt? Recall of confession promotes prosocial behavior. *Religion, Brain and Behavior, 3*(3), 201–209.

McMillen, J. C., Smith, E. M., &. Fisher, R. H. (1997). Perceived benefit and mental health after three types of disaster. *Journal of Consulting and Clinical Psychology, 65*(5), 733–739.

McNamara, P. (2011). *Spirit possession and exorcism: History, psychology, and neurobiology.* Santa Barbara, CA: Praeger.

Mead, N. L., Baumeister, R. F., Gino, F., Schweitzer, M. E., & Ariely, D. (2009). Too tired to tell the truth: Self-control resource depletion and dishonesty. *Journal of Experimental Social Psychology, 45*(3), 594–597.

Medlock, M. M., Rosmarin, D. H., Connery, H. S., Griffin, M. L., Weiss, M. D., Karakula, S. L., et al. (2017). Religious coping in patients with severe substance use disorders receiving acute inpatient detoxification. *American Journal on Addictions, 26*(7), 744–750.

Meisenhelder, J. B., & Marcum, J. P. (2004). Responses of clergy to 9/11: Posttraumatic stress, coping, and religious outcomes. *Journal for the Scientific Study of Religion, 43*(4), 547–554.

Menninger, K. (1963). *The vital balance: The life process in mental health and illness.* New York: Viking.

Mercadante, L. (2020). Spiritual struggles of nones and "spiritual" but not religious (SBNRs). *Religions, 11*(10), 513.

Merton, T. (1948). *The seven storey mountain.* San Diego, CA: Harcourt/HBJ Book.

Mihaljević, S., Aukst-Margetić, B., Vuksan-Ćusa, B., Koić, E., & Milošević, M. (2012). Hopelessness, suicidality, and religious coping in Croatian war veterans with PTSD. *Psychiatrica Danubina, 24*(3), 292–297.

Mikulincer, M., & Shaver, P. R. (Eds.). (2012). *The social psychology of morality: Exploring the causes of good and evil.* Washington, DC: American Psychological Association Books.

Moen, P. (1951). *Peter Moen's diary* (K. Austin-Lund, Trans.). London: Faber and Faber.

Mogenson, G. (1989). *God is a trauma: Vicarious religion and soul-making.* Dallas, TX: Spring.

Mohr, S. (2013). Religion, spirituality, in severe mental disorder. In K. I. Pargament, J. J. Exline, & J. W. Jones (Eds.), *APA handbook of psychology, religion, and spirituality (Vol. 1): Context, theory, and research* (pp. 241–256). Washington, DC: American Psychological Association.

Morgan, K. A. D., Scott, J.-K., Parshad-Asnani, M., Gibson, R. C., O'Garo, K. N., Lowe, G. A., et al. (2014). Associations amongst disease severity, religious coping, and depression in a cohort of Jamaicans with sickle-cell disease. *Mental Health, Religion and Culture, 17*(9), 937–945.

Mother Teresa, & Kolodiejchuk, B. (Ed.). (2007). *Mother Teresa: Come be my light: The private writings of the "Saint of Calcutta."* New York: Doubleday.

Movahedizadeh, M., Sheikhi, M. R., Shahsavari, S., & Chen, H. (2019). The association between religious belief and drug adherence mediated by religious coping in patients with mental disorders. *Social Health and Behavior, 2*(3), 77–82.

Murphy, P. E., Fitchett, G., & Emery-Tiburcio, E. E. (2016). Religious and spiritual struggle: Prevalance and correlates among older adults with depression in the BRIGHTEN program. *Mental Health, Religion and Culture, 19*(7), 713–721.

Murray, H. A. (1938). *Explorations in personality: A clinical and experimental study of 55 men of college age.* New York: Oxford University Press.

Murray-Swank, N. A. (2003). *Solace for the soul: A journey towards wholeness: Treatment manual for female survivors of sexual abuse.* Baltimore: Loyola College.

Murray-Swank, N. A. (2010, November). *Spirituality, religion, and PTSD among survivors of clergy sexual abuse.* Paper presented at the meeting of the International Society for Traumatic Stress Studies, Montreal, Quebec, Canada.

Murray-Swank, N. A., & Murray-Swank, A. B. (2012). Navigating the storm: Helping clients in the midst of spiritual struggles. In J. D. Aten, K. A. O'Grady, & E. L. Worthington, Jr. (Eds.), *The psychology of religion and spirituality for clinicians: Using research in your practice* (pp. 217–244). New York: Routledge.

Murray-Swank, N. A., & Pargament, K. I. (2005). God, where are you? Evaluating a spiritually-integrated intervention for sexual abuse. *Mental Health, Religion and Culture, 8*(3), 191–203.

Murray-Swank, N. A., & Waelde, L. C. (2013). Spirituality, religion, and sexual trauma: Integrating research, theory, and clinical practice. In K. I. Pargament, A. Mahoney, & E. P. Shafranske (Eds.), *APA handbook of psychology, religion, and spirituality (Vol. 2): An applied psychology of religion and spirituality* (pp. 335–354). Washington, DC: American Psychological Association.

Mussett, J. M. (2012). *Spiritual appraisals, spiritual struggles, and growth in parents of children with Down syndrome: A double ABCX hierarchical regression analysis* (Unpublished doctoral dissertation). St. Mary's University, San Antonio, TX.

Neff, K. (2003). Self-compassion: An alternative conceptualization of a healthy attitude toward oneself. *Self and Identity, 2*(2), 85–101.

Neff, K. D., & Germer, C. K. (2013). A pilot study and randomized clinical trial of the mindful self-compassion program. *Journal of Clinical Psychology, 69*(1), 28–44.

Neff, K. D., & Knox, M. C. (2017). Self-compassion. In V. Zeigler-Hill & T. K. Shackelford (Eds.), *Encyclopedia of personality and individual differences* (pp. 1–8). New York: Spring International.

Neimeyer, R. A., & Burke, L. A. (2011). Complicated grief in the aftermath of homicide: Spiritual crisis and distress in an African American sample. *Religions, 2*(2), 145–164.

Neimeyer, R. A., & Burke, L. A. (2017). Spiritual distress and depression in bereavement: A meaning-oriented contribution. *Journal of Rational-Emotive and Cognitive-Behavior Therapy, 35*(1), 38–59.

New World Encyclopedia. (2008). Holy. Retrieved from *www.newworldencyclopedia. org/entry/Holy*.

Nguyen, H. T., Yamada, A. M., & Dinh, T. Q. (2012). Religious leaders' assessment and attribution of the causes of mental illness: An in-depth exploration of Vietnamese American Buddhist leaders. *Mental Health, Religion and Culture, 15*(5), 511–527.

Nicholson, R. A. (1914). *The mystics of Islam*. London: Routledge.

Nielsen, S. L., Johnson, W. B., & Ellis, A. (2001). *Counseling and psychotherapy with religious persons: A rational emotive behavior therapy approach*. Mahway, NJ: Erlbaum.

Norman, M. (1989). *These good men: Friendships forged from war*. New York: Crown.

Nosek, M. A. (1995). The defining light of Vedanta: Personal reflections on spirituality and disability. *Rehabilitation Education, 9*(2), 171–182.

O'Brien, B., Shrestha, S., Stanley, M. A., Pargament, K. I., Cummings, J., Kunik, M. E., et al. (2019). Positive and negative religious coping as predictors of distress among minority older adults. *International Journal of Geriatric Psychiatry, 34*(1), 54–59.

O'Donnell, S. J. (2020). The deliverance of the administrative state: Deep state conspiracism, charismatic demonology, and the post-truth politics of American Christian nationalism. *Religion, 50*(4), 696–719.

Ok, U. (2004). Handling doubt in teaching religion: A Turkish case study. *Teaching Theology and Religion, 7*(4), 201–212.

Olatunji, B. O., Abramowitz, J. S., Williams, N. L., Connolly, K. M., & Lohr, J. M. (2007). Scrupulosity and obsessive–compulsive symptoms: Confirmatory factor analysis and validity of the Penn Inventory of Scrupulosity. *Journal of Anxiety Disorders, 21*(6), 771–787.

Oman, D. (Ed.). (2018). *Why religion and spirituality matter for public health: Evidence, implications, and resources*. Cham, Switzerland: Springer Nature.

Oman, D., Shapiro, S. L., Thoresen, C. E., Flinders, T., Driskill, J. D., & Plante, T. G. (2007). Learning from spiritual models and meditation: A randomized evaluation of a college course. *Pastoral Psychology, 55*(4), 473–493.

Ortberg, J. (2008). *Know doubt: The importance of embracing uncertainty in your faith*. Grand Rapids, MI: Zondervan.

Öst, L.-G. (2014). The efficacy of acceptance and commitment therapy: An updated systematic review and meta-analysis. *Behaviour Research and Therapy, 61*, 105–121.

Otto, R. (1928). *The idea of the holy: An inquiry into the nonrational factor in the idea of the divine and its relation to the rational* (J. W. Harvey, Trans.). London: Oxford University Press. (Originally published in 1917)

Oxhandler, H. K., Parrish, D. E., Torres, L. R., & Achenbaum, W. A. (2015). The integration of clients' religion/spirituality in social work practice: A national survey. *Social Work, 60*(3), 228–237.

Padgett, E., Mahoney, A., Pargament, K. I., & DeMaris, A. (2019). Marital sanctification and spiritual intimacy predicting married couples' observed intimacy skills across the transition to parenthood. *Religions, 10*(3), 177.

Paika, V., Andreoulakis, E., Ntountoulaki, E., Papaioannou, D., Kotsis, K., Siafaka, V., et al. (2017). The Greek-Orthodox version of the Brief Religious Coping (B-RCOPE) instrument: Psychometric properties in three samples and associations with mental disorders, suicidality, illness perceptions, and quality of life. *Annals of General Psychiatry, 16*, 13.

Palmer, P. J. (2004). *A hidden wholeness: The journey toward an undivided life*. New York: Jossey-Bass.

Palmer, P. J. (2008). *The promise of paradox: A celebration of contradictions in the Christian life*. San Francisco: Jossey-Bass.

Pals, J. L., & McAdams, D. P. (2004). The transformed self: A narrative understanding of posttraumatic growth. *Psychological Inquiry, 15*(1), 65–69.

Pargament, K. I. (1997). *The psychology of religion and coping: Theory, research, practice*. New York: Guilford Press.

Pargament, K. I. (1999). The psychology of religion and spirituality? Yes and no. *International Journal for the Psychology of Religion, 9*(1), 3–16.

Pargament, K. I. (2007). *Spiritually integrated psychotherapy: Understanding and addressing the sacred*. New York: Guilford Press.

Pargament, K. I. (2009, October). *Wrestling with the angels: Religious struggles in the context of mental illness*. Paper presented at the American Psychiatric Association Institute for Psychiatric Services, New York, NY.

Pargament, K. I. (2013). Searching for the sacred: Toward a non-reductionistic theory of spirituality. In K. I. Pargament, J. J. Exline, & J. W. Jones (Eds.), *APA handbook of psychology, religion, and spirituality (Vol. 1): Context, theory, and research* (pp. 257–274). Washington, DC: American Psychological Association.

Pargament, K. I., & Exline, J. J. (2021). Religious and spiritual struggles and mental health: Implications for clinical practice. In A. Moreira-Almeida, B. P. Mosqueiro, & D. Bhugra (Eds.), *Spirituality and mental health across cultures*. Oxford, UK: Oxford University Press.

Pargament, K. I., Feuille, M., & Burdzy, D. (2011). The Brief RCOPE: Current psychometric status of a short measure of religious coping. *Religions, 2*(1), 51–76.

Pargament, K. I., Kennell, J., Hathaway, W., Grevengoed, N., Newman, J., & Jones, W. (1988). Religion and the problem-solving process: Three styles of coping. *Journal for the Scientific Study of Religion, 27*(1), 90–104.

Pargament, K. I., Koenig, H. G., & Perez. L. M. (2000). The many methods of religious coping: Development and initial validation of the RCOPE. *Journal of Clinical Psychology, 56*(4), 519–543.

Pargament, K. I., Koenig, H. G., Tarakeshwar, N., & Hahn, J. (2001). Religious struggle as a predictor of mortality among medically ill elderly patients: A 2-year longitudinal study. *Archives of Internal Medicine, 161*(15), 1881–1885.

Pargament, K. I., Koenig, H. G., Tarakeshwar, N., & Hahn, J. (2004). Religious coping methods as predictors of psychological, physical, and spiritual outcomes among medically ill elderly patients: A two-year longitudinal study. *Journal of Health Psychology, 9*(6), 713–730.

Pargament, K. I., Lomax, J. W., McGee, J. S., & Fang, Q. (2014). Sacred moments in psychotherapy from the perspectives of mental health providers and clients: Prevalence, predictors, and consequences. *Spirituality in Clinical Practice, 1*(4), 248–262.

Pargament, K. I., Magyar, G. M., Benore, E., & Mahoney, A. (2005). Sacrilege: A study of sacred loss and desecration and their implications for health and well-being in a community sample. *Journal for the Scientific Study of Religion, 44*(1), 59–78.

Pargament, K. I., & Mahoney, A. M. (2005). Sacred matters: Sanctification as a vital topic for the psychology of religion. *International Journal for the Psychology of Religion, 15*(3), 179–198.

Pargament, K. I., Mahoney, A. M., Exline, J. J., Jones, J. W., & Shafranske, E. P. (2013).

Envisioning an integrative paradigm for the psychology of religion and spirituality. In K. I. Pargament, J. J. Exline, & J. W. Jones (Eds.), *APA handbook of psychology, religion, and spirituality (Vol. 1): Context, theory, and research* (pp. 3–20). Washington, DC: American Psychological Association.

Pargament, K. I., Murray-Swank, N. A., Magyar, G. M., & Ano, G. G. (2005). Spiritual struggle: A phenomenon of interest to psychology and religion. In W. R. Miller & H. D. Delaney (Eds.), *Judeo-Christian perspectives on psychology: Human nature, motivation, and change* (pp. 245–268). Washington DC: American Psychological Association Press.

Pargament, K. I., Murray-Swank, N. A., & Mahoney, A. (2008). Problem and solution: The spiritual dimension of clergy sexual abuse and its impact on survivors. *Journal of Child Sexual Abuse, 17*(3–4), 397–420.

Pargament, K. I., Smith, B. W., Koenig, H. G., & Perez, L. (1998). Patterns of positive and negative religious coping with major life stressors. *Journal for the Scientific Study of Religion, 37*(4), 710–724.

Pargament, K. I., Tarakeshwar, N., Ellison, C. G., & Wulff, K. M. (2001). Religious coping among the religious: The relationships between religious coping and well-being in a national sample of Presbyterian clergy, elders, and members. *Journal for the Scientific Study of Religion, 40*(3), 497–513.

Pargament, K. I., Trevino, K., Mahoney, A., & Silberman, I. (2007). They killed our Lord: The perception of Jews as desecrators of Christianity as a predictor of anti-Semitism. *Journal for the Scientific Study of Religion, 46*(2), 143–158.

Pargament, K. I., Wong, S., & Exline, J. J. (2016). Wholeness and holiness: The spiritual dimension of eudaimonics. In J. Vittersø (Ed.), *Handbook of eudaimonic well-being* (pp. 379–394). New York: Springer.

Pargament, K. I., Wong, S., Pomerleau, J., & Krause, N. (2016). [Landmark Spirituality and Health Study: Spirituality findings.] Unpublished raw data.

Pargament, K. I., Zinnbauer, B. J., Scott, A. B., Butter, E. M., Zerowin, J., & Stanik, P. (1998). Red flags and religious coping: Identifying some religious warning signs among people in crisis. *Journal of Clinical Psychology, 54*(1), 77–89.

Park, C. L. (2005). Religion as a meaning-making framework in coping with life stress. *Journal of Social Issues, 61*(4), 707–729.

Park, C. L. (2013). Religion and meaning. In R. F. Paloutzian & C. L. Park (Eds.), *Handbook of the psychology of religion and spirituality* (2nd ed., pp. 357–379). New York: Guilford Press.

Park, C. L. (2016). Meaning making in the context of disasters. *Journal of Clinical Psychology, 72*(12), 1234–1246.

Park, C. L., & Cho, D. (2017). Spiritual well-being and spiritual distress predict adjustment in adolescents and young adult cancer survivors. *Psycho-Oncology, 26*(9), 1293–1300.

Park, C. L., Cohen, L. H., & Murch, R. L. (1996). Assessment and prediction of stress-related growth. *Journal of Personality, 64*(1), 71–105.

Park, C. L., Currier, J. M., Harris, J. I., & Slattery, J. M. (2017). *Trauma, meaning, and spirituality: Translating research into clinical practice.* Washington DC: American Psychological Association Press.

Park, C. L., Edmondson, D., Hale-Smith, A., & Blank, T. O. (2009). Religiousness/spirituality and health behaviors in young adult cancer survivors: Does faith promote a healthy lifestyle? *Journal of Behavioral Medicine, 32*(6), 582–591.

Park, C. L., & Fenster, J. R. (2004). Stress-related growth: Predictors of occurrence and correlates with psychological adjustment. *Journal of Social and Clinical Psychology, 23*(2), 195–215.

Park, C. L., Groessi, E., Maiya, M., Sarkin, A., Eisen, S. V., Riley, K., et al. (2014). Comparison groups in yoga research: A systematic review and critical evaluation of the literature. *Complementary Therapies in Medicine, 22*(5), 920–929.

Park, C. L., Holt, C. L., Le, D., Christie, J., & Williams, B. R. (2018). Positive and negative religious coping styles as prospective predictors of well-being in African Americans. *Psychology of Religion and Spirituality, 10*(4), 318–326.

Park, C. L., Lim, H., Newlon, M., Suresh, D. P., & Bliss, D. E. (2014). Dimensions of religiousness and spirituality as predictors of well-being in advanced chronic heart failure patients. *Journal of Religion and Health, 53*(2), 579–590.

Park, C. L., Smith, P. H., Le, S. Y., Mazure, C. M., McKee, S. A., & Hoff, R. (2017). Positive and negative religious/spiritual coping and combat exposure as predictors of posttraumatic stress and perceived growth in Iraq and Afghanistan veterans. *Psychology of Religion and Spirituality, 9*(1), 13–20.

Park, C. L., Wortmann, J. H., & Edmondson, D. (2011). Religious struggle as a predictor of subsequent mental and physical well-being in advanced heart failure patients. *Journal of Behavioral Medicine, 34*(6), 426–436.

Park, J., & Baumeister, R. F. (2017). Meaning in life and adjustment to daily stressors. *Journal of Positive Psychology, 12*(4), 333–341.

Parks, S. D. (2000). *Big questions, worthy dreams: Mentoring emerging adults in their search for meaning, purpose, and faith.* San Francisco: Jossey-Bass.

Parrott, W. G. (2014). Feeling, function, and the place of negative emotions in a happy life. In W. G. Parrott (Ed.), *The positive side of negative emotions* (pp. 273–296). New York: Guilford Press.

Patrick, J. H., & Henrie, J. A. (2015). Religious doubt and spiritual growth among adults bereaved of a grandparent. *Journal of Religion, Spirituality and Aging, 27*(2–3), 93–107.

Pearce, M. (2020). *Night bloomers: 12 principles for thriving in adversity.* Mineola, NY: Ixia Press.

Pearce, M. J., & Koenig, H. G. (2016). Spiritual struggles and religious cognitive behavioral therapy: A randomized clinical trial in those with depression and chronic illness. *Journal of Psychology and Theology, 44*(1), 3–15.

Pearce, M. J., Pargament, K. I., Oxhandler, H. K., Vieten, C., & Wong, S. (2019). A novel training program for mental health providers in religious and spiritual competencies. *Spirituality in Clinical Practice, 6*(2), 73–82.

Pearce, M. J., Pargament, K. I., Oxhandler, H. K., Vieten, C., & Wong, S. (2020). Novel online training program improves spiritual competencies in mental health care. *Spirituality in Clinical Practice, 7*(3), 145–161.

Peck, M. S. (1983). *People of the lie: The hope for healing human evil.* New York: Touchstone.

Pedersen, H. F., Pedersen, C. G., Pargament, K. I., & Zachariae, R. (2013). Coping without religion? Religious coping, quality of life, and existential well-being among lung disease patients and matched controls in a secular society. *Research in the Social Scientific Study of Religion, 24*, 163–192.

Pennycook, G., Cheyne, J. A., Seli, P., Koehler, D. J., & Fugelsang, J. A. (2012). Analytic cognitive style predicts religious and paranormal belief. *Science, 123*(3), 335–346.

Perry, S. L. (2018). Pornography use and depressive symptoms: Examining the role of moral incongruence. *Society and Mental Health, 8*(3), 195–213.

Peteet, J. R. (2004). *Doing the right thing: An approach to moral issues in mental health treatment.* New York: American Psychiatric Publishing.

Pew Research Center. (2009). Many Americans mix multiple faiths. Retrieved from *www.pewforum.org/2009/12/09/many-americans-mix-multiple-faiths.*

Pew Research Center. (2017a). *More Americans now say they're spiritual but not religious.* Washington, DC: Author.

Pew Research Center. (2017b). *U.S. Muslims concerned about their place in society, but continue to believe in the American dream: Findings from the Pew Research Center's 2017 survey of U.S. Muslims.* Washington, DC: Author.

Pew Research Center. (2018, November 20). *Where Americans find meaning in life: Findings from the Pew Research Center.* Washington, DC: Author.

Phillips, J. B. (1997). *Your God is too small.* New York: Touchstone Books.

Phillips, R. E., III, Cheng, C. M., Pargament, K. I., Oemig, C., Colvin, S. D., Abarr, A. N., et al. (2009). Spiritual coping in American Buddhists: An exploratory study. *International Journal for the Psychology of Religion, 19*(4), 231–243.

Piaget, J. (1954). *The construction of reality in the child.* (M. Cook, Trans.). New York: Basic Books.

Piderman, K. M. (2015). "Why did God do this to me?" Angela, a 17-year-old girl with spinal injury. In G. Fitchett & S. Nolan (Eds.), *Spiritual care in practice: Case studies in healthcare chaplaincy* (pp. 69–93). London: Jessica Kingsley.

Piderman, K. M., Breitkopf, C. R., Jenkins, S. M., Lapid, M. I., Kwete, G. M., Sytsma, T. T., et al. (2017). The impact of a spiritual legacy intervention in patients with brain cancers and other neurologic illnesses and their support persons. *Psycho-Oncology, 26*(3), 346–353.

Piderman, K. M., Egginton, J. S., Ingram, C., Dose, A. M., Yoder, T. J., Lovejoy, L. A., et al. (2017). I'm still me: Inspiration and instruction from individuals with brain cancer. *Journal of Health Care Chaplaincy, 23*(1), 15–33.

Piedmont, R. L. (1999). Does spirituality represent the sixth factor of personality? Spiritual transcendence and the five-factor model. *Journal of Personality, 67*(6), 985–1013.

Piedmont, R. L. (2012). Overview and development of a trait-based measure of numinous conflicts: The Assessment of Spirituality and Religious Sentiments (ASPIRES) scale. In L. Miller (Ed.), *The Oxford handbook of psychology and spirituality* (pp. 104–122). New York: Oxford University Press.

Piedmont, R. L., & Wilkins, T. A. (2013). Spirituality, religiousness, and personality: Theoretical foundations and empirical applications. In K. I. Pargament, J. J. Exline, & J. W. Jones (Eds.), *APA handbook of psychology, religion, and spirituality (Vol. 1): Context, theory, and research* (pp. 173–186). Washington, DC: American Psychological Association.

Pirutinsky, S., Cherniak, A. D., & Rosmarin, D. H. (2020). COVID-19, mental health, and religious coping among American Orthodox Jews. *Journal of Religion and Health, 59,* 2288–2301.

Pirutinsky, S., Rosmarin, D. H., Pargament, K. I., & Midlarsky, E. (2011). Does negative religious coping accompany, precede, or follow depression among Orthodox Jews? *Journal of Affective Disorders, 132*(3), 401–405.

Pleins, J. D. (2013). *The evolving God: Charles Darwin on the naturalness of religion.* New York: Bloomsbury Academic.

Pomerleau, J. M., Pargament, K. I., Krause, N., Ironson, G., & Hill, P. (2020). Religious and spiritual struggles as a mediator of the link between stressful life events and psychological adjustment in a nationwide sample. *Psychology of Religion and Spirituality, 12*(4), 451–459.

Pomerleau, J. M., Pargament, K. I., & Mahoney, A. (2016). Seeing life through a sacred lens: The spiritual dimension of meaning. In P. Russo-Netzer, S. E. Schulenberg, & A. Batthyany (Eds.), *Clinical perspectives on meaning* (pp. 37–57). Cham, Switzerland: Springer International.

Poole, W. S. (2009). *Satan in America: The devil we know.* Plymouth, UK: Rowman & Littlefield.

Posadski, P., Choi, J., Lee, M. S., & Ernst, E. (2014). Yoga for addictions: A systematic review of randomized clinical trials. *Focus on Alternative and Complementary Therapies, 19*(1), 1–8.

Prager, D., & Telushkin, J. (1983). *Why the Jews? The reason for antisemitism.* New York: Simon & Schuster.

Prati, G., & Pietrantoni, L. (2009). Optimism, social support, and coping strategies as factors contributing to posttraumatic growth: A meta-analysis. *Journal of Loss and Trauma, 14*(5), 364–388.

Preston, J. L., & Ritter, R. S. (2013). Different effects of religion and God on prosociality with the ingroup and outgroup. *Personality and Social Psychology Bulletin, 39*(11), 1471–1483.

Price, P., Kinghorn, J., Patrick, R., & Cardell, B. (2012). "Still there is beauty": One man's resilient adaptation to stroke. *Scandinavian Journal of Occupational Therapy, 19*(2), 111–117.

Prusak, J. (2016). Differential diagnosis of "religious or spiritual problem": Possibilities and limitations implied by the V-code 62.89 in DSM-5. *Psychiatria Polska, 50*(1), 175–186.

Pruyser, P. W. (1968). *A dynamic psychology of religion.* New York: Harper & Row.

Pruyser, P. W. (1974). *Between belief and unbelief.* New York: Harper & Row.

Puffer, K. A., Pence, K. G., Graverson, T. M., Wolfe, M., Pate, E., & Clegg, S. (2008). Religious doubt and identity formation: Salient predictors of adolescent religious doubt. *Journal of Psychology and Theology, 36*(4), 270–284.

Putnam, R. D. (2000). *Bowling alone: The collapse and revival of American community.* New York: Simon & Schuster.

Raines, A. M., Currier, J., McManus, E. S., Walton, J. L., Uddo, M., & Franklin, C. L. (2017). Spiritual struggles and suicide in veterans seeking PTSD treatment. *Psychological Trauma: Theory, Research, Practice, and Policy, 9*(6), 746–749.

Ramirez, S. P., Macêdo, D. S., Sales, P. M. G., Figueiredo, S. M., Daher, E. F., Araújo, S. M., et al. (2012). The relationship between religious coping, psychological distress, and quality of life in hemodialysis patients. *Journal of Psychosomatic Research, 72*(2), 129–135.

Ransom, S., Sheldon, K. M., & Jacobsen, P. B. (2008). Actual change and inaccurate recall contribute to posttraumatic growth following radiotherapy. *Journal of Consulting and Clinical Psychology, 76*(5), 811–819.

Ray, S. D., Lockman, J. D., Jones, E. J., & Kelly, M. H. (2015). Attributions to God and Satan about life-altering events. *Psychology of Religion and Spirituality, 7*(1), 60–69.

Reist Gibbel, M., Regueiro, V., & Pargament, K. I. (2019). A spiritually integrated intervention for spiritual struggles among adults with mental illness: Results of an initial evaluation. *Spirituality in Clinical Practice, 6*(4), 240–255.

Reynolds, N., Mrug, S., Hensler, M., Guion, K., & Madan-Swain, A. (2014). Spiritual coping and adjustment in adolescents with chronic illness: A two-year prospective study. *Journal of Pediatric Psychology, 39*(5), 542–551.

Reynolds, N., Mrug, S., Wolfe, K., Schwebel, D., & Wallander, J. (2016). Spiritual coping, psychosocial adjustment, and physical health in youth with chronic illness: A meta-analytic review. *Health Psychology Review, 10*(2), 226–243.

Richards, P. S., Owen, L., & Stein, S. (1993). A religiously oriented group counseling intervention for self-defeating perfectionism: A pilot study. *Counseling and Values, 37*(2), 96–104.

Richards, T. A., Acree, M., & Folkman, S. (1999). Spiritual aspects of loss among partners of men with AIDS: Postbereavement follow-up. *Death Studies, 23*(2), 105–127.

Rilke, R. M. (2001). *Letters to a young poet: Letter four 16 July 1903* (S. Mitchell, Trans.). Malden, MA: Scriptor Press.

Rio, K., MacCarthy, M., & Blanes, R. (Eds.). (2017). *Pentecostalism and witchcraft: Spiritual warfare in Africa and Melanesia.* London: Palgrave Macmillan.

Rizzuto, A.-M. (1979). *The birth of the living God.* Chicago: University of Chicago Press.

Robatmili, S., Sohrabi, F., Shahrak, M. A., Talepasand, S., Nokani, M., & Hasani, M. (2015). The effect of group logotherapy on meaning in life and depression levels of Iranian students. *International Journal for the Advancement of Counseling, 37*(1), 54–62.

Roberts, L. R., Mann, S. K., & Montgomery, S. B. (2016). Mental health and sociocultural determinants in an Asian Indian community. *Family and Community Health, 39*(1), 31–39.

Robertson, T. M., Magyar-Russell, G. M., & Piedmont, R. L. (2020). Let him who is without sin cast the first stone: Religious struggle among persons convicted of sexually offending. *Religions, 11*(11), 546.

Rockenbach, A. B., Walker, C. R., & Luzader, J. (2012). A phenomenological analysis of college students' spiritual struggles. *Journal of College Student Development, 53*(1), 55–75.

Rogers, M. L. (1992). A call for discernment—natural and spiritual: An introductory editorial to a special issue on SRA. *Journal of Psychology and Theology, 20*(3), 175–186.

Roose, K. (2020, October 19). What is QAnon, the viral pro-Trump conspiracy theory? *New York Times.* Retrived from *www.nytimes.com/article/what-is-qanon.html.*

Rosetti, S. J. (1995). The impact of child sexual abuse on attitudes toward God and the Catholic church. *Child Abuse and Neglect, 19*(12), 1469–1481.

Rosmarin, D. H. (2018). *Spirituality, religion, and cognitive-behavioral therapy: A guide for clinicians.* New York: Guilford Press.

Rosmarin, D. H., Bigda-Peyton, J. S., Öngur, D., Pargament, K. I., & Björgvinsson, T. (2013). Religious coping among psychotic patients: Relevance to suicidality and treatment outcomes. *Psychiatry Research, 210*(1), 182–187.

Rosmarin, D. H., Malloy, M. C., & Forester, B. P. (2014). Spiritual struggle and affective symptoms among geriatric mood disordered patients. *International Journal of Geriatric Psychiatry, 29*(6), 653–660.

Rosmarin, D. H., Pargament, K. I., & Flannelly, K. J. (2009). Do spiritual struggles predict poorer physical/mental health among Jews? *International Journal for the Psychology of Religion, 19*(4), 244–258.

Rotz, E., Russell, C. S., & Wright, D. W. (1993). The therapist who is perceived as "spiritually correct": Strategies for avoiding collusion with the "spiritually one-up" spouse. *Journal of Marital and Family Therapy, 19*(4), 369–375.

Routledge, C., Abeyta, A. A., & Roylance, C. (2016). An existential function of evil: The effects of religiosity and compromised meaning on belief in magical evil forces. *Motivation and Emotion, 40*(5), 681–688.

Ruiz, F. J. (2010). A review of acceptance and commitment therapy (ACT) empirical evidence: Correlational, experimental psychopathology, component and outcome studies. *International Journal of Psychology and Psychological Therapy, 10*(1), 125–162.

Rupp, J. (1997). *The cup of our life: A guide to spiritual growth.* Notre Dame, IN: Ave Maria Press.

Russell, J. B. (1975). The experience of evil. In R. Woods (Ed.), *Heterodoxy, mystical experience, religious dissent and the occult* (pp. 71–83). River Forest, IL: Listening Press.

Russo-Netzer, P. (2019). Prioritizing meaning as a pathway to meaning in life and well-being. *Journal of Happiness Studies, 20*(6), 1863–1891.

Russo-Netzer, P., & Mayseless, O. (2014). Spiritual identity outside institutional religion: A phenomenological exploration. *Identity: An International Journal of Theory and Research, 14*(1), 19–42.

Ryan, R. M., LaGuardia, J. G., & Rawsthorne, L. J. (2005). Self-complexity and the authenticity of self-aspects: Effects on well-being and resilience to stressful events. *North American Journal of Psychology, 7*(3), 431–447.

Sacks, J. (2016, March 12). Don't sit: Walk. *Covenant and Conversation,* 1–4.

Saint Augustine. (1960). *The confessions of St. Augustine* (J. K. Ryan, Trans.). New York: Image Books.

Sampson, E. E. (1977). Psychology and the American ideal. *Journal of Personality and Social Psychology, 35*(11), 767–782.

Sandage, S. J., & Crabtree, S. (2012). Spiritual pathology and religious coping as predictors of forgiveness. *Mental Health, Religion, and Culture, 15*(7), 689–707.

Sandage, S. J., Rupert, D., Stavros, G., & Devor, N. G. (2020). *Relational spirituality in psychotherapy: Healing suffering and promoting growth.* Washington, DC: American Psychological Association Press.

San Roman, L., Mosher, D. K., Hook, J. N., Captari, L. E., Aten, J. D., Davis, E. B., et al. (2019). Religious support buffers the indirect negative psychological effects of mass shooting in church-affiliated individuals. *Psychological Trauma: Theory, Research, Practice, and Policy. 11*(6), 571–577.

Santiago, P. N., & Gall, T. L. (2016). Acceptance and commitment therapy as a spiritually integrated psychotherapy. *Counseling and Values, 61*(2), 239–254.

Saritoprak, S. N., & Exline, J. J. (2021). Applying a mindset of spiritual jihad to religious/ spiritual struggles: The development of a preliminary measure. In A. L. Ai, P. M. Wink, R. F. Paloutzian, & K. A. Harris (Eds.), *Assessing spirituality in a diverse world* (pp. 333–354). Cham, Switzerland: Springer Nature.

Saritoprak, S. N., Exline, J. J., & Abu-Raiya, H. (2020). Spiritual jihad as an emerging psychological concept: Connections with religious/spiritual struggles, virtues, and perceived growth. *Journal of Muslim Mental Health, 14*(2), 109–131.

Saritoprak, S. N., Exline, J. J., Hall, T. W., & Pargament, K. I. (2017, April). *Does God use struggles to transform us? Both Christians and Muslims can approach struggles with a transformational mindset.* Paper presented at a meeting of the Society for the Psychology of Religion and Spirituality, Chattanooga, TN.

Saritoprak, S. N., Exline, J. J., & Stauner, N. (2016). *Religious/spiritual struggles: Differences among U.S. religious affiliations.* Paper presented at the annual meeting of the American Psychological Association, Denver, CO.

Saritoprak, S. N., Exline, J. J., & Stauner, N. (2018). Spiritual jihad among U.S. Muslims: Preliminary measurement and associations with well-being and growth. *Religions, 9*(5), 158.

Sartre, J.-P. (1948). *Being and nothingness* (H. E. Barnes, Trans.). New York: Philosophical Library.

Saunders, S. M., Petrik, M. L., & Miller, M. L. (2014). Psychology doctoral students' perspectives on addressing spirituality and religion with clients: Associations with personal preferences and training. *Psychology of Religion and Spirituality, 6*(1), 1–8.

Sawai, R. P., Noah, S. M., Krauss, S. E., Sulaiman, M., Sawai, J. P., & Safien, A. M. (2017). Relationship between religiosity, shame, and guilt among Malaysian Muslims youth. *International Journal of Academic Research in Business and Social Sciences, 7,* 144–155.

Schaal, S., Heim, L., & Elbert, T. (2014). Posttraumatic stress disorder and appetitive aggression in Rwandan genocide perpetrators. *Journal of Aggression, Maltreatment, and Trauma, 23*(9), 930–945.

Schimmel, S. (1992). *The seven deadly sins: Jewish, Christian, and classical reflections on human nature.* New York: Free Press.

Schmid, K., Hewstone, M., Küpper, B., Zick, A., & Tausch, N. (2014). Reducing aggressive intergroup action tendencies: Effects of intergroup contact via perceived intergroup threat. *Aggressive Behavior, 40*(3), 250–262.

Schnitker, S. A., Currier, J. M., Abernethy, A. D., Witvliet, C. V. O., Foster, J. D., Root Luna, L. M., et al. (2021). Gratitude and patience moderate meaning struggles and suicidal risk in a cross-sectional study of inpatients at a Christian psychiatric hospital. *Journal of Personality.* Advance online publication.

Schuck, K. D., & Liddle, B. J. (2001). Religious conflicts experienced by lesbian, gay, and bisexual individuals. *Journal of Gay and Lesbian Psychotherapy, 5*(2), 63–82.

Schuster, M. A., Stein, B. D., Jaycox, L. H., Collins, R. L., Marshall, G. N., Elliott, M. N., et al. (2001). A national survey of stress reactions after the September 11, 2001 terrorist attacks. *New England Journal of Medicine, 345*(20), 1507–1512.

Sedlar, A. E., Stauner, N., Pargament, K. I., Exline, J. J., Grubbs, J. B., & Bradley, D. F. (2018). Spiritual struggles among atheists: Links to psychological distress and well-being. *Religions, 9*(8), 242.

Segall, M., & Wykle, M. (1988–1989). The black family's experience with dementia. *Journal of Applied Social Sciences, 13*(1), 170–191.

Seldes, G. (1985). *The great thoughts.* New York: Ballantine.

Seligman, M. E. P. (1975). *Helplessness: On depression, development, and death.* San Francisco: Jossey-Bass.

Seligman, M. E. P. (2014). God comes at the end. *Spirituality in Clinical Practice, 1*(1), 67–70.

Senpai Sensei. (2017). Daily affirmation prayer. Retrieved from *http://buddhistfaith.tripod.com/buddhistprayer/id4.html taken on 10/12/17.*

Shafranske, E. P., & Cummings, J. P. (2013). Religious and spiritual beliefs, affiliations, and practices of psychologists. In K. I. Pargament, A. Mahoney, & E. P. Shafranske

(Eds.), *APA handbook of psychology, religion, and spirituality (Vol. 2): An applied psychology of religion and spirituality* (pp. 23–42). Washington, DC: American Psychological Association.

Shakespeare-Finch, J., & Enders, T. (2008). Corroborating evidence of posttraumatic growth. *Journal of Traumatic Stress, 21*(4), 421–424.

Shanshan, L., Stampfer, M. J., Williams, D. B., & VanderWeele, T. J. (2016). Association of religious service attendance with mortality among women. *JAMA Internal Medicine, 176*(6), 777–785.

Shapiro, F. R. (2014, April). Who wrote the Serenity Prayer? *The Chronicle of Higher Education*, 2.

Shariff, A. F., & Norenzayan, A. (2011). Mean gods make good people: Different views of God predict cheating behavior. *International Journal for the Psychology of Religion, 21*(2), 85–96.

Shariff, A. F., & Rhemtulla, M. (2012). Divergent effects of beliefs in heaven and hell on national crime rates. *PLoS One, 7*, e39048.

Shenhav, A., Rand, D. G., & Greene, J. D. (2012). Divine intuition: Cognitive style influences on belief in God. *Journal of Experimental Psychology: General, 141*(3), 423–428.

Sherman, A. C., Plante, T. G., Simonton, S., Latif, U., & Anaissie, E. J. (2009). Prospective study of religious coping among patients undergoing autologous stem cell transplantation. *Journal of Behavioral Medicine, 32*(1), 118–128.

Sherman, A. C., Simonton, S., Latif, U., Spohn, R., & Tricot, G. (2005). Religious struggle and religious comfort in response to illness: Health outcomes among stem cell transplant patients. *Journal of Behavioral Medicine, 28*(4), 359–367.

Sherman, A. C., Simonton-Atchley, S., O'Brien, C. E., Campbell, D., Reddy, R. M., Guinee, B., et al. (2021). Associations between religious/spiritual coping and depression among adults with cystic fibrosis: A 12-month longitudinal study. *Journal of Religion and Health*. Advance online publication.

Sherman, M. D., Harris, J. I., & Erbes, C. (2015). Clinical approaches to addressing spiritual struggles in veterans with PTSD. *Professional Psychology: Research and Practice, 46*(4), 203–212.

Siegel, K., & Schrimshaw, E. W. (2000). Perceiving benefits in adversity: Stress-related growth in women living with HIV/AIDS. *Social Science and Medicine, 51*(10), 1543–1554.

Silver, R. L., & Wortman, C. B. (1980). Coping with undesirable life events. In J. Garber & M. E. P. Seligman (Eds.), *Human helplessness: Theory and applications* (pp. 279–375). New York: Academic Press.

Slater, M. (2009). *Charles Dickens: A life defined by writing*. New Haven, CT: Yale University Press.

Small, J. L., & Bowman, N. A. (2011). Religious commitment, skepticism, and struggle among U.S. college students: The impact of majority/minority religious affiliation and institutional type. *Journal for the Scientific Study of Religion, 50*(1), 154–174.

Smeets, E., Neff, K., Alberts, H., & Peters, M. (2014). Meeting suffering with kindness: Effects of a brief self-compassion intervention for female college students. *Journal of Clinical Psychology, 70*(9), 794–807.

Smigelsky, M. A., Gill, A. R., Foshager, D., Aten, J. D., & Im, H. (2017). "My heart is in his hands": The lived spiritual experiences of Congolese refugee women survivors of sexual violence. *Journal of Prevention and Intervention in the Community, 45*(4), 261–273.

Smith, B. W., Pargament, K. I., Brant, C., & Oliver, J. M. (2000). Noah revisited: Religious coping by church members and the impact of the 1993 Midwest flood. *Journal of Community Psychology, 28*(2), 169–186.

Smith, C., & Exline J. J. (2002, August). Effects of homelessness on a person's perceived relationship with God. Paper presented at the annual meeting of the American Psychological Association, Chicago, IL.

Smith, H. (1958). *The world's religions.* New York: Harper Collins.

Smith, H. A. (1887, October 29). Chief Seattle's message. *Seattle Sunday Star.* Retrieved from *www.halcyon.com/arborhts/chiefsea.html.*

Smith, T. B., McCullough, M. E., & Poll, J. (2003). Religiousness and depression: Evidence for a main effect and the moderating influence of stressful life events. *Psychological Bulletin, 129*(4), 614–636.

Snyder, C. R., Lopez, S. J., Edwards, L. M., & Marques, S. C. (Eds.). (2021). *Oxford handbook of positive psychology* (3rd ed.). New York: Oxford University Press.

Southard, S. (2015). *Nagasaki: Life after nuclear war.* New York: Penguin Books.

Sremac, S., & Ganzevoort, R. R. (2013). Addiction and spiritual transformation: An empirical study on narratives of recovering addicts' conversion testimonies in Dutch and Serbian contexts. *Archive for the Psychology of Religion, 35*(3), 399–435.

Starmans, C., & Bloom, P. (2016). When the spirit is willing, but the flesh is weak: Developmental differences in judgments about inner moral conflict. *Psychological Science, 27*(11), 1498–1506.

Starnino, V. R., Angel, C. T., Sullivan, J. E., Lazarick, D. L., Jaimes, L. D., Cocco, J. P., et al. (2019). Preliminary report on a spiritually-based PTSD intervention for military veterans. *Community Mental Health Journal, 55*(7), 1114–1119.

Stauner, N., Exline, J. J., Grubbs, J. B., Pargament, K. I., Bradley, D. F., & Uzdavines, A. (2016). Bifactor models of religious and spiritual struggles: Distinct from religiousness and distress. *Religions, 7*(6), 68.

Stauner, N., Exline, J. J., Kusina, J. R., & Pargament, K. I. (2019). Religious and spiritual struggles, religiousness, and alcohol problems among undergraduates. *Journal of Prevention and Intervention in the Community, 47*(3), 243–258.

Stauner, N., Exline, J. J., & Pargament, K. I. (2015). *The demographics of religious and spiritual struggles in the USA.* Paper presented at the annual meeting of the American Psychological Association, Provo, UT.

Stauner, N., Exline, J. J., & Pargament, K. I. (2016). Religious and spiritual struggles as concerns for health and well-being. *Horizonte, 14*(41), 48–75.

Stauner, N., Exline, J. J., Pargament, K. I., Wilt, J. A., & Grubbs, J. B. (2019). Stressful life events and religiousness predict struggles about religion and spirituality. *Psychology of Religion and Spirituality, 11*(3), 291–296.

Stauner, N., Wilt, J. A., Exline, J. J., & Pargament, K. I. (2017, April). *Religiousness and spiritual struggles throughout college life.* Presentation at the 97th annual convention of the Western Psychological Association, Sacramento, CA.

Streib, H., & Klein, C. (2014). Religious styles predict interreligious prejudice: A study of German adolescents with the Religious Schema Scale. *International Journal for the Psychology of Religion, 24*(2), 151–163.

Streit-Horn, J. (2011). *A systematic review of research on after-death communication*

(ADC); (Unpublished doctoral dissertation). University of North Texas, Denton, TX.

Stroppa, A., & Moreira-Almeida, A. (2013). Religiosity, mood symptoms, and quality of life in bipolar disorder. *Bipolar Disorders, 15*(4), 385–393.

Strosky, D. G., Wang, D. C., Hill, P. C., Long, J. E., Davis, E. B., & Cuthbert, A. D. (2018). Students in faith-based doctoral psychology programs: Religious/spiritual struggles moderate the effects of distress from clinical work on negative affect. *Journal of Psychology and Theology, 46*(1), 52–66.

Szcześniak, M., Kroplewski, Z., & Szałachowski, R. (2020). The mediating effect of coping strategies on religious/spiritual struggles and life satisfaction. *Religions, 11*(4), 195.

Szcześniak, M., & Timoszyk-Tomczak, C. (2020). Religious struggle and life satisfaction among adult Christians: Self-esteem as a mediator. *Journal of Religion and Health, 59*(6), 2833–2856.

Szcześniak, R. D., Zou, Y., Stamper, S. M., & Grossoehme, D. H. (2017). Spiritual struggle in parents of children with cystic fibrosis increases odds of depression. *Depression Research and Treatment, 2017,* 5670651.

Szymanski, D. M., & Carretta, R. F. (2020). Religious-based sexual stigma and psychological health: Roles of internalization, religious struggle, and religiosity. *Journal of Homosexuality, 67*(8), 1062–1080.

Tajfel, H., & Turner, J. (2001). An integrative theory of intergroup conflict. In M. A. Hogg & D. Abrams (Eds.), *Intergroup relations: Essential readings* (pp. 94–109). New York: Psychology Press.

Tangney, J. P., Stuewig, J., & Masheg, D. J. (2007). Moral emotions and moral behavior. *Annual Review of Psychology, 58,* 345–372.

Tanksley, C. P. (2010). *Decreasing anxiety through training in spiritual warfare* (Unpublished doctoral dissertation). Oral Roberts University, Tulsa, OK.

Tarakeshwar, N., & Pargament, K. I. (2001). Religious coping in families of children with autism. *Focus on Autism and Other Developmental Disabilities, 16*(4), 247–260.

Tarakeshwar, N., Pargament, K. I., & Mahoney, A. (2003). Initial development of a measure of religious coping among Hindus. *Journal of Community Psychology, 31*(6), 607–628.

Tarakeshwar, N., Pearce, M. J., & Sikkema, K. J. (2005). Development and implementation of a spiritual coping group intervention for adults living with HIV/AIDS: A pilot study. *Mental Health, Religion and Culture, 8*(3), 179–190.

Tarakeshwar, N., Vanderwerker, L. C., Paulk, E., Pearce, M. J., Kasl, S. V., & Prigerson, H. G. (2006). Religious coping is associated with the quality of life of patients with advanced cancer. *Journal of Palliative Medicine, 9*(3), 646–657.

Taylor, B. B. (2014). *Learning to walk in the dark.* New York: HarperOne.

Tedeschi, R. G., & Calhoun, L. G. (1995). *Trauma and transformation: Growing in the aftermath of suffering.* Thousand Oaks, CA: SAGE.

Tedeschi, R. G., & Calhoun, L. G. (1996). The Posttraumatic Growth Inventory: Measuring the positive legacy of trauma. *Journal of Traumatic Stress, 9*(3), 455–471.

Tedeschi, R. G., & Calhoun, L. G. (2004). Posttraumatic growth: Conceptual foundations and empirical evidence. *Psychological Inquiry, 15*(1), 1–18.

ten Boom, C. (1971). *The hiding place.* Toronto: Bantam Books.

Teng, E. J., Stanley, M. A., Exline, J. J., & Pargament, K. I. (2016). [Frequency of reports of religious and spiritual growth following religious and spiritual struggles.] Unpublished raw data.

Teng, E. J., Stanley, M. A., Fletcher, T. L., Pargament, K. I., & Exline, J. J. (2015). [Qualitative interviews with veterans experiencing religious and spiritual struggles.] Unpublished raw data.

Thigpen, P. (2014). *Manual for spiritual warfare*. Charlotte, NC: Tan Books.

Thomas, C. A. (2004). *At hell's gate: A soldier's journey from war to peace*. Boston: Shambhala.

Thombre, A., Sherman, A. C., & Simonton, S. (2010). Religious coping and posttraumatic growth among family caregivers of cancer patients in India. *Journal of Psychosocial Oncology, 28*(2), 173–188.

Thuné-Boyle, I. C. V., Stygall, J. A., Keshtgar, M. R. S., Davidson, T. I., & Newman, S. P. (2013). Religious/spiritual coping resources and their relationship with adjustment in patients newly diagnosed with breast cancer in the UK. *Psycho-Oncology, 22*(3), 646–658.

Tick, E. (2014). *Warrior's return: Restoring the soul after war*. Boulder, CO: Sounds True.

Tillich, P. (1948). *The shaking of the foundations*. New York: Scribner's Sons.

Tillich, P. (1957). *Dynamics of faith*. New York: Harper Torchbooks.

Tillich, P. (1975). *Systematic theology* (Vol. 2). Chicago: University of Chicago Press.

Tobin, E. T., & Slatcher, R. B. (2016). Religious participation predicts diurnal cortisol profiles 10 years later via lower levels of religious struggle. *Health Psychology, 35*(12), 1356–1363.

Tolstoy, L. (1983). *Confession* (D. Patterson, Trans.). New York: Norton.

Trevino, K. M., Archambault, E., Schuster, J., Richardson, P., & Moye, J. (2012). Religious coping and psychological distress in military veteran cancer survivors. *Journal of Religion and Health, 51*(1), 87–98.

Trevino, K. M., Balboni, M., Zollfrank, T., Balboni, T., & Prigerson, H. G. (2014). Negative religious coping as a correlate of suicidal ideation in patients with advanced cancer. *Psycho-Oncology, 23*(8), 936–945.

Trevino, K. M., Desai, K., Lauricella, S., Pargament, K. I., & Mahoney, A. (2012). Perceptions of lesbian and gay (LG) individuals as desecrators of Christianity as predictors of anti-LG attitudes. *Journal of Homosexuality, 59*(4), 535–563.

Trevino, K. M., Naik, A. D., & Moye, J. (2016). Perceived and actual change in religion/spirituality in cancer survivors: Longitudinal relationships with distress and perceived growth. *Psychology of Religion and Spirituality, 8*(3), 195–205.

Trevino, K. M., Pargament, K. I., Cotton, S., Leonard, A. C., Hahn, J., Caprini-Faigin, C. A., et al. (2010). Religious coping and physiological, psychological, social and spiritual outcomes in patients with HIV/AIDS: Cross-sectional and longitudinal findings. *AIDS and Behavior, 14*(2), 379–389.

Trevino, K. M., Pargament, K. I., Krause, N., Ironson, G., & Hill, P. (2019). Stressful life events and religious/spiritual struggle: Moderating effects of the general orienting system. *Psychology of Religion and Spirituality, 11*(3), 214–224.

Tsai, J., El-Gabalawy, R., Sledge, W. H., Southwick, S. M., & Pietrzak, R. H. (2015). Posttraumatic growth among veterans in the USA: Results from the National Health and Resilience in Veterans study. *Psychological Medicine, 45*(1), 165–179.

Turner, A. K. (1993). *The history of hell*. New York: Houghton Mifflin Harcourt.

Twenge, J. M., & Campbell, W. K. (2009). *The narcissism epidemic: Living in the age of entitlement.* New York: Free Press.

Twenge, J. M., Campbell, W. K., & Gentile, B. (2012). Increases in individualistic words and phrases in American books, 1960–2008, *PLoS One, 7*(7), e40181.

Twohig, M. P., Crosby, J. M., & Cox, J. M. (2009). Viewing Internet pornography: For whom is it problematic, how, and why? *Sexual Addiction and Compulsivity, 16*(4), 252–266.

Vaaler, M. L., Ellison, C. G., & Powers, D. A. (2009). Religious influences on the risk of marital dissolution. *Journal of Marriage and Family, 71*(4), 917–934.

Vanderbleek, E., & Gilbert, K. (2018). Too much versus too little control: The etiology, conceptualization, and treatment implications of overcontrol and undercontrol. *Behavior Therapist, 41*(3), 125–130.

Van Tongeren, D. R., Aten, J. D., McElroy, S., Davis, D. E., Shannonhouse, L., & Davis, E. B., et al. (2019). Development and validation of a measure of spiritual fortitude. *Psychological Trauma: Theory, Research, Practice, and Policy, 11*(6), 588–596.

Van Tongeren, D. R., Hill, P. C., Krause, N., Ironson, G. H., & Pargament, K. I. (2017). The mediating role of meaning in the association between stress and health. *Annals of Behavioral Medicine, 51*(5), 775–781.

Van Tongeren, D. R., Sanders, M., Edwards, M., Davis, E. B., Aten, J. D., Ranter, J. M., et al. (2019). Religious and spiritual struggles alter God representations. *Psychology of Religion and Spirituality, 11*(3), 225–232.

Van Tongeren, D. R., Worthingon, E. L., Jr., Davis, D. E., Hook, J. N., Reid, C. A., & Garthe, R. C . (2018). Positive religious coping in relationships predicts spiritual growth through communication with the sacred. *Psychology of Religion and Spirituality, 10*(1), 55–62.

van Uden, M. H. F., Pieper, J. Z. T., & Zondag, H. J. (2014). *Knockin' on heaven's door: Religious and receptive coping in mental health.* Aachen, Germany: Shaker Verlag.

Vazquez, C., Cervellón, P., Pérez-Sales, P., Vidales, D., & Gaborit, M. (2005). Positive emotions in earthquake survivors in El Salvador (2001). *Journal of Anxiety Disorders, 19*(3), 313–328.

Vieten, C., & Scammell, S. (2015). *Spiritual and religious competencies in clinical practice: Guidelines for psychotherapists and mental health professionals.* Oakland, CA: New Harbinger.

Vishkin, A., Bigman, Y. E., Porat, R., Solak, N., Halperin, E., & Tamir, M. (2016). God rest our hearts: Religiosity and cognitive reappraisal. *Emotion, 16*(2), 252–262.

Vohs, K. D., Baumeister, R. F., & Schmeichel, B. J. (2012). Motivation, personal beliefs, and limited resources all contribute to self-control. *Journal of Experimental Social Psychology, 48*(4), 943–947.

Wachholtz, A., & Sambamoorthi, U. (2011). National trends in prayer use as a coping mechanism for health concerns: Changes from 2002 to 2007. *Psychology of Religion and Spirituality, 3*(2), 67–77.

Wade, N. G., Worthington, E. L., Jr., & Vogel, D. L. (2007). Effectiveness of religiously tailored interventions in Christian therapy. *Psychotherapy Research, 17*(1), 91–105.

Walker, D. F., Reid, H. W., O'Neill, T., & Brown, L. (2009). Changes in personal religion/spirituality during and after childhood abuse: A review and synthesis. *Psychological Trauma: Theory, Research, Practice, and Policy, 1*(2), 130–145.

Wang, D. C., Aten, J. D., Boan, D., Jean-Charles, W., Griff, K. P, Valcin, V. C., et al. (2016).

Culturally adapted spiritually oriented trauma-focused cognitive-behavioral therapy for child survivors of Restavek. *Spirituality in Clinical Practice, 3*(4), 224–236.

Warner, H. L., Mahoney, A., & Krumrei, E. J. (2009). When parents break sacred vows: The role of spiritual appraisals, coping, and struggles in young adults' adjustment to parental divorce. *Psychology of Religion and Spirituality, 1*(4), 233–248.

Warren, P., Van Eck, K., Townley, G., & Kloos, B. (2015). Relationships among religious coping, optimism, and outcomes for persons with psychiatric disabilities. *Psychology of Religion and Spirituality, 7*(2), 91–99.

Watts, A. (2004). *Out of your mind.* Retrieved from *https://www.organism.earth/library/document/out-of-your-mind-7.*

Webb, M., Charbonneau, A. M., McCann, R. A., & Gayle, K. R. (2011). Struggling and enduring with God, religious support, and recovery from severe mental illness. *Journal of Clinical Psychology, 67*(12), 1161–1176.

Webber, D., & Kruglanski, A. W. (2018). The social psychological makings of a terrorist. *Current Opinion in Psychology, 19*, 131–134.

Weeks, M., & Lupfer, M. B. (2000). Religious attributions and proximity of influence: An investigation of direct interventions and distal explanations. *Journal for the Scientific Study of Religion, 39*(3), 348–362.

Werdel, M. B., Dy-Liacco, G. S., Ciarrocchi, J. W., Wicks, R. J., & Breslford, G. M. (2014). The unique role of spirituality in the process of growth following stress and trauma. *Pastoral Psychology, 63*(1), 57–71.

Wiesel, E. (1972). *The night trilogy.* New York: Hill & Wang.

Wiesel, E. (1979). *The trial of God* (M. Wiesel, Trans.). New York: Random House.

Wiesel, E. (2012). *Open heart* (M. Wiesel, Trans.). New York: Schocken.

Wilt, J. A., Evans, W. R., Pargament, K. I., Exline, J. J., Fletcher, T. L., Teng, E. J., et al. (2019). Predictors of moral struggles among veterans. *Traumatology, 25*(4), 303–315.

Wilt, J. A., Exline, J. J., Grubbs, J. B., Park, C. L., & Pargament, K. I. (2016). God's role in suffering: Theodicies, divine struggle, and mental health. *Psychology of Religion and Spirituality, 8*(4), 352–362.

Wilt, J. A., Grubbs, J. B., Exline, J. J., & Pargament, K. I. (2021). Authenticity, inauthenticity, presence of meaning, and struggles with ultimate meaning: Nuanced between- and within-personal associations. *Journal of Research in Personality.* Advance online publication.

Wilt, J. A., Grubbs, J. B., Lindberg, M. J., Exline, J. J., & Pargament, K. I. (2017). Anxiety predicts increases in struggles with religious/spiritual doubt over two weeks, one month, and one year. *International Journal for the Psychology of Religion, 27*(1), 26–34.

Wilt, J. A., Grubbs, J. B., Pargament, K. I., & Exline, J. J. (2017). Religious and spiritual struggles, past and present: Relations to the Big Five and well-being. *International Journal for the Psychology of Religion, 27*(1), 51–64.

Wilt, J. A., Hall, T., Pargament, K. I., & Exline, J. J. (2017). Trajectories of religious/spiritual struggles between years 1 and 2 of college: The predictive role of religious belief salience. *International Journal for the Psychology of Religion, 27*(4), 172–187.

Wilt, J. A., Pargament, K. I., & Exline, J. J. (2018). The transformative power of the sacred: Social, personal, and religious/spiritual antecedents and consequents of sacred moments during a religious/spiritual struggle. *Psychology of Religion and Spirituality, 11*(3), 233–246.

Wilt, J. A., Pargament, K. I., Exline, J. J., Barrera, T. L., & Teng, E. J. (2019). Spiritual transformation among veterans in response to a religious/spiritual struggle. *Psychology of Religion and Spirituality, 11*(3), 266–277.

Wilt, J. A., Stauner, N., & Exline, J. J. (2020). *Beliefs and experiences involving God, the devil, human spirits, and fate: Social, motivational, and cognitive predictors.* Manuscript submitted for publication.

Wilt, J. A., Stauner, N., Harriott, V. A., Exline, J. J., & Pargament, K. I. (2019). Partnering with God: Religious coping and perceptions of divine intervention predict spiritual transformation in response to religious/spiritual struggle. *Psychology of Religion and Spirituality, 11*(3), 278–290.

Wilt, J. A., Stauner, N., Lindberg, M. J., Grubbs, J. B., Exline, J. J., & Pargament, K. I. (2017). Struggle with ultimate meaning: Nuanced associations with search for meaning, presence of meaning, and mental health. *Journal of Positive Psychology, 13*(3), 240–251.

Wilt, J. A., Takahashi, J. T., Jeong, P., Exline, J. J., & Pargament, K. I. (2020). Open-ended and closed-ended measures of religious/spiritual struggles: A mixed-methods study. *Religions, 11*(10), 505.

Winkelman, W. D., Lauderdale, K., Balboni, M. J., Phelps, A. C., Peteet, J. R., Block, S. D., et al. (2011). The relationship of spiritual concerns to the quality of life of advanced cancer patients: Preliminary findings. *Journal of Palliative Medicine, 14*(9), 1022–1028.

Winter, U., Hauri, D., Huber, S., Jenewein, J., Schnyder, U., & Kraemer, B. (2009). The psychological outcome of religious coping with stressful life events in a Swiss sample of church attendees. *Psychotherapy and Psychosomatics, 78*(4), 240–244.

Wittmeyer, A. P. Q. (2018, October 19). Eight stories of men's regret. *New York Times.* https://www.nytimes.com/interactive/2018/10/18/opinion/men-metoo-high-school.html.

Witvliet, C. V. O., Phipps, K. A., Feldman, M. E., & Beckham, J. C. (2004). Posttraumatic mental and physical health correlates of forgiveness and religious coping in military veterans. *Journal of Traumatic Stress, 17*(3), 269–273.

Wong, P. T. P. (2015). Meaning therapy: Assessments and interventions. *Existential Analysis, 26*(1), 154–167.

Wong, P. T. P. (2017). A decade of meaning: Past, present, and future. *Journal of Constructivist Psychology, 30*(1), 82–89.

Wong, S. (2020). *Cultivating sacred moments: Evaluating a pilot program to foster psychospiritual well-being* (Unpublished doctoral dissertation). Bowling Green State University, Bowling Green, OH.

Wong, S., & Pargament, K. I. (2017). Seeing the sacred: Fostering spiritual vision in counselling. *Counselling and Spirituality, 36*(1–2), 51–69.

Wong, S., & Pargament, K. (2019). Meaning, "maker," and morality: Spiritual struggles as predictors of distress and growth in family caregivers. *International Journal of Existential Positive Psychology, 8*(2), 1–17.

Wood, A. W., & Conley, A. H. (2014). Loss of religious or spiritual identifies among the LGBT population. *Counseling and Values, 59*(1), 95–111.

Wortman, C. B. (2004). Posttraumatic growth: Progress and problems. *Psychological Inquiry, 15*(1), 81–90.

Wortmann, J. H., Eisen, E., Hundert, C., Jordan, A. H., Smith, M. W., & Nash, W. P., et al. (2017). Spiritual features of war-related moral injury: A primer for clinicians. *Spirituality in Clinical Practice, 4*(4), 249–261.

Wortmann, J. H., Park, C. L., & Edmondson, D. (2011). Trauma and PTSD symptoms: Does spiritual struggle mediate the link? *Psychological Trauma: Theory, Research, Practice, and Policy, 3*(4), 442–452.

Yaden, D. B., Haidt, J., Hood, R. W., Jr., Vago, D. R., & Newberg, A. B. (2017). The varieties of self-transcendent experience. *Review of General Psychology, 21*(2), 143–160.

Yalom, I. D. (1980). *Existential psychotherapy.* New York: Basic Books.

Yancey, P. (1977). *Where is God when it hurts?* Grand Rapids, MI: Zondervan.

Yildirim, M., Arslan, G., & Alkahtani, A. M. (2021). Do fear of COVID-19 and religious coping predict depression, anxiety, and stress among the Arab populations during health crisis? *Death Studies.* Advanced online publication.

Zarzycka, B. (2019). Predictors and mediating role of forgiveness in the relationship between religious struggle and mental health. *Polskie Forum Psychologiczne, 24*(1), 93–116.

Zarzycka, B., & Zietek, P. (2019). Spiritual growth or decline and meaning-making as mediators of anxiety and satisfaction with life during religious struggle. *Journal of Religion and Health, 58*(4), 1072–1086.

Zeligman, M., Majuta, A. R., & Shannonhouse, L. R. (2020). Posttraumatic growth in prolonged drought survivors in Botswana: The role of social support and religious coping. *Traumatology, 26*(3), 308–316.

Zornow, G. B. (2014). Recovering the forgotten spirituality of lamentation. *Caregiver Journal, 7*(1), 104–117.

Zuckerman, P. (2012). *Faith no more: Why people reject religion.* Oxford, UK: Oxford University Press.

Author Index

Aarnio, K., 279
Abadi, L., 304
Abeling, S., 69
Abeyta, A. A., 281
Abramowitz, J. S., 7, 247
Abu-Raiya, H., 14, 45, 48, 49, 51, 65, 69, 73, 75, 86, 101, 115, 116, 118, 122, 159, 163, 247, 275, 283, 300, 301, 302, 308, 319
Achenbaum, W. A., 20
Acquah, D., 46
Acree, M., 99
Adom-Fynn, D., 46
Affleck, G., 98
Agbaria, Q., 14
Ahles, J. J., 116
Ahmad, S., 69
Ahmadi, F., 120
Ahrens, C. E., 69, 101
Ai, A. L., 57, 75, 79, 100
Ake, G. S., III, 42, 69, 79
Alayan, R., 318
Alberts, H., 257
Alexander, B. B., 109
Alimujiang, A., 190
Alkahtani, A. M., 57
Allen, J. G., 113
Allport, G. W., 25, 28, 30, 226, 228, 309
Altemeyer, B., 227, 235
Alvaro, C., 97
American Psychological Association., 141
Anaissie, E. J., 67
Anderson, S. R., 299
Anderson-Mooney, A. J., 49
Ano, G. G., 6, 49, 57, 62, 101, 119, 268
Appel, J. E., 173
Archambault, E., 101
Arendt, H., 274, 275
Ariely, D., 253
Armour, M. P., 164
Arslan, G., 57
Asamoah, D., 46
Astin, H. S., 49, 51, 64, 65, 100
Aten, J. D., 100, 300
Aukst-Margetić, B., 71
Avants, S. K., 266, 267
Aveni, A., 213

B

Bader, C. D., 279
Baider, L., 56, 164
Baird, J., 220
Baird, R. M., 231
Bakan, D., 27
Baker, J. O., 270, 279
Balboni, M., 72
Balboni, T. A., 19, 72
Baltazar, T., 224
Baltes, P. B., 126
Barclay, P. A., 71
Baron-Cohen, S., 307, 318
Barrera, T. L., 100
Barrett, J. L., 279
Bartkowski, J. P., 303
Bassett, R. L., 319
Batson, C. D., 21, 30, 50, 131, 219, 220, 224, 225
Baubet, T., 279
Baumann, K., 171
Baumeister, R. F., 44, 190, 242, 245, 251, 252, 253, 275
Bechara, A. O., 78
Beck, J. S., 46
Beck, R., 12, 111, 159, 162, 281, 292
Becker, E., 190
Beckham, J. C., 68
Begelman, D. A., 273, 279
Beitel, M., 266
Belavich, T. G., 173
Benhabib, S., 274
Benjet, C., 33
Benore, E. R., 55, 67, 122, 204
Bentley, D. P., 116
Bentzen, J., 121
Berg, G., 190, 223
Bergin, A. E., 36, 141, 154
Berkman, E. T., 263
Berkovits, E., 32
Bermúdez, J. M., 205
Bermúdez, S., 205
Berry, D. L., 144
Berzengi, A., 69, 71
Berzenji, L., 69
Bhikkhu, S., 106
Bigda-Peyton, J. S., 68
Binau, B. A., 112

Bisonó, A. M., 270
Biswas, B., 131
Bjorck, J. P., 64
Björgvinsson, T., 68
Blackie, L. E. R., 85
Blanes, R., 273
Blank, T. O., 74
Bliss, D. E., 48
Blom, J. D., 278
Bloom, P., 245
Bloomfield, H., 181
Boals, A., 101
Boccaccini, M. T., 49
Bockrath, M. F., 63, 69, 80
Boisen, A. T., 18
Bojuwoye, O., 278
Boland, V., 224
Bolling, S. F., 75
Borowiecki, K. J., 87
Boshan, Y., 215
Bourguignon, E., 273
Bowland, S. E., 131, 160, 314
Bowman, N. A., 51, 219, 225
Bradley, D. F., 15, 167, 218
Bradley, R., 78
Brammer, C., 71
Branigan, C., 118
Brant, C., 167
Breines, J. G., 257
Breitkopf, C. R., 210
Brelsford, G. M., 171, 193, 309
Breuninger, M. M., 45, 96, 242, 249, 275
Brewster, M. E., 307
Bridges, R. A., 51
Brocas, J., 273
Broer, K. A., 176
Brontë, A., 232
Brooks, D., 42, 197, 198
Brown, K. W., 265
Brown, L., 54
Bruce, A. J., 49
Brudek, P., 78
Brunell, A. B., 86
Bryant, A. N., 49, 51, 64, 65, 100, 102
Buber, M., 211
Bull, D. L., 279
Burdzy, D., 64
Burke, L. A., 8, 45, 63, 168
Burley, M., 264
Bushman, B. J., 44
Büssing, A., 171, 264

C

Cahill, S. P., 7
Calhoun, L. G., 85, 88, 96, 98, 113, 131, 225
Campbell, J., 89
Campbell, W. K., 42, 86, 198, 252
Camus, A., 197
Cann, A., 131
Cardell, B., 179
Carey, M. P., 57
Carlson, H., 71
Carpenter, R., 20
Carr, B. I., 77
Carretta, R. F., 303
Carroll, T. D., 54
Carson, V. B., 62
Carter, E. C., 245, 264
Cashwell, C. S., 116
Castaneda, C., 123
Cervellón, P., 165
Chan, C. S., 69, 101

Chapman, H., 243
Charbonneau, A. M., 49, 180
Charbonneau, C., 100, 167
Chardon, M. L., 71
Chatters, L. M., 306
Chatzisarantis, N. L., 253
Chen, H., 68
Chen, S., 257
Chen, Y., 191
Chen, Z. J., 78
Cheng, Z. H., 302
Cherniak, A. D., 77
Cheung, C., 27
Cheyne, J. A., 279
Childs, R. E., 217
Chittister, J. D., 15, 21, 88, 123, 131, 181, 268
Cho, D., 101
Chochinov, H. M., 210
Chodron, P., 235
Choi, J., 264
Chouhoud, Y., 217
Chow, E. O. W., 194
Christie, J., 65
Christopher, A. N., 224
Churchwell, M. C., 193
Ciarrocchi, J. W., 171
Clarke, A., 6
Clements, M., 307
Cloninger, C. R., 27
Coe, G. A., 92
Coffen, R. D., 224
Cohen, A. B., 7
Cohen, L. H., 98
Cole, B. S., 77, 96, 160, 208
Collins, D. J., 273, 274, 278
Conley, A. H., 306
Connery, A. L., 196
Connolly, K. M., 247
Cooper, L. B., 49
Cotton, S., 67
Cowden, R. G., 81
Cox, J. M., 242
Crabtree, S., 49
Creswell, J. D., 265
Croog, S., 98
Crosby, J. M., 242
Crumpler, C. A., 28
Csikszentmihalyi, M., 78
Cummings, J. P., 20, 140
Currier, J. M., 17, 19, 20, 54, 71, 72, 168, 172, 193, 247, 258, 300
Curtis, K. T., 303

D

Dabrowski, K., 36
Damen, A., 15, 67
Davidson, T. I., 176
Davis, C. G., 98
Davis, D. E., 257, 306
Davis, E. B., 78
de Castella, R., 91, 93, 94
De la Cruz, J., 181
Decker, L. R., 82, 243, 256
Dees, M. K., 193
Dein, S., 170, 278
Dekkers, W. J., 193
Del Re, A. C., 140
Delaney, H. D., 270
DeMarco, G. A., 73
DeMaris, A., 309, 317
Desai, K. M., 96, 100, 102, 116, 120, 202, 308, 319
DeShea, L., 257

DeSteno, D., 266
Devor, N. G., 314
DeWall, C. N., 253
Dickens, C., 215
Dillard, A., 216
Dinh, T. Q., 274
Doane, M. J., 302
Dodge, B., 303
Doehring, C., 6, 19, 46, 54, 111, 117, 123, 140, 156, 158, 172
Doheny, K. K., 193
Dollahite, D. C., 300, 301, 305
Done, D., 224, 227, 235
Dostoevsky, F., 215
Dransart, D. A. C., 217
Drescher, K. D., 17, 144, 246
Driscoll, M., 273
Dubow, E. F., 302
Duckitt, J., 307
Durà-Vilà, G., 170
During, E. H., 279
Durkheim, E., 26, 298
Dworsky, C. K. O., 19, 93, 112, 157, 159, 160, 237
Dy-Liacco, G. S., 171

E

Earl, T. R., 273
Eaton, H. S., 159
Ebadi, A., 120
Ecklund, E. H., 270
Edinger-Schons, L. M., 124
Edmond, T., 131, 160
Edmondson, D., 30, 56, 74
Edwards, L. M., 118
Efrati, Y., 263
Egginton, J. S., 91, 94, 210
Einstein, A., 28
Elahi, F. M., 279
Elbert, T., 76
El-Gabalawy, R., 96
Elkins, D. N., 210
Elliott, M., 302
Ellis, A., 109
Ellis, M. R., 110
Ellison, C. G., 16, 64, 65, 116, 168, 190, 218, 221, 223, 226, 231, 303
Emery-Tiburcio, E. E., 15
Emmons, R. A., 26, 27, 28, 32, 43, 191
Enders, T., 98
Engdahl, B. E., 180
Epictetus, 53
Erbes, C. R., 180, 258
Erdrich, L., 236
Erikson, E. H., 17, 34, 87, 124, 218, 224
Ernst, E., 264
Eskin, M., 72
Espnes, G. A., 118
Esposito, J., 307
Evans, T., 293
Evans, W. R., 16, 247, 249, 251
Exline, J. J., 6, 8, 9, 10, 14, 15, 20, 27, 30, 31, 35, 36, 40, 41, 42, 43, 45, 46, 49, 50, 51, 52, 55, 56, 57, 58, 64, 65, 70, 77, 86, 96, 100, 105, 106, 112, 115, 120, 122, 123, 131, 139, 143, 144, 148, 156, 161, 162, 163, 164, 166, 167, 168, 170, 171, 172, 173, 176, 178, 180, 192, 193, 199, 205, 215, 217, 218, 220, 222, 223, 225, 227, 242, 245, 247, 251, 252, 255, 257, 258, 271, 272, 273, 275, 276, 277, 278, 280, 281, 283, 287, 290, 300, 301, 302, 305, 307, 325

F

Falb, M. D., 69, 247
Fallot, R. D., 160, 170
Fang, Q., 116, 205
Fater, K., 54, 303
Feindler, E. L., 170
Feldman, D., 48
Feldman, M. E., 68
Fenster, J. R., 98, 99
Festinger, L., 221
Feuille, M., 64
Fincham, F., 52
Finocchiaro, M. A., 13
Fisher, A. R., 227
Fisher, M. L., 245, 255
Fisher, R. H., 95
Fitchett, G., 15, 41, 49, 52, 57, 67, 73, 144
Flaherty, S. M., 170, 178, 181, 182
Flannelly, K. J., 16, 66, 116, 190, 218, 220, 221, 223, 303
Fleischhack, M., 273
Fletcher, M. A., 75
Fletcher, T. L., 56, 275, 300
Florack, P., 100, 167
Floyd, F. J., 307
Flückiger, C., 140
Flynn, K. A., 301
Folkman, S., 33, 53, 99, 282
Fontana, A., 243
Ford, M. E., 26
Forester, B. P., 15
Foshager, D., 300
Foster, A., 307
Foster, J. D., 86, 193, 247
Foster, K. A., 314
Fowler, J. W., 88, 107, 129, 218, 234, 235
Foy, D. W., 144
Frankel, E., 106, 112, 113, 129, 130, 131, 155, 156, 158, 177, 182, 194, 207, 224, 235, 236, 253
Frankl, V. E., 40, 93, 177, 189, 192, 193, 194, 197, 199, 200, 209
Frantz, C. M., 196
Fraser, G. A., 273
Frazier, A. L., 191
Frazier, P., 98
Fredrickson, B. L., 118
Freud, S., 26
Frick, E., 171
Friedman, T. L., 131
Fromm, E., 26, 275
Frueh, B. C., 247
Fugelsang, J. A., 279
Fujikawa, A. M., 46, 171
Fullilove, M. T., 208
Fullilove, R. E., 208
Funai, A. P., 71
Fundaminsky, S., 166

G

Gaborit, M., 165
Gailliot, M., 253
Galek, K., 190, 218, 223
Galilei, G., 233
Gall, T. L., 17, 100, 119, 167, 170, 327
Gallagher, T. M., 295
Gallup, G., Jr., 116
Gandhi, M., 213, 256
Ganzevoort, R. R., 267, 270
Gauthier, K. J., 224
Gayle, K. R., 180
Gearing, R. E., 279

Gee, C. B., 168
Geertz, C., 26, 213
Gemmill, C., 110
Genia, V., 235
Gentile, B., 42
George, L. S., 190
Gerber, M. M., 101
Germer, C. K., 257
Gervais, W. M., 301
Ghaempanah, Z., 34
Ghanei, M., 120
Gibbons, J. A., 70
Gilbert, K., 252, 267
Gilbert, P., 257
Gill, A. R., 300
Gino, F., 253
Goldberg, P., 181
Goldhagen, D. J., 281
Goodman, M., 109
Gow, K. M., 274
Gramling, S. E., 101
Grand, S., 245
Granqvist, P., 49
Grant, J., 243
Green, C. L., 20
Green, L. L., 208
Greenberg, D., 262, 278
Greene, B., 40
Greene, J. D., 279
Greene, J. M., 14
Griffith, J. L., 18, 19, 43, 150, 157, 168, 169, 314, 318
Griffith, M. E., 150
Groessi, E., 264
Groopman, J., 169
Grossoehme, D. H., 70
Grubbs, J. B., 9, 10, 14, 20, 30, 40, 41, 42, 43, 45, 46,
    47, 49, 50, 55, 56, 64, 65, 105, 112, 139, 143,
    144, 156, 161, 163, 166, 167, 170, 171, 172, 180,
    192, 193, 199, 205, 215, 217, 220, 222, 223, 225,
    242, 243, 251, 272, 275, 276, 278, 283, 300,
    302, 307
Guillory, J. M., 303
Guion, K., 45
Guirguis-Younger, M., 119
Gutierrez, I. A., 168, 243, 247

H
Haar, J. M., 128
Haggar, M. S., 253
Hahn, J., 67, 74
Haidt, J., 28
Haines, S. J., 127
Hale-Smith, A., 30, 74
Hall, D. L., 109
Hall, T. W., 46, 50, 86, 96, 116, 120, 122, 166, 171,
    184
Hanh, T. N., 294
Haque, A., 264
Harari, Y. N., 307
Hardy, A., 122
Harman, M. J., 49
Harriott, V. A., 50, 86, 123, 168, 258, 287
Harris, J. I., 19, 72, 73, 76, 160, 180, 258
Harris, W., 110
Harrison, D. A., 144
Hart, A. C., 105, 116, 118, 128, 131, 225, 325
Hartog, K., 274
Haugen, M. R. G., 99
Haugk, K. C., 140
Hawking, S., 231
Hawkins, D. E., 20
Hayes, J. A., 15

Hayes, S. C., 112, 264
Hayward, R. D., 190, 217, 223, 303
Hecht, J. M., 215, 216, 224
Heckman, J. P., 170
Heim, L., 76
Heintzelman, S. J., 190
Held, P., 246
Helgeson, V. S., 98, 99
Henning, K. R., 247
Henrie, J. A., 226
Hensler, M., 45
Herman, J. L., 18, 19
Hernandez, K. M., 6
Herold, J., 245
Hewstone, M., 316
Hill, P. C., 16, 55, 58, 74, 109, 192, 196
Hinman, J., 69
Hodge, D. R., 150, 248
Hoek, H. W., 278
Hofmann, W., 251
Holeman, V. T., 257
Holland, J. M., 17
Holley, D. M., 215
Holt, C. L., 65
Homolka, S. J., 167, 168, 170, 173
Hood, R. W., Jr., 28, 30
Hopkins, C. M., 77
Hopkins, P., 299
Hornbacher, M., 118
Horen, S. G., 42, 69, 79
Horvath, A. O., 140, 154
Horváth-Szabó, K., 224
Hosseini, S. M., 34
Huang, B., 57, 100
Hudson, M. R., 116
Humphreys, J., 235
Hunsberger, B., 215, 218, 219, 221, 222, 227, 228, 235
Huppert, J. D., 7, 262

I
Idliby, R., 235
Illaiee, A. S., 278
Im, H., 300
Ingber, H., 319
Inglehart, M. R., 131
Ironson, D., 75
Ironson, G. H., 16, 45, 49, 55, 58, 74, 75, 79, 109, 169,
    192, 196, 245
Isaak, S. L., 247
Ishisaka, A., 57

J
Jackson, M., 280
Jacobs, C., 171
Jacobsen, P. B., 99
Jaffe, H., 181
James, F. A., III, 121
James, W., 21, 28, 106, 112, 127, 191, 197, 241, 291
Jankowski, K. R. B., 190
Janoff-Bulman, R., 33, 45, 196
Janu, A., 54
Jayawickreme, E., 85
Jeffries, W. L., IV, 303
Jelinek, C. S., 318
Jensen, L. A., 273, 278
Jeong, P., 275
Jobson, L., 69
Johnson, C. V., 15
Johnson, R. H., 49
Johnson, S. K., 164
Johnson, T. H., 21
Johnson, W. B., 109

Jones, E. J., 273
Jones, J. W., 27, 42, 128, 197, 226
Jones, R. S., 19, 141, 154, 232, 326
Jones, S. L., 36
Joseph, S., 85, 95, 97
Jouriles, E. N., 168, 175
Juergensmeyer, M., 299
Jung, C. G., 159, 275, 294
Jung, J. H., 168

K

Kadim, A., 69
Kam, C. D., 308
Kamble, S., 162, 166
Kane, M. N., 301
Kao, L. E., 168
Kaplan, A., 108
Kaplan, K. J., 139
Karff, S. E., 7, 15, 86, 107, 119, 155, 156, 176, 244
Kashdan, T. B., 130
Kaslow, N. J., 78
Kass, J. D., 183, 210, 265
Kazak, A. E., 71
Kazemnejad, A., 120
Kelly, M. H., 273
Keng, S L., 265
Kesebir, P., 252
Kesebir, S., 252
Keshavarzi, H., 264
Keshtgar, M. R. S., 176
Ketcham, K., 106, 129, 187, 249, 250, 258, 268
Kézdy, A., 224
Khalsa, S. B. S., 264
Khan, Z. H., 67, 76
Kidd, S. M., 156
Kim, E. S., 191
Kimel, S. Y., 318
Kinder, D. R., 308
King, D. E., 62
King, L. A., 126, 190
King, S. D. W., 11, 41, 49, 52, 144
Kinghorn, J., 179
Kirkpatrick, L. A., 49, 173, 294
Kirvan, J., 264
Kitchens, M. B., 114
Klass, D., 204
Klein, C., 319
Klöckner, C. A., 118
Kloos, B., 68
Knox, M. C., 257
Koehler, D. J., 279
Koenig, H. G., 8, 62, 67, 70, 73, 74, 119, 160, 169, 243,
    246, 274, 283, 298, 327
Koh, H. K., 191
Koić, E., 71
Kojetin, B. A., 51, 219, 225
Kolodiejchuk, B., 166
Kooistra, W. P., 214, 215, 217, 222
Kopacz, M. S., 196
Korbman, M. D., 170
Kornfield, J., 157, 235
Kosarkova, A., 54
Krause, N., 16, 45, 47, 48, 49, 55, 58, 65, 74, 79, 109,
    115, 116, 118, 122, 159, 163, 190, 192, 196, 217,
    218, 221, 223, 224, 226, 231, 247, 283, 302,
    303, 306
Krause, S. J., 176
Kremer, H., 74
Kristjansson, E., 167
Krok, D., 78
Kronfol, Z., 75
Kroplewski, Z., 108

Kruglanski, A. W., 198
Krumrei, E. J., 55, 69, 78, 274, 285
Kübler-Ross, E., 324
Kudler, T., 218, 223
Kuhlman, S., 72
Kunda, Z., 281
Kunst, J. R., 318
Küpper, B., 308, 316
Kurtz, E., 106, 129, 187, 249, 250, 258, 268
Kushner, H. S., 116, 180, 181, 182, 244
Kusina, J. R., 247
Kusner, K. G., 317, 318
Kvande, M. N., 118
Kyriakakis, S., 131

L

LaGuardia, J. G., 128
LaMothe, R., 28, 172
Lane, C., 224
Larson, J., 98
Latif, U., 67
Latzer, Y., 71
Lauricella, S. K., 302, 304, 308
Laycock, J. P., 273
Lazarus, R. S., 53, 282
Leaman, S. C., 168
Leavey, G., 270
Le, D., 65
Lee, J., 64, 65, 223
Lee, M., 67
Lee, M. S., 264
Lee, S. A., 70
Lehman, D. R., 102
Lemieux, C. M., 100
Lerner, M., 208
Levin, M. L., 303
Levine, S., 98
Lewis, C. S., 11, 162, 167, 273
Liddle, B. J., 304, 305
Liebert, E., 295
Lim, A., 278
Lim, H., 47
Lin, C. Y., 73
Lindberg, M. J., 42, 223
Lindeman, M., 279
Lindsay, D. M., 116
Lindsay, E. K., 265
Linley, P. A., 85, 95, 97
Lipsyte, R., 40
Litz, B. T., 246, 256, 267
Lobel, M., 171
Lockman, J. D., 273
Loevinger, J., 113
Loewenthal, K. M., 160
Lohr, J. M., 247
Lomax, J. W., 205, 218, 232
Lopez, S. J., 118
Lord, B. D., 101
Luborsky, M., 109
Lucette, A., 74
Lupfer, M. B., 274, 280
Luzader, J., 84
Luzzatto, M. C., 270, 275
Lynberg, M., 199
Lynch, T. R., 251
Lyons, M. E., 170

M

Ma, Y. Y., 113
MacCarthy, M., 273
Madan-Swain, A., 45, 71
Maercker, A., 97, 99

Magyar, G. M., 6, 55, 196, 244, 261
Magyar-Russell, G. M., 16, 49, 55, 68, 78, 101, 165, 205
Mahoney, A. M., 6, 14, 27, 28, 29, 32, 54, 55, 69, 73, 115, 191, 285, 298, 304, 308, 309, 317, 319, 327
Majuta, A. R., 100
Malinakova, K., 54
Malloy, M. C., 15
Maltby, J., 50
Maltby, L. E., 184
Mancuso, R. A., 118
Mandela, N., 203
Mann, S. K., 66
Marcia, J. E., 218
Marcum, J. P., 168, 303
Marek, P., 224
Margolin, A., 266
Markman, H. J., 307
Marks, L. D., 300, 305, 306
Marques, S. C., 118
Martela, F., 190, 191
Martin, J., 125, 209, 300
Martin, P. J., 41, 49, 52
Martínez-Taboas, A., 199
Martos, T., 224
Marty, M. E., 18, 110, 111
Masheg, D. J., 250
Maslow, A. H., 26
Matz, D. C., 109
Maunu, A., 57
May, R., 52, 294
Mayseless, O., 114, 214
McAdams, D. P., 84, 99
McCabe, G., 278
McCann, R. A., 180
McCleary-Gaddy, A. T., 78
McConnell, K. M., 16, 45, 66, 71
McCormick, W. H., 54, 193, 196, 300
McCullough, M. E., 62, 245, 264
McDermott, R. C., 20, 193, 300
McFarland, C., 97
McGee, J. S., 71, 159, 205
McIntosh, D. N., 51, 131, 220
McKay, R., 245
McKenzie, B., 215
McMillan, J., 131
McMillen, J. C., 95, 98
McNamara, P., 273
Mead, N. L., 253
Medlock, M. M., 17
Meisenhelder, J. B., 168
Meltzer, T., 306
Memaryan, N., 34
Mencken, F. C., 279
Menninger, K., 127
Mercadante, L., 14, 323
Merton, T., 112
Mezulis, A. H., 116
Michalsen, A., 264
Midlarsky, E., 68
Mihaljević, S., 71
Mikulincer, M., 275
Milkeris, L., 193
Miller, C. T., 78
Miller, M. L., 5
Miller, W. R., 270
Milošević, M., 71
Moen, P., 242, 243, 249, 250
Mogenson, G., 181
Mohr, S., 69
Moksnes, U. K., 118

Montgomery, S. B., 66
Moreira-Almeida, A., 68
Morgan, D. L., 306
Morgan, K. A. D., 165, 166
Moro, M.-R., 279
Mother Teresa, 166
Mourad, R., 224
Movahedizadeh, M., 68
Moye, J., 98, 101
Mozes, E., 69
Mrug, S., 45, 63
Mullaney, J. A., 54, 303
Murch, R. L., 98
Murphy, P. E., 15, 41, 49, 52, 144
Murray, H. A., 26
Murray-Swank, A. B., 141, 158, 159, 179
Murray-Swank, N. A., 6, 54, 141, 158, 159, 160, 179, 183, 306
Mussett, J. M., 11, 100
Mustafa, F., 69
Mvududu, N., 49
Myers, D. R., 71, 159

N

Naik, A. D., 98
Neff, K. D., 257
Neimeyer, R. A., 45, 63, 168
Nelson-Becker, H., 194
New World Encyclopedia., 106
Newberg, A. B., 28
Newlon, M., 48
Newman, S. P., 176
Nezu, A. M., 67
Nezu, C. M., 67
Nguyen, H. T., 274
Nguyen, X. V., 180
Nicholas, J. J., 73
Nichols, C. W., 26
Nicholson, R. A., 114
Nielsen, S. L., 109
Nolen-Hoeksema, S., 98
Norenzayan, A., 169, 301
Norman M., 19
Nosek, M. A., 120
Novotni, M., 181

O

Oaten, M., 253
O'Brien, B., 120
O'Donnell, S. J., 285
Ok, U., 231
Olatunji, B. O., 247
Oliver, J. M., 167
Oliver, S., 235
Ollier-Malaterre, A., 128
Oman, D., 62, 179, 298
O'Neill, T., 54
Öngur, D., 68
Ortberg, J., 224, 235
Öst, L.-G., 265
Otto, R., 28
Owen, L., 261
Oxhandler, H. K., 5, 20

P

Pacini, R., 131
Padgett, E., 317, 318
Pagano, L. A., Jr., 302
Pai, A. L. H., 71
Paika, V., 72, 73
Pakpour, A. H., 73
Palachy, S., 69

Palmer, P. J., 41, 86, 106, 125, 187, 265, 266
Pals, J. L., 99
Pancer, S. M., 215, 218, 222
Pargament, K. I., 5, 6, 8, 9, 10, 14, 16, 19, 20, 25, 27,
    29, 30, 35, 36, 40, 41, 42, 45, 46, 47, 48, 49, 50,
    51, 52, 54, 55, 56, 57, 58, 63, 64, 65, 67, 68, 69,
    70, 71, 73, 74, 76, 79, 86, 96, 100, 101, 102, 105,
    106, 109, 112, 114, 115, 116, 118, 119, 120, 122,
    123, 128, 131, 140, 142, 143, 144, 145, 150, 159,
    160, 161, 163, 166, 167, 168, 169, 173, 191, 192,
    193, 196, 199, 200, 202, 205, 206, 208, 210, 215,
    217, 218, 220, 222, 223, 225, 232, 242, 244, 247,
    251, 261, 268, 272, 274, 275, 276, 278, 281, 283,
    285, 287, 290, 294, 300, 301, 302, 304, 305,
    307, 308, 309, 317, 319
Park, C. L., 19, 30, 47, 56, 57, 65, 71, 74, 75, 98, 99,
    100, 101, 116, 119, 122, 168, 173, 182, 190, 204,
    216, 258, 264, 279, 281
Park, J., 190
Parks, S. D., 56, 87
Parrish, D. E., 20
Parrott, W. G., 87, 102
Patrick, J. H., 226
Patrick, R., 179
Pearce, M. J., 5, 20, 88, 160, 327
Peck, M. S., 294
Pedersen, C. G., 67
Pedersen, H. F., 67
Peereboom, K. S., 148
Pendleton, S., 67
Pennycook, G., 279
Perez, L. M., 8, 119
Pérez-Sales, P., 165
Perry, S. L., 247, 251
Peteet, J. R., 48, 168
Peters, M., 257
Petersen, R., 181
Petrik, M. L., 5
Pew Research Center, 191, 236, 271
Phillips, J. B., 47, 110, 172
Phillips, R. E., III, 14, 302
Phipps, K. A., 68
Piaget, J., 17, 34, 87, 224
Piderman, K. M., 91, 94, 175, 180, 210
Piedmont, R. L., 8, 27, 28, 68
Pieper, J. Z. T., 68
Pietrantoni, L., 119
Pietrzak, R. H., 96
Pirutinsky, S., 68, 77, 170
Plante, T. G., 67
Pleins, J. D., 13
Poll, J., 62
Pomerleau, J. M., 16, 47, 55, 78, 115, 268
Poole, W. S., 296
Posadski, P., 264
Powers, D. A., 303
Prager, D., 308
Prati, G., 119
Pratt, M., 215, 218, 222
Preston, J. L., 309
Price, P., 179
Prigerson, H. G., 72
Prince-Paul, M., 148
Prusak, J., 224
Pruyser, P. W., 122, 214
Przybeck, T. R., 27
Przeworski, A., 307
Puffer, K. A., 220
Putnam, R. D., 198, 252, 316

Q
Quainoo, E. A., 46

R
Rafieinia, P., 34
Raines, A. M., 168
Ramirez, S. P., 49, 67
Ramsey, C., 126
Rand, D. G., 279
Ransom, S., 99
Rawsthorne, L. J., 128
Ray, S. D., 273, 280
Regueiro, V., 160
Reid, H. W., 54
Reid, R. C., 251
Reist Gibbel, M., 160, 238
Renick, M. J., 307
Reynolds, K. A., 98
Reynolds, N., 45, 63, 119
Rhemtulla, M., 169
Rhodes, J. E., 69, 101
Richards, P. S., 261
Richards, T. A., 99, 122, 204
Richardson, P., 101
Riecken, H. W., 221
Rilke, R. M., 231
Rio, K., 273
Ritter, R. S., 309
Rizzuto, A.-M., 49, 171
Roalson, L. A., 303
Robatmili, S., 209
Roberts, L. B., 70
Roberts, L. R., 66
Robertson, T. M., 68
Robins, C. J., 265
Robinson, M. A., 307
Rockenbach, A. B., 84, 90, 92, 93, 94, 129, 298
Rogers, M. L., 273
Roose, K., 273
Root, B. L., 148
Rosenheck, R., 243
Rosetti, S. J., 54
Rosmarin, D. H., 15, 19, 20, 65, 68, 72, 73, 77, 143,
    170, 269, 325
Ross, J. M., 30
Rottenberg, J., 130
Rotz, E., 312
Routledge, C., 281
Roylance, C., 281
Rubinstein, R. L., 109
Rudin, J., 181
Rudin, M., 181
Ruiz, F. J., 112
Rupert, D., 314
Rupp, J., 156
Russell, C. S., 312
Russell, J. B., 275, 296
Russo, M., 128
Russo-Netzer, P., 114, 203, 214
Ryan, R. M., 128
Rybarczyk, B. D., 73

S
Sabahi, P., 34
Sacks, J., 25
Saffari, M., 73
Saint Augustine., 27
Sambamoorthi, U., 121
Sampson, E. E., 108
Sandage, S. J., 49, 314
Sanders, M., 226
Sanderson, W. C., 8
Sandfort, T. G. M., 303
San Roman, L., 58

Santiago, P. N., 17, 327
Sarell, M., 56, 164
Saritoprak, S. N., 14, 50, 86, 120, 245, 246, 258, 270, 293
Sartre, J.-P., 197
Sasson, T., 69
Saunders, S. M., 5, 20, 140
Sawai, R. P., 251
Scammell, S., 310, 326
Schaal, S., 76
Schachter, S., 221
Schenkel, E., 273
Schimmel, S., 252
Schmeichel, B. J., 252
Schmid, K., 316
Schnitker, S. A., 43, 191, 193
Schoenrade, P., 21
Schrimshaw, E. W., 91, 92
Schuck, K. D., 304, 305
Schuettler, D., 101
Schuster, J., 101
Schuster, M. A., 119
Schutt, W. A., 31
Schwartz, A. C., 78
Schwebel, D., 63
Schweitzer, M. E., 253
Scollon, C. K., 126
Sedlar, A. E., 15, 66, 193, 301
Segall, M., 119
Seldes, G., 128, 215, 251
Seli, P., 279
Seligman, M. E. P., 46, 191
Senpai Sensei., 125
Seymour, E. M., 75
Shafranske, E. P., 20, 27, 140
Shah, S. B., 168
Shahsavari, S., 68
Shakespeare-Finch, J., 98
Shani, M., 318
Shannonhouse, L. R., 100
Shanshan, L., 74
Shapiro, F. R., 127
Shariff, A. F., 169, 301, 302
Shaver, P. R., 275
Sheikhi, M. R., 68
Sheldon, K. M., 99
Shenhav, A., 279
Sherman, A. C., 67, 73, 100, 131, 168
Sherman, J. E., 16
Sherman, K. J., 264
Sherman, M. D., 258
Sibley, C. G., 307
Siegel, K., 91, 92
Siev, J., 262
Sikkema, K. J., 160
Silberman, I., 285
Silton, N. R., 190
Silver, R. L., 33
Simmonds, J. G., 91, 93, 94
Simonton, S., 67, 100
Sims, B. M., 54
Slatcher, R. B., 76
Slater, M., 241
Slattery, J. M., 19
Sledge, W. H., 96
Small, J. L., 51, 219, 225
Smeets, E., 257
Smigelsky, M. A., 300
Smith, B. W., 8, 71, 100, 167
Smith, C., 173
Smith, E. M., 95
Smith, H., 106

Smith, H. A., 115
Smith, M. W., 144
Smith, P. H., 57, 71, 100
Smith, P. N., 72
Smith, T. B., 62, 119
Smoski, M. J., 265
Smyth, J. M., 57, 265
Snyder, C. R., 118
Southard, S., 192
Southwick, S. M., 96
Spearing, A. C., 181
Spilka, B., 51
Spohn, R., 67
Sremac, S., 267, 270
Stamper, S. M., 70
Stampfer, M. J., 74
Stanley, M. A., 56, 96
Stanley, S. M., 307
Starmans, C., 245
Starnino, V. R., 160
Staudinger, U. M., 126
Stauner, N., 14, 31, 46, 49, 50, 52, 55, 56, 58, 65, 86, 123, 128, 162, 190, 193, 197, 202, 218, 220, 225, 247, 258, 271, 276, 277, 280, 305, 307
Stavros, G., 314
Steckler, R. A., 116
Steel, J. L., 77
Steger, M. F., 190, 191
Stein, C. H., 57, 73
Stein, S., 261
Steuden, S., 78
Stiff, C., 253
Streib, H., 319
Streit-Horn, J., 204
Stroppa, A., 68
Strosahl, K. D., 112
Strosky, D. G., 326
Stuetzle, R., 75
Stuewig, J., 250
Stygall, J. A., 176
Sulleiman, R., 101
Sultana, S., 67
Suñe, A., 128
Suresh, D. P., 48
Svrakic, D. M., 27
Symonds, D., 140
Szalachowski, R., 108
Szczesniak, M., 108, 118
Szczesniak, R. D., 70
Szymanski, D. M., 303

T

Taieb, O., 279
Tajfel, H., 308
Takahashi, J. T., 275
Tangney, J. P., 250
Tanksley, C. P., 283
Tarakeshwar, N., 14, 66, 67, 74, 100, 160, 168
Tausch, N., 316
Tavel, P., 54
Taylor, B. B., 110, 112
Taylor, D., 235
Taylor, S., 281, 292
Tedeschi, R. G., 85, 88, 96, 98, 113, 131
Tehrani, K., 27
Telles, S., 264
Telushkin, J., 308
ten Boom, C., 177
Teng, E. J., 56, 96, 100, 306
Tennen, H., 98
Tetteh, S. Q., 46
Thigpen, P., 293

Thomas, C. A., 83
Thombre, A., 100
Thomlinson, P., 110
Thomsen, L., 318
Thuné-Boyle, I. C. V., 176
Thurman, J. W., 64
Tice, T. N., 57, 75, 100
Tick, E., 249
Tillich, P., 27, 42, 82, 86, 114, 197, 214
Timoszyk-Tomczak, C., 118
Tisak, J., 77
Tobin, E. T., 76
Tolin, D. F., 7
Tolliver, D., 280
Tolstoy, L., 13
Tomich, P. L., 98
Torres, L. R., 20
Tourgeman, A., 69
Townley, G., 68
Trevino, K. M., 16, 58, 67, 72, 73, 75, 98, 101, 285, 308, 319
Tricot, G., 67
Tsai, J., 96
Tugade, M. M., 118
Turner, A. K., 296
Turner, J., 308
Twenge, J. M., 42, 198, 252
Twohig, M. P., 242, 263

U

Usset, T. J., 258
Uzdavines, A., 15, 218

V

Vaaler, M. L., 303
Vago, D. R., 28
Van Eck, K., 68
van Schie, H. T., 173
Van Tongeren, D. R., 77, 100, 119, 196, 226
van Uden, M. H. F., 68
van Weel, C., 193
Vanderbleek, E., 252, 267
VanderWeele, T. J., 74, 191
Vasconcelles, E. G., 62, 101, 119
Vazquez, C., 165
Velez, B. L., 307
Ventis, W. L., 21
Vernooij-Dassen, M. J., 193
Vidales, D., 165
Vieten, C., 5, 20, 310, 326
Vishkin, A., 119
Vissers, K. C., 193
Voecks, C. D., 258
Vogel, D. L., 142
Vohs, K. D., 251, 252
Volk, F., 42
Vonasch, A. J., 253
Vosler, A. N., 314
Vuksan-Ćusa, B., 71

W

Wachholtz, A., 121
Wade, N. G., 142
Waelde, L. C., 54
Walker, C. R., 84
Walker, D. F., 54
Wallander, J., 63
Walter, M. I., 224
Wang, D. C., 160
Ward, S. J., 190
Warner, H. L., 69, 303, 306
Warner, P., 235
Warren, P., 68, 118
Watson, P. J., 67

Watts, A., 114
Webb, M., 180
Webb, W., 49
Webber, D., 198
Weeks, M., 274
Weissberger, A., 14, 65, 283, 301
Werdel, M. B., 171
Whitehouse, H., 245
Wicks, R. J., 171
Wiesel, E., 11, 12, 164
Wilkins, T. A., 27
Williams, A. F., 102
Williams, B. R., 65
Williams, D. B., 74
Williams, N. L., 247
Williams, T., 126
Wilson, K. G., 112
Wilt, J. A., 10, 30, 31, 41, 45, 46, 47, 50, 56, 65, 79, 100, 101, 105, 115, 116, 118, 120, 123, 126, 128, 143, 172, 190, 193, 197, 199, 202, 205, 220, 223, 249, 251, 258, 271, 273, 275, 276, 277, 278, 280, 287
Winkelman, W. D., 163, 165, 166, 215
Winskowski, A. M., 180
Winter-Pfändler, U., 57, 100
Wittmeyer, A. P. Q., 247
Witvliet, C. V. O., 68, 71, 194
Witztum, E., 278
Wolfe, K., 63
Wong, P. T. P., 190, 191, 209
Wong, S., 5, 14, 20, 35, 36, 47, 55, 69, 106, 112, 114, 115, 205, 206, 225, 268
Wood, A. W., 306
Wood, C., 253
Wood, W., 109
Worthington, E. L., Jr., 78, 142
Wortman, C. B., 33, 102, 103
Wortmann, J. H., 56, 71, 74, 78, 173, 256
Wright, B. R. E., 168
Wright, D. W., 312
Wulff, K. M., 168, 223, 224
Wykle, M., 119

X

Xu, X., 303

Y

Yaden, D. B., 28, 113
Yali, A. M., 8, 9, 10, 50, 64, 143, 144, 161, 163, 171, 193, 199, 217, 220, 225, 251, 272, 276, 278, 283, 302, 307
Yalom, I. D., 7, 41, 197
Yamada, A. M., 274
Yancey, P., 165, 181
Yarborough, P., 116
Yildirim, M., 57, 69
Young, K. P., 300, 305
Young, S., 265

Z

Zachariae, R., 67
Zarzycka, B., 66, 223, 248, 303, 304
Zeligman, M., 100
Zhao, H. C., 159
Zick, A., 308, 316
Zietek, P., 223, 248
Zinnbauer, B. J., 76, 223, 225
Zoellner, T., 97, 99
Zollfrank, T., 72
Zondag, H. J., 68
Zornow, G. B., 176
Zou, Y., 70
Zuckerman, P., 52, 95, 172, 200, 219, 248, 302

Subject Index

Note. *f* or *t* following a page number indicates a figure or a table.

Abandonment, feelings of, 165–166, 301
Abuse, 131–132, 301. *See also* Child abuse; Sexual abuse/assault; Trauma; Violence
Acceptance
  addressing impulse undercontrol and, 264–265
  addressing moral overcontrol and, 261–262
  doubt-related struggles and, 230–233
  interpersonal struggles and, 318–320
  seeing and accepting the darkness, 110–112
  seeing beneath the surface and, 112–117
  spiritually integrated psychotherapy and, 157–158
  talking about in clinical practice and, 176
  weaving wisdom and, 127
Acceptance and commitment therapy (ACT), 111, 264–265, 327
Activities, meaningful, 202–205, 206*t*
Addiction. *See also* Substance use
  addressing impulse undercontrol and, 262–268
  elevation of preliminary concerns over ultimate concerns and, 42–43
  interpersonal struggles and, 310
  moral struggles and, 252
Adjustment, 87, 101, 127
Affirmation
  assessment and, 150–153
  doubt-related struggles and, 221–222
  overview, 132
  sources of, 119–123
  spiritual support and, 122–123
  wholeness and brokenness and, 117–123
Afterlife, 122
Age, 14–15, 55, 59–60. *See also* Development
Aggression
  demonic struggles and, 285
  implications of spiritual struggles for, 76–77
  interpersonal struggles and, 304, 309
  moral struggles and, 246
Agnosticism, 232, 307, 323–324
Ali, Muhammad, 39–40
Alienation, social, 48–49, 310. *See also* Connectedness
Alienation from God, 8, 8*t*, 165–166. *See also* Anger toward God; Divine struggles; God
All-or-nothing thinking, 187
Altruism, 266
Amends, 256–257

Analytical reasoning styles, 279
Anger, 286, 301, 317
Anger toward God. *See also* Alienation from God; Divine struggles; God
  decline and, 66
  facilitating spiritual connectedness and, 179
  life events and, 170–171
  overview, 163–164
Antisocial attitude and behaviors, 285
Anxiety
  demonic struggles and, 279, 283
  doubt-related struggles and, 222–223
  exploring ultimate meaning struggles and, 202
  interpersonal struggles and, 302, 310
  medical population studies and, 67–68
  moral struggles and, 242–243, 246–247
  overview, 65
  struggles of ultimate meaning and, 193
  studies of people dealing with life stressors, 69–70
Apologies, 256–257
Appraisals
  demonic struggles and, 282, 286
  desecration, 54–55
  exploring benevolent spiritual reappraisals and, 176–178
  moral struggles and, 250
  overview, 53–55
  research regarding growth and, 97
  sacred loss, 53–55
Assessment
  decline and, 63
  demonic struggles and, 272–273, 276, 283, 289, 290–291, 292–293
  doubt-related struggles and, 233–234
  explicit spiritual assessment, 146–150, 147*t*, 150*t*
  implicit spiritual assessment, 145–146, 145*t*
  initial spiritual assessment, 142–144, 142*t*, 144*t*
  interpersonal struggles and, 310–312
  life events and, 56
  overview, 7–9, 8*t*, 161
  research regarding growth and, 97–99
  of spiritual struggles, 9–10, 10*t*, 139–153, 142*t*, 144*t*, 145*t*, 147*t*, 150*t*
  struggles of ultimate meaning and, 200–202
  in the wholeness and growth context, 150–153
Assumptions, 45–47

Assumptive worlds. *See* Orienting system
Atheism
    interpersonal struggles and, 307
    normalizing, accepting, and supporting doubt-
        related struggles, 232
    overview, 323–324
    stories of spiritual struggles among atheists and,
        15
    struggles of ultimate meaning and, 193
Atonement, 256–257
Attachment, 173, 279
Attributions, 250, 280–282, 293–296
Authenticity
    authentic guiding vision and, 124–126
    inauthentic purpose and, 41
    struggles of ultimate meaning and, 199–200
Authoritarian worldview, 307
Authors, 13–14
Avoidance, 111–112, 317–318

B

Balancing, 127–128
Behavioral control
    addressing impulse undercontrol and, 263–
        264
    demonic struggles and, 286
    moral struggles and, 245
Behavioral practices, 47–48
Belief systems, 220–221, 222. *See also* Core beliefs
Belongingness, 221–222
Benevolent spiritual reframing
    exploring benevolent spiritual reappraisals and,
        176–178
    overview, 120–121
    spiritually integrated psychotherapy and, 156–157
Benevolent spirituality, 120–123
Biases of the therapist, 21–23, 289–290. *See also*
        Therapist factors
Blame, 294–295. *See also* Responsibility
Both-and thinking, 187
Boundlessness, 6
Breadth. *See also* Narrowness
    assessment and, 150–153
    doubt-related struggles and, 215, 234–236, 235*t*
    overview, 132
    wholeness and brokenness and, 107–117
Brief Religious Coping scale (Brief RCOPE), 8–9,
        8*t*, 143, 276
Brokenness. *See also* Decline; Dis-integration;
        Outcomes
    assessment and, 142, 150–153
    breadth and depth and, 107–117
    cohesiveness and, 123–132
    conceptual model of spiritual struggles and, 26*f*
    doubt-related struggles and, 222–227
    life affirmation and, 117–123
    meaning of, 35–37, 132–133
    overview, 35–37, 104–107, 132–133
    psychological thought on, 106–107
    reflection and, 158
    religious rituals and, 256–257
    religious thought on, 106
    from spiritual struggles, 18
Buddhism
    addressing moral overcontrol and, 256
    authentic guiding vision and, 124–125
    balance and, 128
    life affirmation and, 119
    moral struggles and, 241, 247
    perspectives on growth and, 86
    wholeness and brokenness and, 106

C

Caregivers
    addressing moral overcontrol and, 260
    moral struggles and, 242, 247
    studies of people dealing with life stressors, 69–70
Catastrophization, 73
Catholicism, 256, 258
Change, 130–132
Character, 198
Child abuse. *See also* Abuse; Clergy, abuse by; Life
        events; Trauma
    interpersonal struggles and, 303
    openness to change and, 131–132
    spiritual struggles and, 54–55
Chittister, Joan, 15–17
Christianity
    benevolent spiritual reframing and, 120–121
    demonic struggles and, 278, 283, 285, 293–294
    interpersonal struggles and, 308
    life affirmation and, 119
    moral struggles and, 241
    perspectives on growth and, 86
    wholeness and brokenness and, 106
Church, the. *See* Religious institutions
Clergy, abuse by. *See also* Child abuse; Religious
        leaders; Sexual abuse/assault
    interpersonal struggles and, 303, 309–322
    spiritual struggles from, 54–55
Clinical interview, 290–291. *See also* Assessment
Clinical practice implications. *See also* Spiritually
        integrated psychotherapy
    assessment and, 139–153, 142*t*, 144*t*, 145*t*, 147*t*,
        150*t*
    concerns regarding addressing spiritual struggles
        and, 325–327
    demonic struggles and, 286–297
    distress, disorientation, and decline, 82–83
    divine struggles and, 174–187, 181*t*
    doubt-related struggles and, 227–239, 235*t*
    how to address spiritual struggles, 153–160
    interpersonal struggles and, 309–322
    intervention programs for spiritual struggles, 160,
        237–239
    moral struggles and, 253–268
    overview, 137
    struggles of ultimate meaning and, 200–211, 206*t*
Cognitive development, 87
Cognitive schemas. *See* Orienting system
Cognitive-behavioral therapy (CBT), 46, 327
Cohesiveness. *See also* Integration; Wholeness
    assessment and, 150–153
    authentic guiding vision and, 124–126
    exploring doubts and, 236–239
    integrating divine struggles into a cohesive whole,
        185–187
    overview, 123–124, 132
    weaving wisdom, 126–132
    wholeness and brokenness and, 123–132
Combat. *See also* Life events; Military veterans
        Posttraumatic stress disorder (PTSD)
    interpersonal struggles and, 300
    moral struggles and, 246–248, 249
    spiritual struggles and, 56–57
Commitment to religious and spiritual beliefs,
        220–221
Commonality with others, 318
Communication skills, 307, 309
Compassion
    addressing impulse undercontrol and, 265–266
    addressing moral overcontrol and, 255–258
    life affirmation and, 117, 118–119

Complex spiritual struggles model, 45. 63, 70, 72, 80–81, 148, 223, 247
Compulsive disorders, 252. *See also* Obsessive–compulsive disorder (OCD); Obsessive–compulsiveness
Conceptual model of spiritual struggles. *See also* Search for significance
    distress, disorientation, and decline, 77–79
    divine struggles and, 170–173
    growth and/or decline and, 34–35, 88–89
    orienting system and, 29–31
    overview, 25, 26*f*, 37
    primary, secondary, and complex, 45, 63
    processes that guide the search for significance, 32–34
    spirituality embedded in significance and, 27–29
    stressful life events and, 31–34
    wholeness and brokenness and, 35–37
Conflicting evidence, 217
Conflicts with others, 300–301, 302, 310, 320–322
Connectedness. *See also* Relationship functioning
    conceptual model of spiritual struggles and, 26
    doubt-related struggles and, 221–222
    facilitating in clinical practice, 178–181, 181*t*
    overview, 48–49
    spiritually integrated psychotherapy and, 159
    working on reconnection with other people, 316–322
Consequences. *See also* Outcomes; Spiritual growth
    demonic struggles and, 283–286
    divine struggles and, 167–169
    doubt-related struggles and, 222–227
    interpersonal struggles and, 302–305
    moral struggles and, 244–248
    of ultimate meaning struggles, 193–195
Contradiction, 128–130
Coping
    access to resources and tools for living, 108–110
    assessment and, 8–9
    decline and, 66
    doubt-related struggles and, 223–224
    explicit spiritual assessment and, 147*t*, 148
    life affirmation and, 117–123
    openness to change and, 130–131
    orienting system and, 47–48
    research regarding growth and, 97, 98
    spiritual orienting system and, 30
Core beliefs. *See also* Belief systems
    demonic struggles and, 296–297
    doubt-related struggles and, 215–216
    overview, 45–47
Crises, 196–197. *See also* Life events; Stressful life events; Trauma
Critical self-awareness, 157–158. *See also* Self-awareness
Cultural factors
    authentic guiding vision and, 125–126
    interpersonal struggles and, 308
    moral struggles and, 252
    research regarding growth and, 97

D

Damnation, 284–285
Darkness, 110–112
Death, 56, 204–205, 206*f. See also* Fear of death; Life events; Spirits of people who have died
Decision making, 284, 296–297
Decline. *See also* Brokenness; Disorientation; Distress; Outcomes; Problems
    associations of spiritual struggles with, 62–76
    clinical practice implications, 82–83

conceptual model of spiritual struggles and, 26*f*, 34–35, 77–79
    demonic struggles and, 283–285
    divine struggles and, 167–169
    doubt-related struggles and, 222–227
    interpersonal struggles and, 302–304
    moral struggles and, 244–248
    overview, 61–62, 80–83
    spiritually integrated psychotherapy and, 139
    spiritual struggles in general and, 62–77, 324
    struggles of ultimate meaning and, 193–194
    studies of serious psychological problems, 70–76
    studies of social problems, 76–77
Defense mechanisms, 97, 98
Delusions, 279
Demographics, 14–15, 49. *See also* Statistics regarding spiritual struggle
Demonic struggles. *See also* Devil; Evil forces; Supernatural evil agents
    attributional processes and, 276–283, 293–296
    consequences of, 283–286
    decline and, 283–285
    existential concerns and questions and, 7
    growth and, 285–286
    initial spiritual assessment and, 144*t*
    meaning of, 271–275
    mental illness lens and approach to, 290–292
    overview, 7, 9, 10*t*, 270–286, 297
    prevalence of, 270–271, 275–276
    psychological lens and approach to, 21–22, 292–297
    roots of, 276–283
    spiritually integrated psychotherapy and, 286–297
Depression
    associations of spiritual struggles with, 62–63
    demonic struggles and, 279, 283
    doubt-related struggles and, 222–223
    exploring ultimate meaning struggles and, 202
    initial spiritual assessment and, 144
    interpersonal struggles and, 302, 310
    medical population studies and, 67–68
    moral struggles and, 246–247
    overview, 65, 66
    struggles of ultimate meaning and, 193
    studies of people dealing with life stressors, 69–70
Depth
    assessment and, 150–153
    exploring doubts, 234–236, 235*t*
    overview, 43, 132
    of spiritual commitment, 116–117
    wholeness and brokenness and, 107–117
Desecration, 54–55
Desires, 251–252
Development
    doubt-related struggles and, 217–218, 220
    growth and, 87, 88
    psychological approach to supernatural beliefs and, 21
    spiritual struggles and, 55, 59–60
    from struggles, 17
    struggles of ultimate meaning and, 198–199
Devil. *See also* Demonic struggles; Evil forces; Supernatural evil agents
    attributions regarding, 294–295
    belief in, 277–278
    initial spiritual assessment and, 144*t*
    psychological lens and approach to, 21–22, 292–297
Dialogue, 209
Differences, intolerance of, 307–309

Disappointments, 217, 317
Disconnection, 107
Discrimination, 31, 55, 285, 301–303. *See also*
　　Marginalized groups; Prejudice
Disengagement, spiritual, 107
Dis-integration, 104. *See also* Brokenness; Outcomes
Disorientation. *See also* Decline; Orienting system
　　associations of spiritual struggles with, 62–70
　　clinical practice implications, 82–83
　　conceptual model of spiritual struggles and, 26*f*,
　　　77–79
　　divine struggles and, 167–169
　　doubt-related struggles and, 222–227
　　explicit spiritual assessment and, 147, 147*t*
　　moral struggles and, 247
　　overview, 80–83
　　spiritually integrated psychotherapy and, 160–
　　　161
Dispositions, 278–279
Dissonance, 221
Distress. *See also* Decline
　　associations of spiritual struggles with, 62–70
　　clinical practice implications, 82–83
　　conceptual model of spiritual struggles and, 26*f*,
　　　77–79
　　demonic struggles and, 283–285
　　divine struggles and, 167–169
　　doubt-related struggles and, 222–227
　　emotion regulation and, 45
　　interpersonal struggles and, 302–304
　　moral struggles and, 247
　　overview, 80–83
　　struggles of ultimate meaning and, 193–194
Disunity of purpose, 43
Divine, 243–244
Divine compassion, 257–258. *See also* Compassion
Divine punishment. *See* Punishment, divine
Divine spark, 199–200. *See also* Authenticity
Divine struggles
　　anger at God and, 163–164
　　conceptual model of spiritual struggles and,
　　　170–173
　　distress, disorientation, and consequences and,
　　　167–169
　　initial spiritual assessment and, 144*t*
　　isolation from God and, 165–166
　　negative emotions and, 163–167
　　overview, 9, 10*t*, 162–173, 188
　　potential benefits from, 169–170
　　prevalence of, 163–166
　　punishment from God and, 164–165
　　roots of, 170–173
　　subtypes of, 163–166
　　spiritually integrated psychotherapy and, 174–187,
　　　181*t*
　　waterfall visualization, 183
Divorce, 55, 69–70, 78. *See also* Marriage
Dogma, 7
Domestic violence. *See* Intimate partner violence
Doubt-related struggles
　　growth and decline and, 222–227
　　initial spiritual assessment and, 144*t*
　　as natural part of life, 218, 237, 240
　　overview, 9, 10*t*, 213–227, 239–240
　　prevalence of, 215, 217, 231
　　sources of, 216–222
　　spiritually integrated psychotherapy and, 227–239,
　　　235*t*
　　Winding Road program, 227–239
Dramatic experiences, 273
Duration of spiritual struggles, 10–12
Dysregulation, 44–45

E

Einstein, Albert, 28
Embarrassment, 254
Embeddedness in secure relationships, 221–222
Emerging adulthood, 55
Emotion regulation, 44–45, 87
Emotional abuse, 131–132. *See also* Abuse
Emotional disorders, 87
Employment, 6, 55
Empowerment, 286
Empty-chair technique, 179
End-of-life legacy programs, 209–210
Enlightenment, 106
Equilibrium, 160–161
Evil, conceptions of, 272–275
Evil forces. *See also* Demonic struggles; Devil;
　　　Supernatural evil agents
　　ascribed to humans, 274–275
　　attributions regarding, 293–296
　　doubt-related struggles and, 217
　　existential concerns and questions and, 7
　　initial spiritual assessment and, 144*t*
　　psychological lens and approach to, 21–22,
　　　292–297
Existential concerns and questions
　　breadth and depth and, 110–112
　　moral struggles and, 249
　　overview, 6–7, 323–324
　　struggles of ultimate meaning and, 196–197
Experience, 21, 32–34. *See also* Life events
Explicit spiritual assessment, 146–150, 147*t*, 150*t*. *See*
　　　also Assessment
Exploratory spiritual questions, 146–149, 147*t*
Exposure to diverse groups and people, 219–220
Expulsion, 285
Extremism, 128
Extrinsic religious orientation, 220–221
Eye movement desensitization and reprocessing
　　　(EMDR) therapy, 160

F

Faith, 220–221, 226–227, 300
Family conflicts, 310
Famous people, 13–14
Fanaticism, 128
Fear, 8, 8*t*, 87. *See also* Fear of divine retribution
Fear of death, 67–68, 74–76. *See also* Death
Fear of divine retribution. *See also* Punishment, divine
　　addressing moral overcontrol and, 259–260
　　demonic struggles and, 282
　　moral struggles and, 250–251
　　normalizing, accepting, and supporting doubt-
　　　related struggles and, 230–233
Fears of rejection. *See* Rejection
Forgiveness
　　addressing moral overcontrol and, 255–258
　　conceptual model of spiritual struggles and, 78
　　decline and, 66
　　interpersonal struggles and, 304
　　moral struggles and, 242, 254
Forrest Gump, 53
From Vice to Virtue intervention, 268
Fundamentalism, 278

G

Gateway to Wholeness program, 265, 266
Gender, 14–15, 49, 182–183
General population studies, 64–66. *See also* Research
Gestsalt psychology, 179

Goals
  conceptual model of spiritual struggles and, 26–27
  search for significance and, 32
  spirituality embedded in significance and, 27–28
  spiritually integrated psychotherapy and, 154
  struggles of ultimate meaning and, 191–192
God. *See also* Relationship with God
  alienation from, 8, 8*t*
  anger toward, 66, 163–164, 170–171, 179
  balance and, 128
  core beliefs and, 46–47
  decline and, 66
  explicit spiritual assessment and, 150*t*
  feeling abandoned by, 165–166
  feeling punished by, 164–165, 171
  isolation from, 165–166
  overview, 7
  psychological approach to, 21–22
  self-reflection and, 114
  small gods and, 47, 172–173
  spiritual support and, 121–122
  spirituality embedded in significance and, 27–28
  talking about in clinical practice and, 174–176
Gods, 21–22, 47, 172–173
Gratitude, 266
Grief, 204–205, 206*f*
Group support and intervention
  exploring doubts and, 237–239
  exploring ultimate meaning struggles and, 209
  moral struggles and, 268
  spiritually integrated psychotherapy and, 159
Growth. *See also* Outcomes; Recovery; Resilience;
    Transformation; Wholeness
  assessment and, 150–153
  conceptual model of spiritual struggles and,
    26–27, 26*f*, 34–35
  definition of, 85
  demonic struggles and, 285–286, 292–297
  divine struggles and, 169–170
  doubt-related struggles and, 222–227
  facilitators of struggle-related, 104–123
  interpersonal struggles and, 304–305
  moral struggles and, 244–248
  narrative accounts of, 89–95
  openness to change and, 130–131
  overview, 84–85, 101–103
  predictors of struggle-related, 104–133
  prevalence, 95–97
  psychological perspectives on, 87–89
  religious perspectives on, 85–86
  research on struggles predicting, 95–101
  spiritual, 115–116, 118, 121, 123, 126, 128, 131,
    227, 246, 261, 264, 283, 285, 304
  spiritually integrated psychotherapy and, 139,
    154
  struggles of ultimate meaning and, 194
  through struggles, 17, 324
  validity of self-reports of, 97–100
Guardian angels, 122
Guide role of therapist, 153–154
Guiding vision, 124–126
Guilt
  addressing moral overcontrol and, 254–255, 257
  divine struggles and, 167
  moral struggles and, 241–243, 245, 250, 254
  normalizing, accepting, and supporting doubt-
    related struggles and, 230–233

H

Hallucinations, 279
Happiness, 223

Hate crimes, 300, 301
Health, mental. *See* Mental health
Health, physical. *See* Physical health
Higher purpose, 199–200. *See also* Significant
    purpose.
Higher self, 265–267
Hinduism
  addressing impulse undercontrol and, 264
  addressing moral overcontrol and, 256
  decline and, 66
  life affirmation and, 119
  moral struggles and, 241
Historical figures, 12–14. *See also* Religious figures
HIV/AIDS, 75–76
Homicide, 284
Hope, 117, 202
Hostility, 223, 285
Human creator belief, 217
Hypocrisy, 301

I

The Idea of the Holy (Otto), 28–29
Identity
  demonic struggles and, 284
  interpersonal struggles and, 302, 316–317
  moral struggles and, 245
  overview, 6–7
Imbalance, 127–128
Immaturity, 17
Immigrants, 285
Implications for clinical practice. *See* Clinical
    practice implications
Implicit spiritual assessment, 145–146, 145*t*. *See also*
    Assessment
Impulse undercontrol, 251–253, 262–268
Impulse-control disorders, 252
Impulsive behaviors
  addressing impulse undercontrol and, 262–268
  moral struggles and, 245, 249–253, 268–269
  overcontrol and, 249–251
  undercontrol and, 251–253
Inauthentic purpose, 41, 199–200. *See also*
    Significant purpose
Incongruity, 128–130
Individualism, 108, 299
Inflexibility, 131
Initial spiritual assessment, 142–144, 142*t*, 144*t*. *See*
    also Assessment
Insecure attachment, 279
Integration, 104, 236–239. *See also* Cohesiveness;
    Outcomes; Wholeness
Interaction between psychological and spiritual
    struggles, 5
Interests, 198
Internalizing problems, 63
Interpersonal spiritual struggles. *See also*
    Relationship functioning
  consequences of, 302–305
  initial spiritual assessment and, 144*t*
  overview, 7, 9, 10*t*, 298–309, 322
  prevalence and types of, 299–301
  roots of, 305–309
  spiritually integrated psychotherapy and, 309–
    322
Intimacy, 317–318. *See also* Relationship functioning
Intimate partner violence, 78, 79, 304. *See also*
    Violence
Intolerance of differences, 307–309. *See also*
    Prejudice
Intrapersonal spiritual struggles, 7
Intuitive reasoning styles, 279

Islam. *See also* Muslim
  addressing impulse undercontrol and, 264
  demonic struggles and, 278, 293–294
  life affirmation and, 119
  moral struggles and, 245–246
  perspectives on growth and, 86

J

Jihad, 245–246, 293–294
Judaism
  addressing moral overcontrol and, 256, 261–
    262
  demonic struggles and, 285
  interpersonal struggles and, 300–301, 308
  life affirmation and, 119

K

Kintsugi, 36

L

Learning, 17, 21
Legacy programs, 209–210
Letting go, 206–211
LGBT (lesbian, gay, bisexual, and transgender)
    individuals
  demonic struggles and, 285
  interpersonal struggles and, 302–303, 304–305,
    306, 307, 308
  spiritual struggles and, 54–55
Life affirmation
  assessment and, 150–153
  overview, 132
  sources of, 119–123
  spiritual support and, 122–123
  wholeness and brokenness and, 117–123
Life events. *See also* Experience; Stressful life
    events; Transitions; Trauma
  conceptual model of spiritual struggles and, 26*f*,
    77–79
  demonic struggles and, 273–274, 278–279,
    280–282
  distress, disorientation, and decline and, 77–79
  divine struggles and, 170–171
  interpersonal struggles and, 305–306
  moral struggles and, 246–248, 249
  orienting system and, 55–58
  search for significance and, 32–34
  spiritual coping practices and, 47–48
  spiritual struggles from, 52–60, 59*t*
  struggles of ultimate meaning and, 196–197
  studies of people dealing with life stressors, 69–
    70
Life satisfaction, 118, 223
Literature, 13–14
Loneliness, 48–49. *See also* Connectedness
Loss. *See also* Life events
  doubt-related struggles and, 217
  exploring ultimate meaning struggles and,
    204–205, 206*f*
  spiritual struggles and, 56
Love, 257–258

M

Marginalized groups
  connectedness and, 49
  demonic struggles and, 285
  interpersonal struggles and, 302–303, 306–307
  spiritual struggles and, 54–55

Marriage. *See also* Relationship functioning
  conceptual model of spiritual struggles and, 78
  decline and, 66
  as an example of sacredness, 6
  interpersonal struggles and, 309, 310
  spiritual struggles and, 55
  studies of people dealing with life stressors, 69–70
Meaning. *See also* Orienting system; Struggles of
    ultimate meaning
  meaning making, 57, 206–211, 213, 281
  overview, 190–191
  questioning, 6–7, 33, 42–43, 144*t*
Medical population studies, 66–68. *See also* Research
Medical problems, 290–292. *See also* Physical health
Medications, 148, 157
Meditation
  addressing impulse undercontrol and, 266–267
  exploring ultimate meaning struggles and, 205,
    206*f*
  facilitating spiritual connectedness and, 179–180
Memories, 205, 206*f*
Mental health. *See also* Psychological problems
  addressing impulse undercontrol and, 264
  addressing moral overcontrol and, 258
  attending to spiritual struggles in treatment and,
    20
  avoidance and, 112
  demonic struggles and, 279, 283
  distress, disorientation, and decline and, 80–83
  doubt-related struggles and, 223
  growth and, 87–88
  moral struggles and, 246
  psychological approach to supernatural beliefs
    and, 21–22
  struggles of ultimate meaning and, 193–194
  studies of people with psychological problems
    and, 68–69
  working with demonic struggles through a mental
    illness lens and, 290–292
Mental illness lens and approach, 22, 279, 290–292
Military veterans. *See also* Combat
  growth and decline, 96, 98, 100–101,116, 118,
    120, 128
  interpersonal struggles, 300
  moral struggles, 242–243, 247, 249
  roots of spiritual struggles, 45, 56–57, 71–72
  spiritual assessment, 144
  spiritual struggles interventions, 16, 258
Mindfulness
  addressing impulse undercontrol and, 264–265,
    266–267
  facilitating spiritual connectedness and, 179–180
  normalizing, accepting, and supporting doubt-
    related struggles and, 231–232
Moderation, 128
Moral boundaries, 286
Moral compass, 265–267, 295–296
Moral decision making, 284
Moral injury, 246–248
Moral overcontrol
  clinical practice implications, 254–262, 267–268
  moral struggles and, 249–251
Moral perfectionism
  addressing moral overcontrol and, 259–262
  demonic struggles and, 284
  overview, 250–251
Moral struggles
  demonic struggles and, 284
  growth and decline and, 244–248
  initial spiritual assessment and, 144*t*
  overview, 9, 10*t*, 241–253, 268–269
  prevalence of, 242

roots of, 248–253
spiritually integrated psychotherapy and, 253–268
Moral transgressions, 274–275
Moral vision, 259–262
Mortality, 74–76, 283
Motivation
    conceptual model of spiritual struggles and, 26–27
    demonic struggles and, 281–282
    elevation of preliminary concerns over ultimate concerns and, 42–43
    psychological approach to supernatural beliefs and, 21
    spiritual orienting system and, 30
    spirituality embedded in significance and, 27
Muslim. *See also* Islam
    addressing impulse undercontrol and, 264
    benevolent spiritual reframing and, 120–121
    exploring doubts in clinical practice, 234–236, 235*t*
    interpersonal struggles and, 300–301, 308
    moral struggles and, 245–246
    normalizing, accepting, and supporting doubt-related struggles and, 231

N

Naming spiritual struggles, 156–157
Narrowness, 43, 109–110, 132. *See also* Breadth; Brokenness
Native American cultures, 125
Nature, 122
Negative emotions
    divine struggles and, 163–167, 170–171
    growth and, 87
    talking about in clinical practice and, 174–176
Negative religious coping. 8–9. *See also* Coping; Spiritual struggles in general
Net wholeness, 36. *See also* Wholeness
Night (Wiesel), 10–12
Normalizing spiritual struggles, 156–157, 230–233

O

Obsessive–compulsive disorder (OCD), 247, 261–262
Obsessive–compulsiveness, 223
One-upmanship, 309
Open Heart (Wiesel), 12
Openness to change, 130–132
Organized religious life, 7, 300. *See also* Religious dogma; Religious institutions
Orienting system. *See also* Disorientation; Significant purpose; Worldviews
    authentic guiding vision and, 124–126
    behavioral practices and, 47–48
    conceptual model of spiritual struggles and, 26*f*, 77–79
    core beliefs and, 45–47
    distress, disorientation, and decline and, 77–79
    divine struggles and, 171–173
    doubt-related struggles and, 216–217, 219–222
    emotion regulation and, 44–45
    explicit spiritual assessment and, 150*t*
    exploring doubts in clinical practice, 234
    growth and decline and, 244
    interpersonal struggles and, 306–309
    life events and, 55–58
    moral struggles and, 249
    relational connectedness and, 48–49
    search for significance and, 29–31, 32–34
    spiritual struggles from, 44–52, 59–60, 59*t*

spiritually integrated psychotherapy and, 139, 160–161
struggles of ultimate meaning and, 198–200
Outcomes. *See also* Brokenness; Consequences; Decline; Dis-integration; Growth; Integration; Spiritual growth; Treatment outcomes; Wholeness
    demonic struggles and, 283–286
    divine struggles and, 167–169
    doubt-related struggles and, 222–227
    facilitators of positive, 104–123
    interpersonal struggles and, 302–305
    moral struggles and, 244–248
    openness to change and, 130–132
    overview, 104–107, 132–133
    predictors of, 104–133
    research regarding growth and, 98
    social problems, 76–77
    spiritual struggles in general and, 62–77
    studies of serious psychological problems and, 70–76
    of ultimate meaning struggles, 193–195
Overcertainty, 131
Overcontrol. *See* Moral overcontrol

P

Pain, 73, 199. *See also* Pain in spiritual struggles
Pain in spiritual struggles
    acceptance and, 110–112
    breadth and depth and, 110–112
    clinical practice implications, 82–83
    interpersonal struggles and, 301
    life events and, 54
    moral struggles and, 242
    overview, 15–17
Paradoxes, 128–130
Paranoid ideation, 223
Pathology, 17, 291–292
Penn Inventory of Scrupulosity, 7–8
Perceived stress, 65
Perceptions, 112–117, 308
Perfectionism, 250–251, 259–262
Personal experiences, 278–279. *See also* Life events
Personal responsibility, 294–295. *See also* Responsibility
Perspectives, 113–114
Pervasiveness of spiritual struggles, 12–15
Philosophies of life. *See* Orienting system
Phobic anxiety, 223
Physical abuse, 131–132. *See also* Abuse
Physical health
    addressing impulse undercontrol and, 264
    associations of spiritual struggles with, 63
    distress, disorientation, and decline and, 80–83
    doubt-related struggles and, 223
    medical population studies and, 66–68
    moral struggles and, 246
    pain involved in spiritual struggles and, 16–17
    research regarding growth and, 98, 100–101
    spiritual coping practices and, 47–48
    studies of serious psychological problems and, 73–74, 75–76
    suicidality and, 72–73
Pivotal times, 17–18, 35, 132, 137, 248, 253, 325
Plausibility structures, 280. *See also* Orienting system
Pollution, 55
Pornography, 262–268
Positive disintegration, 36
Possession, demonic, 273
Posttraumatic growth, 88. *See also* Growth

Posttraumatic Growth Inventory (PTGI), 96, 97–98
Posttraumatic stress disorder (PTSD)
    conceptual model of spiritual struggles and, 78
    doubt-related struggles and, 223
    interpersonal struggles and, 310
    moral struggles and, 243, 246–247
    overview, 19
    studies of people with psychological problems
        and, 68–69
    studies of serious psychological problems and,
        71–72
    suicidality and, 73
Power, 17–18
Prayer, 121, 209, 264
Prejudice, 78, 109, 198, 281, 285, 307–309, 316, 319.
    See also Intolerance of differences.
Preliminary concerns, 42–43
Presence, silence of, 155–156
Prevalence of spiritual struggles
    demonic struggles and, 270–271, 275–276
    divine struggles and, 163–166
    doubt-related struggles and, 215, 217
    growth and, 95–97
    interpersonal struggles and, 299–301
    moral struggles and, 242
    overview, 12–15
    struggles of ultimate meaning and, 192–193
Primary appraisals, 53–55. See also Appraisals
Primary spiritual struggles model, 45, 63, 65, 67, 71,
    73–74, 80–81, 148, 194, 310–312
Problems, 127. See also Decline; Mental health;
    Physical health; Psychological problems
Psychological lens and approach, 21–24, 160,
    292–297
Psychological problems. See also Mental health
    associations of spiritual struggles with, 62–63
    conceptual model of spiritual struggles and, 78
    demonic struggles and, 278–279, 283–285
    distress, disorientation, and decline and, 80–83
    doubt-related struggles and, 223
    explicit spiritual assessment and, 148
    interpersonal struggles and, 302–303, 310–312
    pain involved in spiritual struggles and, 16–17
    research and, 68–69
    statistics regarding spiritual struggle and, 14–15
    studies of serious psychological problems, 70–76
    suicidality and, 72–73
    trauma and, 18–19
    working with demonic struggles through a
        psychological lens and, 292–297
Psychosis, 279
Psychosocial crises, 87
Psychotherapy, 138–139, 228–230, 325–327. See also
    Spiritually integrated psychotherapy
Punishment, divine. See also Divine struggles; Fear
    of divine retribution
    addressing moral overcontrol and, 259–260
    demonic struggles and, 282
    normalizing, accepting, and supporting doubt-
        related struggles and, 230–233
    overview, 164–165
Purpose, sense of. See also Significant purpose
    addressing moral overcontrol and, 259
    life affirmation and, 117–123
    moral struggles and, 245
    seeing and accepting the darkness and, 110–112
    seeing beneath the surface and, 112–117
    strength of purpose, 40–41
    stressful events and, 33
    struggles of ultimate meaning and, 194, 196,
        197–198, 199–200, 211–212
    values and, 42

Q
Quality of life, 63, 66, 76–77
Quest orientation, 50–51, 130–131, 219. See also
    Orienting system

R
Racial discrimination. See Discrimination
Rape, 54–55, 94, 105, 170, 184, 303, 306. See also
    Sexual assault, Trauma; Violence.
Readings
    exploring doubts and, 234–235, 235t
    facilitating spiritual connectedness and, 180, 181t
Reappraisals, 176–178
Reasoning styles, 279, 280
Reconnection, 316–322
Recovery. See Growth; Resilience
Redemption, 251, 255–258
Reflection, 113, 157–158, 205, 206f. See also Self-
    reflection
Reframing spiritual struggles, 156–157
Regret, 247–248
Rejection, 260–261, 301, 317
Relational connectedness. See Connectedness
Relationship functioning, 221–222, 260–261. See
    also Connectedness; Interpersonal spiritual
    struggles; Marriage
Relationship with God. See also God
    addressing moral overcontrol and, 260–262
    balance and, 128
    demonic struggles and, 283
    divine struggles and, 171–173
    facilitating spiritual connectedness and, 178–181,
        181t
Relativism, 217
Religious and spiritual change, 99, 114, 304–305
Religious and Spiritual Struggles (RSS) Scale
    demonic struggles and, 272–273, 276, 283
    initial spiritual assessment and, 143
    items from, 10, 10t
    overview, 56, 63, 65
Religious communities, 300, 302–303
Religious Coping scale (RCOPE), 276
Religious Crisis Scale, 8
Religious disaffiliation, 95, 143
Religious dogma, 7
Religious figures
    divine struggles and, 167, 169–170
    moral struggles and, 241
    pain involved in spiritual struggles and, 17
    stories of spiritual struggles among, 12–14, 18
Religious institutions. See also Organized religious
    life
    addressing spiritual struggles and, 327–328
    interpersonal struggles and, 300
    overview, 7
    spiritual orienting system and, 30
Religious leaders, 300. See also Clergy, abuse by
Religious passivity, 66
Religious rifts, 8, 8t
Religious Strain Scale, 8, 8t, 63
Remorse, 245
Reorientation, 26f
Research
    clinical and stressed population studies, 66–70
    general population studies, 64–66
    growth and, 95–101
    medical population studies, 66–68
    overview, 14–15
    psychological approach to supernatural beliefs
        and, 23
    social problems and, 76–77

studies of people dealing with life stressors, 69–70
studies of people with psychological problems, 68–69
studies of serious psychological problems, 70–76
Resilience, 55–56, 257. *See also* Growth; Recovery
Resources for living, access to, 108–110, 158–160, 245
Responsibility
  addressing moral overcontrol and, 255–256, 257, 259–262
  demonic struggles and, 294–295
  moral struggles and, 242
Rifts, religious. *See* Religious rifts
Rigidity, 131
Rituals
  authentic guiding vision and, 125
  doubt-related struggles and, 217
  exploring ultimate meaning struggles and, 208–209
  letting go and, 208–209
  spiritual support and, 122

S

Sacred lens, 6, 114–115
Sacred loss, 53–55
Sacred moments reflection/meditation, 205, 206*f*
Sacred purpose, 41, 150*t*. *See also* Sacredness; Significant purpose
Sacred spark, 318–319
Sacredness
  addressing moral overcontrol and, 261
  breadth and depth and, 109–110
  facilitating spiritual connectedness and, 178–179
  interpersonal struggles and, 318–319
  life events and, 55
  moral struggles and, 243–244
  openness to change and, 131–132
  overview, 6
  perception of, 6, 114–115
  spiritual orienting system and, 30–31
  spiritual support and, 122
  spirituality embedded in significance and, 27–29
Safety, 312–314, 316–318
Salvation, 117–123
Sanctification, 6, 114–115
Satan. *See* Demonic struggles; Devil; Evil forces
Satisfaction, 66
Scarred by Struggle (Chittister), 15–17
Scientists, 13–14, 28
Screening, 142–144, 142*t*, 144*t*
Scrupulosity, 261, 284–285
Search for significance. *See also* Significant purpose
  authentic guiding vision and, 124–126
  moral struggles and, 249
  orienting system and, 29–31
  overview, 25–27, 26*f*
  path or journey of, 31
  processes that guide, 32–34
  spirituality embedded in, 27–29
  wholeness and brokenness and, 35–37
Secondary spiritual struggles model, 45, 63, 68, 71–72, 80–82, 148, 157, 310–312
Secular patients, 143, 218
Self-attributions, 250
Self-awareness, 141, 157–158
Self-compassion, 257–258. *See also* Compassion
Self-contempt, 254
Self-control
  addressing impulse undercontrol and, 263–264
  demonic struggles and, 286
  moral struggles and, 245, 251–253
Self-control training methods, 263–264
Self-criticism, 108–110
Self-disclosure, 156
Self-efficacy, 198–199
Self-esteem, 118
Self-evaluation, 242–243
Self-punitiveness, 257
Self-reflection. *See also* Reflection
  seeing beneath the surface and, 114
  spiritually integrated psychotherapy and, 157–158
Self-regulation, 245
Self-reports, 97–99
Self-worth, 97, 167
Sexual abuse/assault. *See also* Abuse; Child abuse; Clergy, abuse by; Rape, Trauma; Violence
  considering new ways to understand the divine, 182–183
  interpersonal struggles and, 303, 309–322
  openness to change and, 131–132
  research regarding growth and, 101
  spiritual struggles from, 54–55
  studies of people dealing with life stressors, 69–70
Shallowness, 109–110, 132. *See also* Brokenness
Shame
  addressing moral overcontrol and, 257
  divine struggles and, 167
  moral struggles and, 241–243, 250, 254
Significance, search for. *See* Search for significance
Significant purpose. *See also* Orienting system; Purpose, sense of; Search for significance
  addressing moral overcontrol and, 259
  authentic guiding vision and, 124–126
  divine struggles and, 171–173
  doubt-related struggles and, 219–222
  growth and decline and, 244
  sacred spark, 318–319
  search for significance and, 32–34
  spiritual struggles from, 39–44, 59–60, 59*t*
Silence of presence, 155–156
Sin
  addressing moral overcontrol and, 257–258, 261–262
  demonic struggles and, 284
  moral struggles and, 254
Social alienation, 48–49, 310. *See also* Connectedness
Social connections, 180–181, 221–222. *See also* Connectedness
Social identity, 221–222
Social problems, 76–77
Social support, 49, 282. *See also* Connectedness; Support
Socialization, 21, 278
Sociocultural context, 26*f*, 37
Socratic dialogue, 209
Somatization, 223
Soul, 122
Spirits, evil. *See* Evil forces; Supernatural evil agents
Spirits of people who have died. *See also* Death
  doubt-related struggles and, 218
  normalizing, accepting, and supporting doubt-related struggles and, 232
  psychological approach to, 21–22
  spiritual support and, 122
Spiritual commitment, 116–117
Spiritual competencies of therapists, 5, 20, 320
Spiritual connections, 222
Spiritual goals, 191–192. *See also* Goals
Spiritual growth, 115–116, 118, 121, 123, 126, 128, 131, 227, 246, 261, 264, 283, 285, 304
Spiritual history, 149–150, 150*t*, 278, 306

Spiritual life of the client
    demonic struggles and, 277–278
    doubt-related struggles and, 226–227
    explicit spiritual assessment and, 149–150, 150*t*
    interpersonal struggles and, 306
Spiritual one-upmanship, 309
Spiritual orientation, 30–31, 50, 110, 149, 150, 227,
        266, 299, 301
Spiritual orienting system, 30–31, 33, 79, 182
Spiritual roots of spiritual struggles, 46–51
Spiritual self-schema (3-S+) therapy, 266–267
Spiritual struggles in general. *See also* Demonic
        struggles; Divine struggles; Doubt-related
        struggles; Interpersonal spiritual struggles;
        Moral struggles; Struggles of ultimate meaning
    attending to in treatment, 19–21
    characteristics of, 12–18
    conceptual model of spiritual struggles and,
        26*f*
    definition of, 5–7
    diversity of, 7–12, 8*t*, 10*t*
    example of, 3–4
    as forks in the road, 17–18, 35, 132, 137, 248, 253,
        325
    future directions for practice, 326–327
    intervention programs, 160, 237–239
    as mediators of orienting system and decline,
        79
    as mediators of stressful life events and decline,
        77–78
    mental illness lens and approach to, 22
    as natural parts of life, 17, 20, 34, 82, 139, 218,
        237, 240, 323
    overview, 5–7, 20–21, 104–105, 323–328
    prevalence of, 12–15
    psychological lens and approach to, 22
    roots of, 38–60
    supernatural lens and approach to, 22
    therapist's presence to, 155–156
    uneasiness of working with clients dealing with,
        4–5, 325–326
Spiritual warfare, 283, 293–294
Spirituality
    definition and meaning of, 27–29
    orienting system and, 30, 49–51
    overview, 323–324
    search for significance and, 27–29
    seeing beneath the surface and, 114–116
    wholeness and brokenness and, 35
Spiritually integrated psychotherapy. *See also*
        Clinical practice implications
    assessment and, 139–153, 142*t*, 144*t*, 145*t*, 147*t*,
        150*t*, 289, 310–312
    being transparent with methods and values of,
        228–230
    client interest in, 20
    concerns regarding addressing spiritual struggles
        and, 325–327
    conservation and, 202–205, 206*t*
    considering new ways to understand the divine,
        181–185
    creating a safe space, 312–314
    discovering new ultimate meaning through,
        206–211
    exploring beliefs about evil, 289
    exploring benevolent spiritual reappraisals and,
        176–178
    exploring doubts, 233–237, 235*t*
    exploring ultimate meaning struggles in, 200–202
    facilitating spiritual connectedness, 178–181, 181*t*
    holding on to ultimate meaning, 202–205, 206*t*
    how to address spiritual struggles, 153–160

    impulse undercontrol and, 262–268
    integrating divine struggles into a cohesive whole,
        185–187
    intervention programs for spiritual struggles, 160,
        237–239
    letting go, 206–211
    moral overcontrol and, 254–262
    normalizing, accepting, and supporting doubt-
        related struggles in, 230–233
    overview, 137–139, 160–161
    processing interpersonal struggles in, 314–316
    talking about God, 174–176
    training in, 5, 20, 290
    transformation and, 206–211
    working on reconnection with other people
        through, 316–322
    working with demonic struggles through a mental
        illness lens and, 290–292
    working with demonic struggles through a
        psychological lens and, 292–297
Standards, moral, 243–244, 250–251
Stressful life events. *See also* Life events
    acceptance and, 110–112
    conceptual model of spiritual struggles and, 77–79
    demonic struggles and, 273–274, 278–279,
        280–282
    distress, disorientation, and decline and, 77–79
    divine struggles and, 170–171
    doubt-related struggles and, 216–218
    interpersonal struggles and, 305–306
    moral struggles and, 246–248, 249
    search for significance and, 32–34
    spiritual struggles from, 52–60, 59*t*
    struggles of ultimate meaning and, 196–197
    studies of people dealing with, 69–70
Stress-related disorders, 310
Struggles, 110–112
Struggles of ultimate meaning. *See also* Meaning
    consequences of, 193–195
    elevation of preliminary concerns over ultimate
        concerns and, 42–43
    initial spiritual assessment and, 144*t*
    overview, 9, 10*t*, 189–200, 211–212
    prevalence of, 192–193
    roots of, 195–200
    seeing and accepting, 110–112
    seeing beneath the surface and, 112–117
    spiritually integrated psychotherapy and, 200–211,
        206*t*
Struggles with doubt. *See* Doubt-related struggles
Substance use, 48, 246. *See also* Addiction
Suffering
    seeing and accepting, 110–112
    seeing beneath the surface and, 112–117
    struggles of ultimate meaning and, 199
    talking about in clinical practice and, 174–176
Suicidality
    demonic struggles and, 284
    divine struggles and, 168
    moral struggles and, 246, 247
    studies of serious psychological problems and,
        72–73, 75
Supernatural evil agents, 7, 21–22, 272–274, 277–278,
        297. *See also* Devil; Evil forces
Supernatural spiritual struggles, 7, 9
Support
    addressing impulse undercontrol and, 264
    doubt-related struggles and, 221–222, 230–233
    life affirmation and, 117, 118
    spiritual support, 121–123
    spiritually integrated psychotherapy and, 159
Surrender, 127

T

Taoism, 128
Temperament, 21
Temptation, 294–295
Tension, 320–322
Terrorism, 299–300
Therapeutic relationship. *See also* Therapist factors
  assessment and, 140–142
  concerns regarding addressing spiritual struggles and, 325–327
  creating a safe space and, 312–314
  importance of, 153–154
  interpersonal struggles and, 312–314
Therapist factors. *See also* Spiritually integrated psychotherapy; Therapeutic relationship
  assessment and, 140–142
  being transparent with methods and values of psychotherapy and, 228–230
  concerns of regarding addressing spiritual struggles, 325–327
  helping clients find forgiveness for themselves, 255–258
  how to address spiritual struggles, 153–160
  moral struggles and, 253–254
  therapist's presence to spiritual struggles and, 155–156
  training and, 5, 20, 290
  working with demonic struggles and, 289–290
Threat appraisals, 282, 286. *See also* Appraisals
3-S+ (spiritual self-schema) therapy, 266–267
Tools for living, access to, 108–110, 158–160, 245
Transcendence, 6, 18, 191–192
Transformation. *See also* Growth
  considering new ways to understand the divine, 183–184
  exploring ultimate meaning struggles and, 206–211
  growth and, 88
  letting go and, 208–209
  spiritually integrated psychotherapy and, 139
  struggles of ultimate meaning and, 194
  weaving wisdom and, 127
Transitions. *See also* Life events
  divine struggles and, 170–171
  doubt-related struggles and, 217–218
  search for significance and, 32–34
  spiritual struggles from, 52–59
  struggles of ultimate meaning and, 196–197
Trauma. *See also* Life events; Stressful life events
  conceptual model of spiritual struggles and, 78
  considering new ways to understand the divine, 182–183
  duration of spiritual struggles and, 10–12
  growth and, 87–88
  interpersonal struggles and, 301
  moral struggles and, 241–242, 246–248
  openness to change and, 130–132
  research regarding growth and, 101
  role of in psychological problems, 18–19
  spiritual struggles from, 52–59
Treasure Chest Meditation, 205, 206*f*
Treatment implications. *See* Clinical practice implications
Treatment outcomes, 16–17, 20. *See also* Clinical practice implications; Outcomes
Treatment plan, 152–153
Trust, 316–317
Truth, 21–22

12-step approaches, 267
Types of spiritual struggle. *See also* Demonic struggles; Divine struggles; Doubt-related struggles; Interpersonal spiritual struggles; Moral struggles; Struggles of ultimate meaning
  explicit spiritual assessment and, 147, 147*t*
  initial spiritual assessment and, 143, 144*t*
  overview, 9–10, 10*t*, 161

U

Ultimate concerns, 6, 42–43. *See also* Meaning; Struggles of ultimate meaning
Undercontrol. *See* Impulse undercontrol

V

Values
  demonic struggles and, 286
  elevation of preliminary concerns over ultimate concerns and, 42–43
  existential concerns and questions and, 7
  moral struggles and, 243–244
  purpose and, 42
  struggles of ultimate meaning and, 198
Victimhood, 285
Violence. *See also* Rape; Sexual Abuse; Trauma
  conceptual model of spiritual struggles and, 78
  implications of spiritual struggles for, 76–77
  interpersonal struggles and, 299–300, 301
Virtue, 243–244, 245, 252
Virtuous deeds, 266
Visualization, 178–179, 266
Vulnerability, 57–58

W

Weakness, 17, 59–60
Weaving wisdom, 126–132, 150–153
Well-being
  addressing moral overcontrol and, 257
  conceptual model of spiritual struggles and, 78
  doubt-related struggles and, 223
  life affirmation and, 118, 119
Well-organized life, 123–124. *See also* Cohesiveness
Wholeness. *See also* Growth; Integration; Outcomes
  assessment and, 150–153
  breadth and depth and, 107–117
  cohesiveness and, 123–132
  conceptual model of spiritual struggles and, 26*f*
  demonic struggles and, 284, 292–297
  doubt-related struggles and, 222–227
  growth and decline and, 244–248
  ingredients of, 104–123
  integrating divine struggles into, 185–187
  life affirmation and, 117–123
  meaning of, 35, 105–107
  overview, 35–37, 104–107, 132–133, 325
  psychological thought on, 106–107
  religious thought on, 106
Wiesel, Elie, 10–12
Winding Road program, 237–239
Wisdom, 126–132
Wisdom of weaving, 126–132, 150–153
Work, 6, 55
Working models. *See* Orienting system
Worldviews, 277–279, 280–282. *See also* Orienting system

Y

Yoga, 264